中醫五臟

Pathomechanisms of the Five Viscera

Zhōng Yī Wǔ Zàng Bìng Jī Xué

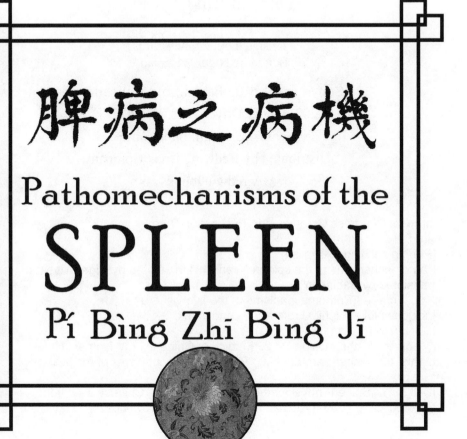

脾病之病機

Pathomechanisms of the

SPLEEN

Pí Bìng Zhī Bìng Jī

Yán Shí-Lín

Edited by Nigel Wiseman and Eric Brand
Translated by Sabine Wilms

Paradigm Publications

Taos, New Mexico 2009

Pathomechanisms of the Five Viscera

Volume 3:
Pathomechanisms of the Spleen

Yán Shí Lín 严石林

Translated by Sabine Wilms
Edited by Nigel Wiseman

Copyright © 2009 Paradigm Publications
202 Bendix Drive, Taos, NM 87571
www.paradigm-pubs.com
Distributed by Redwing Book Company
www.redwingbooks.com

Library of Congress Cataloging-in-Publication Data:
Yan, Shi-Lin, 1943-
[Pí bìng zhi bing ji. English]
Pathomechanisms of the spleen / Yan Shi Lin ; edited by Nigel Wiseman ;
translated by Sabine Wilms.
    p. ; cm. -- (Pathomechanisms of the five viscera ; v. 3)
Includes bibliographical references and index.
ISBN 978-0-912111-84-1 (pbk.)
1. Spleen--Pathophysiology. 2. Medicine, Chinese. I. Wiseman, Nigel.
II. Title. III. Series: Yan, Shi Lin, 1943- Pathomechanisms of the five
viscera ; v. 3.
[DNLM: 1. Spleen--physiopathology. 2. Medicine, Chinese Traditional.
 WH 600 Y21p 2009a] RC645.Y3613 2009 616.4'107--dc22
                    2009034388

Library of Congress Number: 2009034388
International Standard Book Number (ISBN-13): 9780912111841
Printed in the United States of America

Table of Contents

Council of Oriental Medical Publishers Designation   v

Introduction   1

     1. Breakdown of Movement and Transformation 运化障碍   2

     2. Fluid Imbalances 水液失调   3

     3. Disordered Qì Dynamic 气机紊乱   3

     4. Impaired Movement of Blood 血液失运   4

     5. Insecurity of External Defense 卫外不固   5

     6. Malnutrition 营养缺乏   5

     Summary of the Pathomechanisms of Spleen Disease   9

PART ONE: Pathomechanisms of Spleen Repletion 脾实的病机   11

Introduction: Spleen Repletion 脾实   13

Chapter 1: Spleen Qì Depression 脾气郁滞   17

     Literature Review of Thought & Preoccupation Stagnating the Spleen 文献评述   22

     Summary of Thought and Preoccupation Stagnating the Spleen   22

     Literature Review of Cold-Damp Encumbering the Spleen 文献评述   29

     Summary of Cold-Damp Encumbering the Spleen   30

     Literature Review of Phlegm Turbidity Obstructing the Spleen 文献评述   34

     Summary of Phlegm-Turbidity Obstructing the Spleen   35

     Literature Review of Food and Drink Damaging the Spleen 文献评述   38

     Summary of Food and Drink Damaging the Spleen   39

     Literature Review of Static Blood Accumulating in the Spleen 文献评述   43

     Summary of Static Blood Accumulating in the Spleen   44

Chapter 2: Spleen Fire Exuberance 脾火亢盛   45

     Literature Review of Spleen Channel Repletion Fire 文献评述   53

     Summary of Spleen Channel Repletion Fire   54

     2.2.1 Impairment of Splenic Movement and Transformation 脾失健运   58

     2.2.2 Earth Congestion and Wood Depression 土壅木郁   61

     2.2.3 Damp-Heat Lying Depressed and Steaming 湿热郁蒸   63

     Literature Review of Damp-Heat Brewing in the Spleen 文献评述   65

     Summary of Damp-Heat Brewing in the Spleen   66

PART TWO: Pathomechanisms of Spleen Vacuity 脾虚的病机   71

Introduction: Spleen Vacuity 脾虚   73

Chapter 1: Spleen Qì Vacuity 脾气虚   79

1.1.1 Grain and Water Movement Failure 水谷失运   85

1.1.2 Water-Damp Failing to Transform 水湿不化   86

Literature Review of Spleen Vacuity Movement Failure 文献评述   94

Summary of Spleen Vacuity Movement Failure 脾虚失运   95

1.2.1 Spleen Qì Failing to Bear Upward 脾气不升   100

1.2.2 Center Burner Qì Stagnation 中焦气滞   104

1.2.3 Falling of the Qì Dynamic 气机下陷   109

Literature Review of Spleen Qì Fall 文献评述   113

Summary of Spleen Qì Fall 脾气下陷   115

Literature Review of Spleen Failing to Control Blood 文献评述   120

Summary of Spleen Failing to Control Blood 脾不统血   121

1.4.1 Improper Nourishment of the Body 形体失养   125

1.4.2 Improper Nourishment of the Offices and Orifices 官窍失养   131

Literature Review of Spleen Qì Failing to Provide Luxuriance 文献评述   136

Summary of Spleen Qì Failing to Provide Luxuriance 脾气不荣   138

Literature Review of Qì Vacuity Heat Effusion 文献评述   141

Summary of Qì Vacuity Heat Effusion 气虚发热   141

Chapter 2: Spleen Yáng Vacuity 脾阳虚   **149**

Literature Review of Grain and Water Failing to Move 文献评述   161

Summary of Grain and Water Failing to Move 水谷失运   162

Literature Review of Water-Damp Failing to Transform 文献评述   171

Summary of Water-Damp Failing to Transform 水湿不化   172

Literature Review of Impaired Warming 文献评述   180

Summary of Impaired Warming 温煦失职   181

Chapter 3: Spleen Yīn Vacuity 脾阴虚   **183**

Literature Review of Breakdown of Movement and Transformation 文献评述   191

Summary of Breakdown of Movement and Transformation 运化失职   192

Literature Review of Loss of Nourishment 文献评述   196

Summary of Loss of Nourishment 失于滋养   197

Literature Review of Internal Generation of Vacuity Heat 文献评述   201

Summary of Internal Generation of Vacuity Heat 虚热内生   202

Index   **203**

Council of Oriental Medical Publishers

Designation

This work is a whole-text translation of the Chinese text, *Pí Bìng Zhī Bìng Jī* 脾 病 之病 机 by Yán Shí Lín 严石林. English terminology conforms to Wiseman and Féng, *Practical Dictionary of Chinese Medicine,* published by Paradigm Publications.

Introduction

Pathomechanisms of Spleen Disease
脾病的病机

The spleen belongs to earth and its nature belongs to yīn. Located at the top of the abdominal cavity and below the diaphragm, it is connected with the stomach and diaphragm and stands in an interior-exterior relationship with the stomach. The spleen holds the office of the granaries. As such, it moves and transforms water and grain and the fluids. Through transformation, it engenders construction, defense, qì, and blood. It manages the center in order to irrigate the four sides; it fills and nourishes the five viscera and six bowels, flesh, sinews, five offices and nine orifices, and the four limbs and hundred bones. The spleen governs upbearing of the clear and the ascent of enrichment to the heart, lungs, head, and eyes; it keeps the internal organs in a permanent and fixed location; and it controls blood, containing blood in the channels and guarding against blood spilling outside the vessels. Thus, it constitutes the mainstay for the upbearing and downbearing of the qì dynamic, provides assistance in the movement of blood, safeguards fluids, and is the source for the formation of qì and blood. It is therefore extremely important for the healthy performance of vital activities in the human body.

The spleen is closely linked to many aspects of physiology. When it is affected by disease, this can therefore easily lead to many kinds of pathological changes like breakdown of movement and transformation, fluid imbalances, disordered qì dynamic, impaired movement of blood, insecurity of external defense, or general malnutrition.

脾属土而性属阴，位于腹腔之上，膈膜之下，与胃隔膜相连，互为表里。脾为仓廪之官，运化水谷津液，化生营卫气血，执中央以灌四旁，充养五脏六腑、肌肉、筋膜、五官九窍、四肢百骸。脾主升清而上滋心肺头目，保持内脏位置恒定，主统血而摄血归经，防止血溢脉外，为气机升降之枢纽，血液运行之辅佐，水液代谢之保证，气血生化之本源，对人体生命活动的正常进行有十分重要的意义。

·脾与人体多方面生理功能有密切的关系，发生病变时，病理上易引起运化障碍，水液失调，气机紊乱，血液失运，卫外不固，全身营养缺乏等多种变化。

1. Breakdown of Movement and Transformation

The spleen governs movement and transformation. It has the ability to digest, absorb, and distribute the essence of grain and water and thereby nourish the whole body. Various kinds of disease causes can lead to a failure of the spleen to move and transform, to disordered digestive functions, to nontransformation of food, and to impaired distribution of essence. As a result, one tends to observe such manifestations as torpid intake and absence of hunger, reduced eating and difficult transformation, distention and fullness in the stomach duct and abdomen, abdominal pain and rumbling intestines, diarrhea and dysentery, sloppy stool or constipation, and scant or frequent urination.

运化障碍

运化障碍：脾主运化，能消化、吸收、输布水谷精微，营养全身。各种病因可使脾失健运，消化功能紊乱，饮食不化，精微失布，易见纳呆不饥、食少难化、脘腹胀满、腹痛肠鸣、腹泄下痢、便溏或便秘、尿少或频多等表现。

2. Fluid Imbalances

While the spleen moves and transforms the essence of grain and water, it simultaneously absorbs and distributes the fluids. This function allows water and liquid to be distributed everywhere, the five channels to work in tandem, the waterways to flow freely, and the fluids to be balanced. When the spleen fails to move and transform, earth fails to dam water. The distribution of water and liquid is impaired, the fluids collect and stagnate, water qì floods, and rheum and phlegm are engendered, giving rise to the problem of dampness gathering. As a result, one tends to observe such manifestations as damp turbidity, phlegm-rheum, water swelling, drum distension, obesity, cough and panting, and vaginal discharge.

水液失调

脾在运化水谷精微的同时，亦吸收、输布水液，使水津四布，五经并行，水道通调，水液平衡。脾失健运，土不制水，水津失布，水液停滞，水气泛溢，化饮生痰，聚湿为患，易见湿浊、痰饮、水肿、鼓胀、肥胖、咳喘、带下等表现。

3. Disordered Qì Dynamic

The proper direction for spleen qì to move is to rise and upbear. Spleen qì upbears the clear and leads the upward movement of the qì dynamic in the whole body. Complementing the function of stomach qì to downbear turbidity, it constitutes the mainstay for regulating the upbearing and downbearing activity of the qì dynamic in the whole body. When spleen qì is damaged and fails to govern the upbearing of the clear but bears downward instead, this can cause an imbalance and disorder in the up-bearing and downbearing of the qì dynamic of the whole body.

When spleen qì fails to bear upward, the essence of grain and water cannot be transported up to the heart, lungs, head, face, ears, and eyes, and the clear orifices are deprived of nourishment. This manifests as dizzy head and vision, a pale white facial complexion, and inhibited mouth and pharynx.

When spleen qì does not downbear, qì can stagnate in the center burner, manifesting as distention and fullness in the stomach duct and abdomen, torpid intake and reduced eating, and nontransformation of food.

When spleen qì falls downward, the qì dynamic sags down and its uplifting lacks strength. This can result in such manifestations as sagging heaviness in the stomach duct and abdomen, frequent desire to defecate, enduring diarrhea and disinhibition, sagging heaviness in the anus, and prolapse of the rectum and other organs.

气机紊乱

脾气以上升为顺，脾气升清，带动全身气机上行，与胃气降浊相互为用，成为调节全身气机升降运动之枢纽。脾气受伤，不主升清，反而下降，可使全身气机升降失调而紊乱。脾气不升，水谷精微不能上输心肺头面耳目，清窍失养，而见头目眩晕、面色淡白、口咽不利；脾气不降，气滞中焦，而见脘腹胀满、纳呆食少、饮食不化；脾气下陷，气机下坠，升举乏力，可致脘腹重坠、便意频数、久泻久利、肛门重坠或脱肛、内脏下垂等表现。

4. Impaired Movement of Blood

The spleen stores construction and transforms and engenders construction-blood. The spleen engenders qì. When qì is effulgent, it manages and contains blood so that it moves ceaselessly, circulates inside the vessels, and does not spill to the outside. When spleen qì is vacuous, its managing and containing function breaks down, and blood fails to stay in the channels. This can result in blood spilling to the outside, blood desertion, or frenetic movement of blood. When the spleen fails to manage blood in the upper body, blood can spill in the upper body, manifesting as nosebleed, expectoration of blood, or blood ejection. When the spleen fails to manage blood in the lower body, blood flows downward. This can cause bloody urine, bloody stool, profuse menstruation, flooding and spotting, and bloody stool. When the spleen fails to manage blood in the skin, blood will exit from the skin, causing spontaneous bleeding of the flesh. When a failure of the spleen to manage blood causes blood to spill to the outside of the vessels and to collect in the tissue of the bowels and viscera, it can form static blood and transform into pathogenic evil qì, resulting in even more complex pathomechanisms.

血液失运

脾藏营，化生营血。脾生气，气旺统摄血液，运行不息，循环脉内，而不外溢。脾气虚弱，统摄无权，血不归经，可致血液外溢，血脱妄行。脾不统血于上，血从上溢，而见衄血、咯血、吐血；脾不统血于下，血向下流，则为尿血、便血、月经过多、崩漏下血；脾不统血于肌肤，血从皮出，则为肌衄。脾不统血，血溢脉外，停留脏腑组织局部，可成瘀血，转化为病理性致病邪气，引起更为复杂病机变化。

5. Insecurity of External Defense

The chapter, "Five Types of Dribbling Urinary Stoppages" in the *Líng Shū* ("The Magic Pivot"), states: "The spleen constitutes defense." The chapter, "Successive Diseases in the Bowels and Viscera and Channels and Network Vessels" in the *Jīn Guì Yào Lüè* ("Essential Prescriptions of the Golden Coffer") contains the following statement: "When the spleen is effulgent in the four seasons, [the body] does not contract evil." Both of these quotes point out that spleen qì has the function of defending and fighting against evil.

When spleen qì is effulgent, it transforms and engenders ancestral qì, enriches and engenders defense qì, protects and defends the fleshy exterior, and fights and resists external evil. If spleen qì is vacuous, however, it is unable to engender defense qì, causing an insufficiency of defense yáng. The interstices are not closed tightly and are unable to provide a secure external defense. This can easily result in an invasion of external evil, leading to a common cold. It manifests in such recurrent symptoms as spontaneous sweating, aversion to wind, nasal congestion and clear snivel, and fatigued spirit and lack of strength. At the same time, the insufficiency at the source of transformation causes qì and blood to be depleted, the functions of the whole body and the viscera and bowels to be impaired, and the resistance to disease to be weakened, making diseases continuous and difficult to treat.

卫外不固

《灵枢•五癃津液篇》云："脾为之卫"。《金匮要略•脏腑经络先后病》有"四季脾旺不受邪"之说，均指出脾气具有防卫抗邪的功能。脾气旺盛，化生宗气，滋生卫气，护卫肌表，抗御外邪。若脾气虚弱，不能化生卫气，卫阳不足，腠理不密，不能卫外为固，易致外邪入侵，引起感冒，表现为自汗、恶风、鼻塞清涕、神疲乏力、反复发作等症。同时因其化源不足，气血亏虚，全身脏腑功能低下，抗病力减弱，使疾病缠绵难愈。

6. Malnutrition

The spleen is the root of the acquired constitution and the source of qì and blood formation. It is able to engender qì and blood and the fluids, to convert kidney essence, to enrich spirit qì, and to nourish the whole body. When spleen qì is damaged, the source of engendering transformation is deficient. As a result, the organism lacks the provision of such fundamental substances as qì, blood, essence, spirit, and fluids, the functions and activities of the bowels and viscera are impaired, and the whole body presents with nutritional insufficiency. This leads to symptoms of vacuity such as emaciation of the body, fatigued spirit and lack of strength, shortage of qì and laziness to speak, fatigue and somnolence, heart palpitations, insomnia, and a pale white and lusterless facial complexion.

营养缺乏

脾为后天之本，气血生化之源，能化生气血，生成津液，转化肾精，滋生神气，营养全身。脾气受伤，生化之源匮乏，机体缺乏

气、血、精、神、津液等基础物质的供养，脏腑功能活动衰退，全
身呈现营养不足而致的形体消瘦、神疲乏力、少气懒言、困倦嗜
卧、心悸失眠、面色淡白无华等虚羸症状。

The following can become pathogenic factors in the formation of spleen
disease: An external contraction of the six excesses (wind, cold, summerheat, damp, dryness, fire); internal damage from the seven affects
(joy, anger, anxiety, thought, sorrow, fear, fright); dietary irregularities;
excessive taxation fatigue; an untimely way of living; an internal collection of phlegm-damp and nontransformation of water qì; blood or food
and drink collecting, stagnating, and causing internal blockage; prolonged or severe illness, or lack of or inappropriate treatment; constitutional insufficiency; and shift from another disease.

外感六淫，风寒湿热；内伤七情，忧思抑郁；饮食不节，饥饱失
宜；劳倦过度，起居不时；痰湿内停，水气不化；瘀血饮食，停滞
内阻；久病重病，失治误治；禀赋不足，疾病传变，均可成为脾病
的致病因素。

The spleen and stomach are both located in the central region and are intimately related to each other. Beginning with the *Nèi Jīng* ("Inner
Canon"), the spleen and stomach are often discussed together. The
"Chapter on Greater Yīn and Yáng Brightness Diseases" in the *Sù Wèn*
("Plain Questions") states: "When the yáng pathways are replete, the yīn
pathways are vacuous." In later times, the saying, "Repletion indicates
yáng brightness, and vacuity indicates greater yīn" became popular. This
further emphasizes the pathological tendency of spleen disease towards
vacuity and of stomach disease towards repletion. In fact, spleen and
stomach diseases should be discussed separately, and spleen diseases are
not limited primarily to vacuity patterns, but also manifest as repletion
patterns.

    The *Nèi Jīng* ("Inner Canon") not only mentions the expression
"spleen vacuity" directly, but also describes its pathomechanisms and
manifestations. In the "Treatise on Showing Breadth of Vision" in the
Sù Wèn ("Plain Questions"), we find statements like the following:
"Liver vacuity, kidney vacuity, and spleen vacuity all cause heaviness
of the body, vexation, and low spirits," and "The spleen is spongy and
unsolid, like the lung." While it does not yet mention the term "spleen
repletion," it contains such descriptions as "exuberant spleen qì," "generalized pain and heaviness of the body in spleen disease," (*Sù Wèn,*
"Treatise on the Tip and Root and on Passage of Disease") as well as

the statement, "Superabundance of body and qì results in abdominal distention and inhibited urination" (*Sù Wèn*, "Treatise on Regulating the Channels"). These established the foundation for the pathomechanism of spleen repletion.

In the chapter, "On Calming the Pulse" in the *Shāng Hán Lùn* ("On Cold Damage"), Zhāng Zhòngjǐng elaborated on the main ideas in the *Nèi Jīng* ("Inner Canon"), statiing:

> "When the instep yáng pulse is slippery and tight…this tightness indicates a strong spleen qì, with persistent repletion and strong attack, and pain returning to hurt oneself."

This text thus added a description of the pathomechanism of spleen repletion on the basis of the pulse manifestation.

Carrying on the scholarship and thinking of the *Nèi Jīng* ("Inner Canon"), Wáng Shū-Hé clearly expounded the terms and pathomechanisms of spleen repletion and spleen vacuity. In the chapter, "Calming the Pulse at Man's Prognosis, Spirit Gate, and Qì Opening" in the *Mài Jīng* ("Pulse Canon"), he explained:

> "In cases of spleen repletion, the patient suffers from cold in the feet, heat in the lower legs, abdominal fullness and distention, vexation and harassment, and inability to lie down."

> "In cases of spleen vacuity, the patient will suffer from outpour diarrhea, abdominal fullness and qì counterflow, cholera and vomiting, jaundice, heart vexation and inability to lie down, and rumbling intestines."

In the *Zhōng Zàng Jīng* ("Central Treasury Canon"), Huá Tuó not only turned the pathomechanisms of spleen vacuity and repletion into specialized chapter titles, but also carried out an in-depth discussion. In the "Methods for Discussing Vacuity and Repletion, Cold and Heat, Life and Death, and Favorable and Unfavorable Shifts in the Spleen," he stated:

> "Spleen repletion causes frequent dreams of structures ,walls, and covered rooms. Exuberance causes dreams of singing and joy.

> "In cases of spleen vacuity, essence fails to overcome the loss of original qì, the patient is unable to control urination, and the pulse arrives like running water."

The pediatric treatise, *Xiǎo Ér Yào Zhèng Zhí Jué* ("Key to Diagnosis and Treatment of Children's Diseases"), which is an expert source on bowel and visceral pattern identification, introduced *xiè huáng sǎn* (Yellow-Draining Powder) and *qī wèi bái zhú sǎn* (Seven-Ingredient White Atractylodes Powder) and established the treatment of spleen disease based on pattern identification of vacuity and repletion pathomechanisms. Highly commended by Zhāng Jié-Gǔ, it stated:

"The spleen… is like no other pattern. In cases of vacuity, [treat with] Dr. Qián's *yì huáng sǎn* (Transforming Yellow Powder); in cases of repletion, with *xiè huáng sǎn* (Yellow-Draining Powder)."

The "Heart-Approach to the Main Treatments" in the *Yī Xué Qǐ Yuán* ("Expounding the Origin of Medicine") further strengthened the role of vacuity-repletion pattern identification in the treatment of spleen disease.

Most later medical texts like the *Tài Píng Shèng Huì Fāng* ("Great Peace Sagacious Benevolence Formulary"), *Dān-Xī Shǒu Jìng* ("Dān-Xī's Hand Mirror"), and *Bǐ Huā Yī Jìng* ("Bihua's Medical Mirror") emphasize a clear differentiation between the pathomechanisms of spleen vacuity and spleen repletion in the pattern identification of spleen disease. The chapter, "Vacuity and Repletion in the Five Viscera" in the *Dān-Xī Shǒu Jìng* ("Dān-Xī's Hand Mirror"), explains:

"Spleen vacuity: Inability to lift the limbs, nontransformation of food, acid swallowing or inability to get food down, vomiting after eating, abdominal pain and rumbling intestines, sloppy stool and diarrhea, and a deep, fine, soft, or weak pulse.

Spleen repletion: Heart and chest vexation and oppression, dry mouth and generalized heat effusion, swollen cheeks, heaviness of the body, abdominal distention, cold and hunger, swollen root of the tongue, fatigued and falling limbs, diarrhea, and a tight, urgent, and replete pulse."

This text not only provided the most precise description of and elaboration on vacuity and repletion pathomechanisms of spleen disease; it also played a deeply influential role in the birth of pattern discrimination in spleen disease. It received close attention from the medical world, and has continued to be used up to the present day.

脾胃同处中州，关系密切。从《内经》开始，常把脾胃相提并论。在《素问·太阴阳明病篇》中有："阳道实，阴道虚"之说。后世更有"实则阳明，虚则太阴"之论，提出了脾病多虚，胃病多实的病理趋向。实际上脾与胃病应分开而论，脾病不仅虚证居多，实证亦并非少见。《内经》中不仅直接点出"脾虚"的名称，还阐述其病机和表现。如《素问·示从容论》中说："肝虚、肾虚、脾虚，皆令人体重烦冤"，"夫脾虚浮似肺"等说法。虽未提出"脾实"之名，但有"脾气盛"，"脾病身痛体重"(《素问·标本病传论》)和"形气有余则腹胀，泾溲不利"(《素问·调经论》)等论述，为"脾实"病机奠定了基础。张仲景秉承《内经》旨意，在《伤寒论·平脉篇》中说："趺阳脉，滑而紧…紧则脾气强，持实击强，痛还自伤。"从脉象上对"脾实"的病机加以阐述。王叔和在继承和发扬《内经》学术思想中明确提出"脾实"、"脾虚"的名称和病机。如《脉经·平人迎神门气口前后脉》说："脾实，病苦足寒，胫热，腹胀满，烦扰不得卧。""脾虚，病苦泄注，腹满气逆，霍乱呕吐，黄疸，心烦不得卧，肠鸣。"华佗《中藏经》不仅把脾脏虚实病机专列篇名，还作了深入的探讨。如《论脾脏虚实寒热生死逆顺之法》说："脾实则时梦筑墙盖屋，盛则梦歌乐"。"脾虚则精不胜元气之失，溺不能自持，其脉来似水流。"擅长脏腑辨证的儿科专著《小儿药证直诀》创立了泻黄散，七味白术散，开始了对脾病虚实病机的辨证治疗，被张洁古崇赞为"脾…如无他证，虚则以钱氏益黄散，实则泻黄散"(《医学启源•主治心法》)， 更加巩固了虚实辨证在脾病中的地位。后世许多医著如《太平圣惠方》、《丹溪手镜》、《笔花医镜》对脾病辨证时都十分重视脾虚和脾实病机的鉴别。如《丹溪手镜•五脏虚实》所说："脾虚：四肢不举，饮食不化，吞酸或不下食，食则呕吐，腹痛肠鸣，溏泄，脉沉细软弱。脾实：心胸烦闷，口干身热，颊肿，体重，腹胀寒饥，舌根肿，四肢怠堕，泄下利，脉紧急实。"不仅对脾病虚实病机作了最精辟的论述和发挥，也对脾病的辨证产生深远影响，而颇受医界关注，沿用至今。

Summary of the Pathomechanisms of Spleen Disease

1. Digestive Disorders

   Torpid intake and absence of hunger, reduced eating and difficult transformation, distention and fullness in the stomach duct and abdomen, abdominal pain and intestinal rumbling, diarrhea, sloppy stool or constipation, scant or frequent urination.

2. Fluid Imbalances

   Damp turbidity, phlegm-rheum, water swelling, drum distention, obesity, cough and panting, vaginal discharge.

3. Disordered Qì Dynamic

   Spleen qì failing to upbear: Dizzy head and vision, pale white facial complexion, inhibited mouth and pharynx.

   Qì stagnation in the center burner: Distention and fullness in the stomach duct and abdomen, torpid intake and reduced eating, non-transformation of food.

   Downward fall of spleen qì: Sagging heaviness in the stomach duct and abdomen, frequent desire to defecate, enduring diarrhea, sagging heaviness in the anus, prolapse of the rectum and other organs.

4. Impaired Movement of Blood

Blood spilling out from the top: Nosebleed, expectoration of blood, blood ejection.
Blood flowing downward: Bloody urine, bloody stool, profuse menstruation, flooding and spotting, descent of blood.
Blood exiting from the skin: Spontaneous bleeding of the flesh.
Blood spilling to the outside of the vessels: Blood stasis.

5. Insecurity of External Defense

Spontaneous sweating, aversion to wind, nasal congestion and clear snivel, fatigued spirit and lack of strength, recurrent attacks.

6. Malnutrition

Emaciation of the body, fatigued spirit and lack of strength, shortage of qì and laziness to speak, fatigue and somnolence, heart palpitations, insomnia, pale white lusterless facial complexion.

脾病病机

1、消化障碍——纳呆不饥，食少难化，脘腹胀满，腹痛肠鸣，腹泄下痢，便溏或便秘，尿少或频多。

2、水液失调——湿浊，痰饮，水肿，鼓胀，肥胖，咳喘，带下。
脾气不升——头目眩晕，面色淡白，口咽不利。

3、气机紊乱 中焦气滞——脘腹胀满，纳呆食少，饮食不化。
脾气下陷——脘腹重坠，便意频数，久泻久利，肛门重坠或脱肛，内脏下垂。

血从上溢——衄血，咯血，吐血。

血下下流——尿血，便血，月经过多，崩漏下血。

4、血液失运

血从皮出——肌衄。

血溢脉外——瘀血。

5、卫外不固——自汗，恶风，鼻塞清涕，神疲乏力，反复发作。

6、营养缺乏——形体消瘦，神疲乏力，少气懒言，困倦嗜卧，心悸失眠，面色淡白无华。

脾

PART ONE

Pathomechanisms of Spleen Repletion

脾实的病机

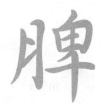

Spleen Repletion
脾实

The most important physiological function of the spleen is that of governing movement and transformation. This is closely linked to the digestion, absorption, and distribution of food and fluids, and to the formation and movement of qi, blood, and fluids. Damage to the spleen can be caused by pathological changes due to an invasion of external evils, damage from food and drink, malfunctions in the movement of the essence of grain and water and of fluids, disorders in the upbearing and downbearing activity of the qì dynamic, poor blood flow or blood stasis, or the retention of pathogenic substances.

When the spleen's movement is encumbered, spleen qì becomes congested, evil and right engage in violent struggles, and exuberance becomes superabundant. This leads to the pathomechanism of spleen repletion. It should be mentioned that spleen disease is mostly associated with vacuity, which is a reflection of the dominant pathological trend. However, the tendency of spleen qì to be encumbered leads to repletion, a situation that is in fact not infrequently observed in clinical practice. The statement in the "Great Treatise on the Essentials of Supreme Truth" in the *Sù Wèn* ("Plain Questions"), "All cases of dampness, swelling, and fullness are associated with the spleen," is the earliest description of the pathomechanism of spleen repletion.

The pathomechanism and transmutations of spleen repletion are portrayed even more succinctly in the "Treatise on Tip and Root and on Passage of Disease" in the same text: "Spleen disease: generalized pain and heaviness of the body, followed by distention after one day, pain in the lesser abdomen and lumbar spine and aching of the lower legs after two days, pain in the back and paravertebral sinews and urinary block after three days, and, if the patient fails to recover, death after ten days."

"The Sixteenth Difficult Issue" in the *Nàn Jīng* ("Classic of Difficult Issues") elaborates on these ideas:

> "Suppose one detects a spleen pulse, its external signs are a yellow face and a tendency to belching, over-mentation, and [dislike of] strong flavors, and its internal sign is the presence of stirring qì right on the umbilicus that feels firm and painful when pressed. The disease manifests as abdominal distention and fullness, failure to disperse food, heaviness of the body and joint pain, fatigue and somnolence, and loss of use of the limbs."

This further expands on the manifestation of the pathomechanism of spleen repletion.

The chapter, "Dual Repletion of Spleen and Stomach" in the *Qiān Jīn Yào Fāng* ("A Thousand Gold Pieces Prescriptions") points out unequivocally:

> "When the bar pulse on the right hand indicates a dual repletion of yīn and yáng, this is a case of dual repletion of the foot greater yīn and the yáng brightness channels. The patient will suffer from spleen distention and abdominal hardness, prodding pain under the rib-side, nonconversion of stomach qì, difficult defecation sometimes alternating with diarrhea, and pain in the abdomen...This is called dual repletion of spleen and stomach."

Summarizing the experience of his predecessors, Qián Yǐ condensed the pathomechanism of spleen repletion into three words: "Spleen governs encumbrance." Mirroring this concept, Qián Yǐ, in his pediatric masterpiece, *Xiǎo Ér Yào Zhèng Zhí Jué* ("Key to Diagnosis and Treatment of Children's Diseases"), "Governings of the Five Viscera," regarding spleen disease in the separate treatment of the five viscera, states: "Repletion causes sleep encumbrance, generalized heat, and drinking of water."

Wàn Mì-Zhāi expanded on this idea, believing that the quality of repletion in "encumbrance" referred to spleen qì being encumbered by disease evil. Therefore, one would frequently observe clinical manifestations of evil repletion encumbrance and obstruction such as torpid and encumbered stomach intake, no desire for food and drink, heavy cumbersome limbs, encumbered sleep and laziness to speak, and generalized encumbrance and fatigue. He portrayed a pathological trend in spleen disease that existed in addition to vacuity detriment, stressing that the pathomechanism of spleen repletion was widely present and not to be overlooked.

With the rise of the Warm Disease School, it was stated that the evil qì of the six excesses, such as wind-damp, damp-heat, summerheat-damp, and cold-damp, could easily invade the spleen and encumber and obstruct spleen qì. This would cause the pathomechanisms of spleen repletion to become even more complex and varied. Nonetheless, when we concentrate on the mutations of spleen yáng qì, the pathomechanisms of spleen repletion can be summed up in the two categories of spleen qì depression and spleen fire (yáng) exuberance.

It is important to note that the pathomechanisms of spleen repletion and spleen vacuity cannot be narrowly distinguished. According to the principle, "for evil to encroach, qì must be vacuous," an evil encumbrance of the spleen will invariably damage the spleen. When the spleen is vacuous, movement and transformation become forceless. This can in turn add to and extend the accumulation of evil qì and pathological substances, aggravating the pathomechanism of spleen repletion. Analyzed from the standpoint of theory, spleen repletion, no matter how severe, includes the pathomechanism of spleen vacuity and manifests only in rare exceptions exclusively in patterns of spleen repletion. However, from the perspective of clinical practice, as long as evil repletion is the chief and vacuity the assistant, evil repletion represents the important aspect of this contradiction. Such cases can therefore all be regarded as pathomechanisms of spleen repletion.

脾的主要生理功能是主运化，与饮食水液的消化、吸收、输布，气血津液的化生、运行有密切关系。发生病理变化时，外邪的侵犯，饮食的损伤，水谷精微、津液运行障碍，气机升降运动失常，血行不畅瘀滞，病理产物贮留，均会伤脾。脾运受困，脾气壅滞，邪正剧烈相争，亢盛有余，引起脾实的病机。应当说脾病多虚，反映了病理趋势的主流。但脾气易困致实，临床确实并非少见。《素问•至真要大论》说："诸湿肿满，皆属于脾"，是对脾实病机最早的描述。该书《标本病传论》："脾病身痛体重，一日而胀，二日少腹腰脊痛，胫酸，三日背月吕筋痛，小便闭，十日不已，死。"更为准确地反映了脾实的病机和传变。《难经•十六难》发挥其旨说："假令得脾脉，其外证面黄，善噫，善思，善味；其内证当齐（脐）有动气，按之牢若痛，其病腹胀满，食不消，体重节痛，怠惰嗜卧，四肢不收。"进一步阐述了脾实的病机表现。《千金要方•脾胃俱实》明确指出："右手关上脉阴阳俱实者，足太阴与阳明经俱实也。病苦脾胀腹坚，抢胁下痛，胃气不转，大便难，时反泄利，腹中痛…名曰脾胃俱实也。"钱乙在总结前人经验的基础上把脾实的病机高度概括为"脾主困"三个字，反映在他的儿科名著《小儿药证直诀•五脏所主》中，按照五脏分治，提出脾病"实则困睡，身热，饮水。"万密斋申明其义，认为"困"的实质是脾气为病邪所困。故临床多见胃纳呆困，不欲饮食，肢体困重，困睡懒言，身体困倦等一派邪实困阻的表现。反映了脾病除虚损外另一类病理趋势，说明脾实病机广泛存在，不容忽视。温病学派兴起，揭示风湿、湿热、暑湿、寒湿等六淫邪气容易犯脾，困阻脾气，使脾实的病机更为复杂多变。不过归纳起来，以脾的阳气变化为中心，脾实的病机可概括为脾气郁滞和脾火（阳）亢盛两大方面。

值得注意，脾实与脾虚的病机不可截然分开。根据"邪之所凑，其气必虚"的原理，脾为邪困，总会伤脾。脾虚运化无力，又可助长邪气和病理产物的停留，加重脾实的病机。从理论分析，脾实之中或多或少包含脾虚的病机，极少单纯见到脾实之证。但从临床实践而言，只要以邪实为主，虚为辅，邪实代表矛盾的主要方面，都可视为脾实的病机。

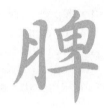

Chapter 1

Spleen Qì Depression
脾气郁滞

Spleen qì represents the functional activity of the spleen, being the driving force behind the spleen's governing of movement and transformation, upbearing of the clear, and controlling blood. Under normal physiological conditions, spleen qì is abundant and thus able to guarantee the healthy development of all the functional activities of the spleen. When evil qì invades the spleen and spleen qì becomes exuberant, this is not at all a case of abundant spleen qì but rather of a sudden encumbrance by disease evil or pathological substances and a depression of spleen qì. It is called spleen qì depression. Not only is depressed spleen qì unable to reinforce the healthy functional activities of the spleen and stomach, but its hyperactivity causes damage and results in functional abnormalities of the spleen.

The *Líng Shū* ("Magic Pivot"), "Chapter on Dreams Caused by Excesses and Evils" explains: "When spleen qì is exuberant, [the patient] dreams of singing and joy," a condition that can cause a disquieted spirit and ethereal soul. The chapter, "Symptoms of Spleen Disease" in the *Zhū Bìng Yuán Hòu Lùn* ("Origin and Indicators of Disease") also explains: "When spleen qì is exuberant, it causes a superabundance of the physical body and the conditions of abdominal distention, inhibited urination, generalized heaviness and hunger, wilting and loss of use of the legs, frequent tugging in the shins, and pain in the underside of the foot. These indicate spleen qì repletion." Both these quotations explain that an exuberance of spleen qì prevents it from governing movement and transformation and from reaching the flesh and limbs. This can result in malfunctions in digestion and physical movement.

Anxiety and preoccupation, the disease evils of cold and damp, phlegm-rheum and water qì, and food and drink-related blood stasis are most likely to depress spleen qì. Depending on the different pathogenic factors, the pathomechanisms of spleen repletion due to spleen qì exuberance can be divided into the following aspects: Thought and preoccupation stagnating the spleen; cold-damp encumbering the spleen; phlegm turbidity obstructing the spleen; food and drink damaging the spleen; and static blood accumulating in the spleen.

脾气代表脾的功能活动，是脾主运化、升清、统血的原动力。生理状态下，脾气充沛，可保证脾的各种功能活动正常发挥。邪气犯脾，脾气亢盛，并非脾气充沛，而是病邪或病理产物困顿、郁滞脾气，称为脾气郁滞。不仅不能加强脾胃正常的功能活动，亢则为害，反致脾的各种功能失常。如《灵枢•淫邪发梦篇》说："脾气盛，则梦歌乐"，可致神魂不安。《诸病源候论•脾病候》亦说："脾气盛，为形有余则病腹胀，泾溲不利，身重苦饥，足痿不收，胻善瘈，脚下痛， 是为脾气之实也。"均说明脾气亢盛，不主运化及肌肉、四肢，可致消化、运动等功能障碍。忧愁思虑、寒湿病邪、痰饮水气、饮食瘀血最易郁滞脾气。根据致病原因的不同，脾气亢盛而致脾实的病机可分为思虑滞脾，寒湿困脾，痰浊阻脾，饮食伤脾，瘀血积脾等几个方面。

1.1 Thought and Preoccupation Stagnating the Spleen

Under normal physiological conditions, thought is said to be an aspect of the spleen. Internal damage from the seven affects or depression related to excessive anxiety and thought can damage spleen qì.

The "Great Treatise on the Correspondences and Manifestations of Yīn and Yáng" in the *Sù Wèn* ("Plain Questions") states, "Thought damages the spleen." "Treatise on Pain" in the same text states, "Thought causes qì to bind." Zhāng Jǐng Yuè further developed this idea: "However, difficulty in relinquishing thoughts causes damage to the spleen," stressing that excessive thought and preoccupation can result in spleen qì depression.

The spleen governs movement and transformation. Thus, when anxiety and thought cause qì to bind, movement and transformation break down, food enters but is difficult to digest and instead collects and binds below the heart, and qì stagnates in the center burner. This can lead to torpid stomach intake, absence of hunger with inability to eat, and low food intake and difficult transformation. When the spleen fails to upbear the clear, the stomach has difficulty in downbearing the turbid, and qì binds in the center burner; this process results in symptoms such as oppression in the heart, glomus in the stomach duct and abdominal distention, abdominal pain and fecal qì (flatus), sloppy and thin stool, white and somewhat slimy tongue fur, and a stringlike pulse.

The "Treatise on the Treatment of Internal Causes; Patterns and Treatments of the Seven Qì" in the *Sān Yīn Jí Yī Bìng Zhèng Fāng Lùn* ("A Unified Treatise on Diseases, Patterns, and Remedies According to the Three Causes") explains:

> "Thought damages the spleen. [As a result,] qì lodges and fails to move, causing accumulations and gatherings in the middle stomach duct, abdominal fullness and distention from food and drink, and fatigue of the four limbs. Therefore, it is said that thought causes qì to bind."

This is an accurate description of the process by which thought and preoccupation damaging the spleen and depressing spleen qì results in the pathomechanism of spleen repletion.

The chapter on "Menstruation" in the *Fù Kē Yù Chǐ* ("Jade Cubit of Gynecology") states:

> "Anxiety and preoccupation damage heart qì, resulting in improper nourishment of spleen qì, binding depression and stoppage, putrefying transformation and lack of movement, and reduced intake of food and drink."

This quotation points out that excessive thought and preoccupation can, when the damage extends from the heart to the spleen, result in spleen qì depression and the formation of spleen repletion patterns in the body.

This condition is treated by moving qì and opening depression, and by moving the spleen and dispersing stagnation. The recommended formula is *píng wèi sǎn* (Stomach-Calming Powder) from the *Tài Píng Huì Mín Hé Jì Jú Fāng* ("Tài-Píng Imperial Grace Pharmacy Formulas") with additions.

Píng Wèi Sǎn 平胃散 Stomach-Calming Powder

chén pí (陈皮 tangerine peel, Citri Reticulatae Pericarpium)
hòu pò (厚朴 officinal magnolia bark, Magnoliae Officinalis Cortex)
cāng zhú (苍术 atractylodes, Atractylodis Rhizoma)
gān cǎo (甘草 licorice, Glycyrrhizae Radix)
Plus:
mù xiāng (木香 costusroot, Aucklandiae Radix)
dà fù pí (大腹皮 areca husk, Arecae Pericarpium)
wū yào (乌药 lindera, Linderae Radix)
xiāng fù zǐ (香附子 cyperus, Cyperi Rhizoma)

If the affect-mind is depressed, ideation can be cramped and the depression of the liver can affect the spleen. Alternatively, if liver qì is effulgent and invades the spleen, spleen qì fails to bear upward, stomach qì fails to bear downward, and the qì dynamic can congest. These situations can also result in spleen qì depression. They manifest as fullness and oppression in the chest and rib-side, frequent sighing, abdominal distention and fullness, abdominal pain with diarrhea, reduced pain after voiding, recurrent attacks, white tongue fur, stringlike pulse, and other symptoms of liver-spleen disharmony.

The chapter, "Swelling and Distention" in the *Lín Zhèng Zhǐ Nán Yī Àn* ("A Clinical Guide with Case Histories") states:

> "The spleen and stomach govern qì. Anger and depression invariably stir the liver and liver-wood then rebels against earth. Thus, the spleen and stomach suffer damage, and chronic depression prevents qì from turning comfortably."

The "Section on the Liver" in the *Bǐ Huā Yī Jìng* ("Bihua's Medical Mirror") also explains:

> "Repletion of the liver causes fullness of qì and internal wind there, and the left bar pulse must be stringlike and surging. Its symptoms consist of pain in the left rib-side, headache, abdominal and smaller-abdominal pain, accumulations and gatherings, mounting qì, cough, and diarrhea."

These quotations clearly describe the pathomechanism by which liver qì exploiting the spleen can cause spleen qì depression, resulting in abdominal pain and diarrhea.

This condition is treated by coursing the liver and opening depression, and by rectifying qì and moving the spleen. The recommended formula is *tòng xiè yào fāng* (Pain and Diarrhea Formula) from the *Jǐng Yuè Quán Shū* ("Jǐng-Yuè's Complete Compendium") with additions.

Tòng Xiè Yào Fāng 痛泻要方 Pain and Diarrhea Formula

fáng fēng (防风 saposhnikovia, Saposhnikoviae Radix)
bái sháo yào (白芍药 white peony, Paeoniae Radix Alba)
chén pí (陈皮 tangerine peel, Citri Reticulatae Pericarpium)
bái zhú (白术 white atractylodes, Atractylodis Macrocephalae Rhizoma)
Plus:
mù xiāng (木香 costusroot, Aucklandiae Radix)
hòu pò (厚朴 officinal magnolia bark, Magnoliae Officinalis Cortex)
xiāng yuán (香橼 citron, Citri Fructus)

思虑滞脾

正常生理状态下，思为脾志。若七情内伤，过度忧思抑郁，可伤及脾气。如《素问•阴阳应象大论》说："思伤脾"。《素问•举痛论》说："思则气结"。张景岳进一步指出："但苦思难释则伤脾"，都强调思虑太过，可致脾气郁滞。脾主运化，忧思气结，运化失司，食入难消，停结心下，气滞中焦，可致胃纳呆滞、不饥不食、食少难化；脾不升清，胃浊难降，气结中焦，则为心中郁闷、脘痞腹胀、腹痛矢气、大便溏稀，苔白略腻，脉弦等症。《三因极—病证方论•内所因治论•七气证治》说："思伤脾，气留而不行，积聚在中脘，饮食腹胀满，四肢怠惰，故经曰思则气结。"是对思虑伤脾，脾气郁滞而引起脾实病机的精辟阐述。《妇科玉尺•月经》云："忧愁思虑，心气受伤，则脾气失养，郁结不通，腐化不行，饮食减少。"指出思虑过度，伤心及脾，可致脾气郁滞，形成脾之实证。治宜行气开郁，运脾消滞。方选《和剂局方》平胃散（陈皮、厚朴、苍术、甘草）加木香、大腹皮、台乌、香附。

若情志抑郁，曲意难伸，肝郁及脾，或肝气旺盛，肝气犯脾，脾气不升，胃气不降，气机壅滞，亦可导致脾气郁滞。表现为胸胁满闷，善太息，腹胀腹满，腹痛作泄，泻后痛减，反复发作，苔白，脉弦等肝脾不调的症状。正如《临证指南医案•肿胀》所云："脾胃主气，愤怒怫郁，无不动肝。肝木侮土，而脾胃受伤，郁久气不转舒。"《笔花医镜•肝部》亦说："肝之实，气与内风充之也，脉左关必弦而洪。其症为左胁痛，为头痛，为腹痛，小腹痛，为积聚，为疝气，为咳嗽，为泄泻。"清楚阐明肝气乘脾，可致脾气郁滞而引起腹痛泄泻的病机。治宜疏肝开郁，理气运脾。方选《景岳全书》痛泻要方（防风、白芍、陈皮、白术）加木香、厚朴、香橼。

Literature Review of Thought & Preoccupation Stagnating the Spleen

📖 *Líng Shū* ("Magic Pivot"), "On Distention"

> "Spleen distension manifests in frequent retching, vexation in the limbs, heaviness of the body with inability to bear the weight of clothing, and unquiet sleep."

This quotation discusses the pathomechanism by which a depression of spleen qì and stagnation of qì in the center burner, when preventing it from carrying out movement and transformation, leads to distention in the stomach duct and abdomen that likes pressure, frequent belching, heaviness of the body, and inability to lie flat.

文献评述

《灵枢•胀论》：”脾胀者，善哕，四肢烦悗，体重不能胜衣，卧不安。”论述脾气郁滞，气滞中焦，运化失职，引起脘腹胀满，嗳气频作，身体沉重，不能平卧的病机。

Summary of Thought and Preoccupation Stagnating the Spleen

1. Qì Binding in the Center Burner

   Torpid stomach intake, absence of hunger and inability to eat, low food intake and difficult transformation, oppression in the heart, glomus in the stomach duct and abdominal distention, abdominal pain and fecal qì, sloppy and thin stool.

2. Liver Qì Invading the Spleen

   Fullness and oppression in the chest and rib-side, frequent sighing, abdominal distention and fullness, abdominal pain with diarrhea, reduced pain after voiding, recurrent attacks.

思虑滞脾

气结中焦——胃纳呆滞，不饥不食，食少难化，心中郁闷，脘痞腹胀，腹痛矢气，大便溏稀。

肝气犯脾——胸胁满闷，善太息，腹胀腹满 ，腹痛作泄，泻后痛减，反复发作。

1.2 Cold-Damp Encumbering the Spleen

Greater yīn spleen-earth is in charge of water-damp, moves by the power of yáng qì, and likes dryness and is averse to dampness. Dampness is a yīn evil and tends to damage yáng qì and obstruct the qì dynamic. It stands in a particularly close relationship with the spleen, and spleen-earth is therefore susceptible to disorders from harassment by the evil of cold-damp.

External dampness is contracted by getting soaked in the rain or wading through water, by living in damp places, by veiling damage from fog or dew, or by working in the water. Internally generated dampness is obtained by indulgent consumption of gourds and fruits, predilection for tea and liquor, or by a loss of movement due to spleen vacuity and the spontaneous production of internal dampness.

External dampness and internal dampness stand in a mutual cause-and-effect relationship and both tend to damage the spleen. A disorder of cold-dampness is most likely to encumber spleen qì and injure spleen yáng. Encumbrance of spleen qì causes a failure of the movement and transformation functions, problems with digesting water and grain, and qì obstruction in the center burner. Consequently, one observes glomus in the stomach duct and abdominal distention, torpid and reduced food intake, upflow nausea and desire to vomit, abdominal pain and intestinal rumbling, diarrhea and sloppy stool, a pale and enlarged tongue with a slimy white tongue fur, and a soggy and moderate pulse.

When water-damp fails to transform, it floods into the skin and flesh where it causes puffy swelling and fatness. When water-damp flows downward, it prevents the girdling vessel from ensuring retention, which causes white turbidity and vaginal discharge. Dampness by nature is heavy and turbid and, when it traps spleen qì, causes inhibition in the channels and vessels. The result is aching and heaviness of the head and body and a fatigued and cumbersome spirit. When spleen dampness is overly exuberant, the dampness of the earth causes wood to be depressed, liver qì fails to outthrust, the gallbladder looses its ability to course freely, and bile seeps to the outside. This results in yīn jaundice and a darkened face, eyes, skin, and flesh, as if they had been fumigated.

When spleen yáng is devitalized, dampness forms under the influence of cold, and the warming and propelling functions fail. Consequently one observes such manifestations as fear of cold and cold limbs, a devitalized essence-spirit, and a pale white and lusterless facial complexion. The chapter on the "Source of Damp Disease" in the *Zá Bìng Yuán Liú Xī Zhú* ("Incisive Light on the Source of Miscellaneous Disease") states:

> "It is said that all dampness with swelling and fullness is ascribed to spleen-earth. This explains that excessive earth-damp generates the diseases of glomus, blockage, swelling, and fullness. Hence it is also said that the various diseases of tetany and rigidity, accumulation of rheum and glomus in the diaphragm, fullness and vomiting in the center and cholera diarrhea below, generalized heaviness and skin swelling, and mud-like flesh that fails to rise when pressed, all are ascribed to dampness. Now greater yīn, dampness, and earth are in fact the qì of the spleen and stomach."

This quotation explains that dampness encumbering spleen qì and impairing splenic movement and transformation can lead to the various symptoms of glomus and fullness, swelling and distension, and vomiting and diarrhea.

The "Treatise on Damp Qì" in the *Yī Yuán* ("Origin of Medicine") also explains:

"[Owing to] internal damage from cold-damp…spleen and stomach yáng is damaged, water is excessive, and earth inundated. When spleen yáng is damaged, one observes patterns with such symptoms as glomus in the stomach duct and abdominal distention, abdominal pain and swelling, sloppy stool and throughflux diarrhea, and triple yīn malaria."

This quotation stresses that cold and damp congealing and encumbering spleen qì can result in an overgrowth of glomus, fullness, swelling, and diarrhea.

The chapter on "Jaundice" in the *Lín Zhèng Zhǐ Nán Yī Àn* ("A Clinical Guide with Case Histories") explains:

"Yīn jaundice works like this: Dampness is formed from cold and water. When spleen yáng is unable to transform dampness and bile is obstructed by dampness, it soaks the spleen, oozes into the flesh, and spills into the skin, causing a smoky yellow complexion."

This source elaborates in detail on the pathomechanism of yīn jaundice due to cold-damp encumbering the spleen, which causes earth to be congested, wood to be depressed, and the gallbladder to fail to course freely.

To sum up, the most important pathomechanisms of cold-damp encumbering the spleen are spleen qì encumbrance, damage to yáng qì, impaired splenic movement, and internal exuberance of yīn cold. Its diseases are ascribed to repletion.

This condition is treated by warming the center and transforming qì, and by drying dampness and moving the spleen. Conditions mainly characterized by spleen qì encumbrance with glomus in the stomach duct, torpid intake, diarrhea, and soupy stool are treated with the formula *píng wèi sǎn* (Stomach-Calming Powder) from the *Tài Píng Huì Mín Hé Jì Jú Fāng* ("Tài-Píng Imperial Grace Pharmacy Formulas") with additions. An alternative choice is *wèi líng tāng* (Stomach-Calming Poria Five Decoction) from the *Fù Rén Dà Quán Liáng Fāng* ("Compendium of Good Remedies for Women") with the addition of *cǎo dòu kòu* (Alpiniae Katsumadai Semen), or *hòu pò wēn zhōng tāng* (Official Magnolia Bark Center-Warming Decoction) from the *Nèi Wài Shāng Biàn Huò Lùn* ("Clarification of Perpexities about Internal and External Damage").

Píng Wèi Sǎn 平胃散
Stomach-Calming Powder

cāng zhú (苍术 atractylodes, Atractylodis Rhizoma)
hòu pò (厚朴 officinal magnolia bark, Magnoliae Officinalis Cortex)
chén pí (陈皮 tangerine peel, Citri Reticulatae Pericarpium)
gān cǎo (甘草 licorice, Glycyrrhizae Radix)
Plus:

fù zǐ (附子 aconite, Aconiti Radix Lateralis Praeparata)
gān jiāng (干姜 dried ginger, Zingiberis Rhizoma)

Wèi Líng Tāng 胃苓汤
Stomach-Calming Poria Five Decoction

cāng zhú (苍术 atractylodes, Atractylodis Rhizoma)
hòu pò (厚朴 officinal magnolia bark, Magnoliae Officinalis Cortex)
chén pí (陈皮 tangerine peel, Citri Reticulatae Pericarpium)
guì zhī (桂枝 cinnamon twig, Cinnamomi Ramulus)
zé xiè (泽泻 alisma, Alismatis Rhizoma)
zhū líng (猪苓 polyporus, Polyporus)
bái zhú (白术 white atractylodes, Atractylodis Macrocephalae Rhizoma)
fú líng (茯苓 poria, Poria)
gān cǎo (甘草 licorice, Glycyrrhizae Radix)
Plus:
cǎo dòu kòu (草豆蔻 Katsumada's galangal seed, Alpiniae Katsumadai Semen)

Hòu Pò Wēn Zhōng Tāng 厚朴温中汤
Officinal Magnolia Bark Center-Warming Decoction

hòu pò (厚朴 officinal magnolia bark, Magnoliae Officinalis Cortex)
gān jiāng (干姜 dried ginger, Zingiberis Rhizoma)
chén pí (陈皮 tangerine peel, Citri Reticulatae Pericarpium)
fú líng (茯苓 poria, Poria)
cǎo dòu kòu (草豆蔻 Katsumada's galangal seed, Alpiniae Katsumadai Semen)
mù xiāng (木香 costusroot, Aucklandiae Radix)
gān cǎo (甘草 licorice, Glycyrrhizae Radix)

For conditions mainly characterized by nontransformation of water-damp with puffy swelling and vaginal discharge, recommended formulas are *shí pí sǎn* (Spleen-Firming Powder) from the *Jì Shēng Fāng,* or *wán dài tāng* (Discharge-Ceasing Decoction) from the *Fù Qīng Zhǔ Nǚ Kē* ("Fù Qīng-Zhǔ's Gynecology") with the addition of *gān jiāng* (Zingiberis Rhizoma).

Shí Pí Sǎn 实脾散
Spleen-Firming Powder

hòu pò (厚朴 officinal magnolia bark, Magnoliae Officinalis Cortex)
bái zhú (白术 white atractylodes, Atractylodis Macrocephalae Rhizoma)

mù guā (木瓜 chaenomeles, Chaenomelis Fructus)
mù xiāng (木香 costusroot, Aucklandiae Radix)
cǎo guǒ (草果 tsaoko, Tsaoko Fructus)
bīng láng (槟榔 areca, Arecae Semen)
pào fù zǐ (炮附子 blast-fried aconite, Aconiti Radix Lateralis Tosta)
bái fú líng (白茯苓 white poria, Poria Alba)
pào jiāng (炮姜 blast-fried ginger, Zingiberis Rhizoma Praeparatum)
zhì gān cǎo (炙甘草 mix-fried licorice, Glycyrrhizae Radix cum
    Liquido Fricta)

Wán Dài Tāng 完带汤
Discharge-Ceasing Decoction

bái zhú (白术 white atractylodes, Atractylodis Macrocephalae Rhizoma)
cāng zhú (苍术 atractylodes, Atractylodis Rhizoma)
shān yào (山药 dioscorea, Dioscoreae Rhizoma)
rén shēn (人参 ginseng, Ginseng Radix)
bái sháo yào (白芍药 white peony, Paeoniae Radix Alba)
chē qián zǐ (车前子 plantago seed, Plantaginis Semen)
chái hú (柴胡 bupleurum, Bupleuri Radix)
jīng jiè (荆芥 schizonepeta, Schizonepetae Herba)
gān cǎo (甘草 licorice, Glycyrrhizae Radix)
Plus:
gān jiāng (干姜 dried ginger, Zingiberis Rhizoma)

For conditions mainly characterized by inhibited channels and aching pain in the head and body, the recommended formula is *píng wèi sǎn* (Stomach-Calming Powder) in combination with *qiāng huó shèng shī tāng* (Notopterygium Dampness-Overcoming Decoction) from the *Nèi Wài Shāng Biàn Huò Lùn* ("Clarification of Perpexities about Internal and External Damage").

Píng Wèi Sǎn 平胃散
Stomach-Calming Powder

cāng zhú (苍术 atractylodes, Atractylodis Rhizoma)
hòu pò (厚朴 officinal magnolia bark, Magnoliae Officinalis Cortex)
chén pí (陈皮 tangerine peel, Citri Reticulatae Pericarpium)
gān cǎo (甘草 licorice, Glycyrrhizae Radix)

Qiāng Huó Shèng Shī Tāng 羌活胜湿汤
Notopterygium Dampness-Overcoming Decoction

qiāng huó (羌活 notopterygium, Notopterygii Rhizoma et Radix)
dú huó (独活 pubescent angelica, Angelicae Pubescentis Radix)
fáng fēng (防风 saposhnikovia, Saposhnikoviae Radix)
gǎo běn (藁本 Chinese lovage, Ligustici Rhizoma)
chuān xiōng (川芎 chuanxiong, Chuanxiong Rhizoma)
màn jīng zǐ (蔓荆子 vitex, Viticis Fructus)
zhì gān cǎo (炙甘草 mix-fried licorice, Glycyrrhizae Radix cum
   Liquido Fricta)

For failure of the gallbladder to course freely and for yīn jaundice, the formula is *yīn chén zhú fù tāng* (Virgate Wormwood, Atractylodes, and Aconite Decoction) from the *Yī Xué Xīn Wù* ("Medical Insights"), with the addition of *fú líng* (Poria) and *zé xiè* (Alismatis Rhizoma).

Yīn Chén Zhú Fù Tāng 茵陈术附汤
Virgate Wormwood, Atractylodes, and Aconite Decoction

yīn chén hāo (茵陈蒿 virgate wormwood, Artemisiae Scopariae Herba)
fù zǐ (附子 aconite, Aconiti Radix Lateralis Praeparata)
gān jiāng (干姜 dried ginger, Zingiberis Rhizoma)
bái zhú (白术 white atractylodes, Atractylodis Macrocephalae Rhizoma)
zhì gān cǎo (炙甘草 mix-fried licorice, Glycyrrhizae Radix cum
   Liquido Fricta)
Plus:
fú líng (茯苓 poria, Poria)
zé xiè (泽泻 alisma, Alismatis Rhizoma)

寒湿困脾

太阴脾土，主司水湿，得阳始运，喜燥恶湿。湿为阴邪，易伤阳气，阻遏气机，与脾有特殊的亲和性，故脾土易被寒湿之邪犯扰为患。湿之外受，得之于淋雨涉水，居处潮湿，冒伤雾露，水中作业；湿之内生，得之于恣食瓜果，嗜茶好酒，或因脾虚失运，内湿自生。外湿内湿，互为因果，均易伤脾。寒湿为患，最易困顿脾气，损伤脾阳。脾气困顿，运化失职，水谷难消，气阻中焦，则见脘痞腹胀、纳呆食少、泛恶欲吐、腹痛肠鸣、腹泄便溏、舌淡胖、苔白腻、脉濡缓。水湿不化，泛溢肌肤，而为浮肿肥胖。水湿下流，带脉失约，而为白浊带下。湿性重浊，脾气被遏，经脉不利，而为头身酸重、神疲困倦。脾湿过盛，土湿木郁，肝气不达，胆失疏泄，胆汁外溢，发为阴黄，面目肌肤晦暗如烟熏。脾阳不振，湿从寒化，失于温煦、推动，则见畏寒肢冷，精神不振，面色淡白无华等表现。《杂病源流犀烛•湿病源流》云："经曰：诸湿肿满，皆属脾土。此言土湿过甚，则痞塞肿满之病生。经故又曰：诸痉强直，积饮痞膈，中满吐下霍乱，体重跗肿，肉如泥，按之不起，皆属于湿也。盖太阴湿土，乃脾胃之气。"说明湿困脾气，脾失健运，可致痞满、肿胀、吐泻诸症。《医原•湿气论》亦说："内伤寒湿…脾胃阳伤，水多土溢。脾阳伤，则见脘痞腹胀，腹痛肿胀，便溏洞泄，三阴痎疟症等证。"指出寒与湿凝，困滞脾气，可致痞满肿泻丛生。《临证指南医案•黄疸》说："阴黄之作，湿从寒水，脾阳不能化湿，胆液为湿所阻，渍于脾，浸淫肌肉，溢于皮肤，色如熏黄。"详细阐明了寒湿困脾，土壅木郁，胆失疏泄而致阴黄的病机。概括而言，寒湿困脾，主要病机为脾气受困，阳气受伤，脾运失职，阴寒内盛，其病属实。

治宜温中化气，燥湿运脾。脾气困顿，脘痞纳呆，腹泻便溏为主，用《和剂局方》平胃散（苍术、厚朴、陈皮、甘草）加附子、干姜，或用《妇人大全良方》胃苓汤（苍术、厚朴、陈皮、桂枝、泽泻、猪苓、白术、茯苓、甘草）加草豆蔻，或用《内外伤辨惑论》厚朴温中汤（厚朴、干姜、橘皮、茯苓、草豆蔻、木香、甘草）；水湿不化，浮肿带下为主，用《济生方》实脾散（厚朴、白术、木瓜、木香、草果仁、大腹子、炮附子、白茯苓、炮干姜、炙甘草）或《傅青主女科》完带汤（白术、苍术、山药、人参、白芍、车前子、柴胡、荆芥、甘草）加干姜；经脉不利，头身酸痛为主，用平胃散合《内外伤辨惑论》羌活胜湿汤（羌活、独活、防风、藁本、川芎、蔓荆子、炙甘草）；胆失疏泄，阴黄，用《医学心悟》茵陈术附汤（茵陈、附子、干姜、白术、炙甘草）加茯苓、泽泻。

Literature Review of Cold-Damp Encumbering the Spleen

📖 *Líng Shū* ("Magic Pivot"), "Chapter on the Five Colors"

> "When the evil is located in the spleen and stomach... the resulting insufficiency of yáng qì and superabundance of yīn qì will cause cold stroke, intestinal rumbling, and abdominal pain."

This quotation points out that vacuity cold in the spleen viscus causes movement and transformation failures and an internal collection of cold dampness. This can create the pathomechanism of abdominal pain and intestinal rumbling.

📖 *Shāng Hán Zhǐ Zhǎng* ("A Guidebook on Cold Damage"), "Damp-ness Symptoms"

"In cases of cold-damp, the pulse is deep, slow, and soggy, the body lacks heat, and the patient suffers from vomiting and diarrhea but without thirst, clear and disinhibited urine, generalized pain and heaviness, or perhaps swelling and pain in the hands and feet."

This describes how cold-damp damaging the spleen, externally obstruct-ing the channels, and inhibiting the flow of qì in the channels results in soreness, heaviness, swelling, and pain in the head and body.

📖 *Yī Chún Shèng Yì* ("Refined and Surplus Meanings in Medicine"), "Various Pains"

"The spleen is rooted in dampness and earth. When cold evil exploits it and cold congeals with dampness, this constitutes a case of double yīn. The stomach duct descends to the umbilicus, causing distention that likes pressure and pain."

This quotation describes how external cold and internal dampness bind together and encumber and obstruct spleen qì, resulting in the pathome-chanism of abdominal distention and pain.

📖 *Shāng Hán Lùn* ("On Cold Damage"), "Identifying Yáng Brightness Disease Pulses and Patterns, and their Treatment"

"In cold damage, promoting sweating results in generalized yellowing, including the eyes. This happens because there is unresolved cold-damp in the interior. It is assumed that [in this situation] one cannot precipitate, [but should] seek [to treat the disease by addressing] cold and dampness."

This quotation points out that cold-damp in the spleen and splenic movement and transformation failure can lead to jaundice.

📖 *Lèi Zhèng Zhì Cái* ("Systematized Patterns with Clear-Cut Treat-ments"), "Jaundice"

"Yīn jaundice is tied to cold-damp in the spleen and lack of movement, causing bile to spread and soaks out into the flesh, erupting as jaundice."

This quotation describes the pathomechanism by which jaundice erupts, when spleen yáng is devitalized and dampness forms with cold, congest-ing earth and depressing wood, so that bile spills outward.

文献评述

《灵枢•五色篇》："邪在脾胃...阳气不足，阴气有余，则寒中肠鸣腹痛。"指出脾脏虚寒，运化失职，寒湿内停，可形成腹痛肠鸣的病机。

《伤寒指掌•湿证》：”寒湿，脉沉迟而濡，身无热，但吐泻，口不渴，小水清利，身痛重着，或手足肿痛者，寒湿。”阐述寒湿伤脾，外阻经脉，经气不通，可致头身酸重肿痛。

《医醇剩义•诸痛》：”脾本湿土，寒邪乘之，寒与湿凝，是为重阴，脘下至脐，胀满作痛。”阐述外寒内湿，相互结合，困阻脾气，引起腹胀作痛的病机。

《伤寒论•辨阳明病脉证并治》：”伤寒发汗已，身目发黄。所以然者，以寒湿在里，不解故也，以为不可下也，于寒湿中求治，”指出寒湿在脾，脾失健运，可致黄疸。

《类证治裁•黄疸》：”阴黄系脾脏寒湿不运，与胆液浸淫，外渍肌肉，则发为黄。”阐述脾阳不振，湿从寒化，土壅木郁，胆汁外溢，发为黄疸的病机。

Summary of Cold-Damp Encumbering the Spleen

1. Spleen Qì Encumbrance

Glomus in the stomach duct and intestinal distention, torpid and reduced food intake, upflow nausea and desire to vomit, abdominal pain and intestinal rumbling, diarrhea and sloppy stool.

2. Water-Damp Failing to Transform

Puffy swelling and fatness, white turbidity and vaginal discharge.

3. Cold-Damp Encumbering the Spleen and Inhibition in the Channels

Aching and heaviness of the head and body, fatigued and cumbersome spirit.

4. Gallbladder Losing its Ability to Course Freely

Yīn jaundice, darkened face, eyes, skin, and flesh as if they had been fumigated.

5. Loss of Warmth

Fear of cold and cold limbs, devitalized essence-spirit, pale white and lusterless complexion.

寒湿困脾

脾气困顿——脘痞腹胀，纳呆食少，泛恶欲吐，腹痛肠鸣，腹泄便溏。

水湿不化——浮肿肥胖，白浊带下。

经脉不利——头身酸重，神疲困倦。

胆失疏泄——阴黄，面目肌肤晦暗如烟熏。

失于温煦——畏寒肢冷，精神不振，面色淡白无华。

1.3 Phlegm Turbidity Obstructing the Spleen

The chapter, "Source of Phlegm-Rheum" in the *Zá Bìng Yuán Liú Xī Zhú* ("Incisive Light on the Source of Miscellaneous Disease"), states:

> "Phlegm-rheum is a dampness disease. It is said that when greater yīn is at the spring, dampness excess is prevalent and the people suffer from rheum accumulation.' Again, it is said that 'when earth is depressed and greater yīn recurs, patients will all suffer from rheum eruption.' In all discussions of phlegm-rheum in the *Nèi Jīng,* [phlegm-rheum] is caused by damp earth. From the very beginning of a person's life to their imminent death, whenever phlegm is present, it is always formed in the spleen and gathers in the stomach."

This statement reinforces the significance of the spleen and stomach in the formation of phlegm. In spite of the fact that the lung, spleen, and kidneys are all closely tied to the formation of phlegm turbidity, the spleen resides in the central region and governs movement to the four sides. If the spleen fails to move dampness, earth fails to dam water and water-damp stops and accumulates, which can easily lead to the formation of phlegm turbidity. For this reason, the ancients already had the expression, "The spleen is the source of phlegm formation."

Moreover, once phlegm turbidity is formed, it is a pathological product that becomes a secondary cause of disease. Pathologic substances can injure the spleen and stomach, suddenly encumber the movement and transformation functions of spleen qì, obstruct the ascending and descending functions of the qì dynamic, and aggravate the depression of spleen qì. In addition to panting and cough and oppression in the chest with copious phlegm that is slippery, disinhibited, and easy to expectorate, the condition will manifest primarily as symptoms of spleen qì depression, such as glomus in the stomach duct and abdominal distention, torpid and reduced food intake, bland taste in the mouth, rumbling intestines with diarrhea, fatigue and lack of strength, obesity, and a pale and fat tongue with white, thick and slimy fur.

In the chapter, "Treatise on Exuberance and Debilitation of the Spleen and Stomach" in the *Pí Wèi Lùn* ("On the Spleen and Stomach"), Lǐ Dōng-Yuán states: "Fatness in spite of reduced eating and inability to lift the limbs in spite of fatness is probably a sign of spleen repletion and exuberance of evil qì." "Spleen repletion" refers to a congestion and repletion of spleen qì. "Exuberance of evil qì" indicates an internal exuberance of phlegm-damp. Thus, patients of this type eat and drink very little, but their body is fat and their limbs lack strength in spite of the fatness. This quotation describes the pathomechanism of phlegm turbidity obstructing the spleen comprehensively.

Further, the *Yī Xué Rù Mén* ("Gateway to Medicine") "Section on Phlegm" states:

> "[Phlegm] is formed in the spleen and primarily [manifests in] fatigued limbs, sometimes with abdominal pain, swelling, and distention, and diarrhea. The pulse is moderate, and it is predominant in fat people. It is called damp phlegm."

The chapter, "The Source of Phlegm-Rheum" in the *Zá Bìng Yuán Liú Xī Zhú* ("Incisive Light on the Source of Miscellaneous Disease"), also explains:

> "In the spleen, it is called damp phlegm. Its color is yellow and it is slippery and easy to expectorate. [It manifests as] tendency to fatigue, limpness with a tendency to lie down, abdominal distention and food stagnation, a pulse that must be moderate, sometimes complicated by vacuity, diet, summerheat, or fright. In each case, it should be treated from the spleen aspect."

This quotation explains in detail the manifestations of the pathomechanism of phlegm turbidity obstructing the spleen.

This condition is treated by moving the spleen and eliminating dampness, and by rectifying qì and transforming phlegm. The recommended formula is a modified version of *èr chén tāng* (Two Matured Ingredients Decoction) from the *Zhāng Shì Yī Tōng* ("Zhang's Clear View of Medicine").

Èr Zhú Èr Chén Tāng 二术二陈汤
Two Atractylodes and Two Matured Ingredients Decoction

chén pí (陈皮 tangerine peel, Citri Reticulatae Pericarpium)
bàn xià (半夏 pinellia, Pinelliae Rhizoma)
fú líng (茯苓 poria, Poria)
shēng jiāng (生姜 fresh ginger, Zingiberis Rhizoma Recens)
dà zǎo (大枣 jujube, Jujubae Fructus)
cāng zhú (苍术 atractylodes, Atractylodis Rhizoma)
bái zhú (白术 white atractylodes, Atractylodis Macrocephalae Rhizoma)

痰浊阻脾

《杂病源流犀烛·痰饮源流》云："痰饮，湿病也。经曰：太阴在泉，湿淫所胜，民病饮积。…又曰：土郁之发，太阴之复，皆病饮发。<内经>论痰饮，皆因湿土，以故人自初生，以至临死，皆有痰，皆生于脾，聚于胃。"强调脾胃在生痰中的重要意义。虽然肺、脾、肾与痰浊生成均有密切关系，但因脾居中州，主运四旁，脾不运湿，土不制水，水湿停聚，易生痰浊，故古人早有"脾为生痰之源"之说。痰浊已成，又可作为继发致病因素—病理产物，损害脾胃，困顿脾气运化，阻滞气机升降，加重脾气郁滞。除见咳嗽气喘、胸闷痰多、滑利易咯外，表现有较多的脾气郁滞症状：如脘痞腹胀，纳呆食少，口淡无味，肠鸣腹泻，身倦乏力，形体肥胖，舌淡胖，苔白厚腻等。东垣《脾胃论•脾胃胜衰论》说："少食而肥，虽肥而四肢不举，盖脾实而邪气盛也。""脾实"是指脾气壅实，"邪气盛"是指痰湿内盛。故这种人饮食很少，反而体胖，虽胖而四肢无力，充分阐述了痰浊阻脾的病机。又如《医学入门•痰门》说："生于脾，多四肢倦怠，或腹痛肿胀，泄泻，其脉缓，肥人多有之，名曰湿痰。"《杂病源流犀烛•痰饮源流》亦说："在脾曰湿痰，其色黄，滑而易出，多倦怠，软弱喜卧，腹胀食滞，脉必缓，或挟虚、挟食、挟暑、挟惊，各宜从脾分治。"均详细说明了痰浊阻脾的病理表现。治宜运脾除湿，理气化痰。方选《张氏医通》二术二陈汤（二陈汤加苍术、白术）加减。

Literature Review of Phlegm Turbidity Obstructing the Spleen

📖 *Zhōng Zàng Jīng* ("Central Treasury Canon"), "Methods for Discussing Vacuity and Repletion, Cold and Heat, Life and Death, and Favorable and Unfavorable Aspects in the Organ of the Spleen"

> "As for repletion, it means a stiff tongue, no pleasure in eating, retching counterflow, and slackness of the four limbs."

> "In excessive cases, it causes people to suffer from heaviness of the four limbs and sluggish and inhibited speech."

Spleen repletion refers to the fact that the spleen is encumbered by phlegm turbidity. Counterflow ascent of phlegm and qì causes vomiting and lack of appetite. Phlegm turbidity stagnating in the root of the tongue causes stiffness of the tongue and unclear speech. Phlegm turbidity flowing into the limbs causes heaviness of the four limbs.

📖 *Bìng Jī Huì Lùn* ("Collection of Pathomechanisms,") "Phlegm-Rheum"

> "What is the cause for the presence of phlegm-rheum? When the six qì invade from the outside, when the seven affects cause internal turmoil, or when fatty or sweet foods or liquor or dampness injure the spleen and stomach, the qì pathways are congested, the flow in the channels and network vessels is stopped, and the fluids congeal, gather, and turn into vanquished turbidity. This results in phlegm-rheum."

This quotation explains how various types of disease causes can injure the spleen so that the spleen fails to transform fluids and phlegm-rheum is generated. When phlegm-rheum collects internally and obstructs the qì pathways and channels and network vessels, it can lead to many kinds of pathologies.

📖 *Zhāng Shì Yī Tōng* ("Zhang's Clear View of Medicine"), "Phlegm-Rheum"

"In the discussions of the former sages, the spleen is the source of phlegm formation, and the lung the receptacle that holds phlegm. Again, it is said that if you treat phlegm without rectifying the spleen and stomach, you will not treat it effectively. When spleen-earth is vacuous, the clear becomes difficult to upbear and turbidity difficult to downbear. Consequently, they remain in the center and obstruct the diaphragm, stagnate, and form phlegm… When phlegm is located in the spleen channel, it is called damp phlegm. It manifests in a moderate pulse, yellow face, heavy limbs, craving for sleep without closing [the eyes], and abdominal distention and food stagnation. This type of phlegm is slippery and easy to expectorate. Treat it with *èr chén tāng* (Two Matured Ingredients Decoction) plus *zhǐ shí* (Aurantii Fructus Immaturus) and *bái zhú* (Atractylodis Macrocephalae Rhizoma)."

When the spleen fails to upbear the clear, and the stomach fails to downbear turbidity, dampness collects in the center burner and transforms into phlegm turbidity. Phlegm turbidity encumbers the spleen, resulting in symptoms like slippery and easily expectorated phlegm, abdominal distention, and heavy limbs.

📖 *Bù Jū Jí* ("Non-limitation Collection"), "Phlegm-Rheum"

"The spleen and stomach constitute the granaries and therefore are responsible for absorbing grain. If the spleen because of weakness is unable to move and provide nourishment for blood and qì, the result is impaired circulation in the pathways of qì, stagnation in the center burner, and inability to decompose grain. Consequently, it will collect and stagnate, forming phlegm-rheum. Its pathologies include cold or heat, panting or coughing, vomiting or stomach reflux, and swelling and fullness… in unlimited forms that are all pathologies of phlegm. Its root cause lies in a stoppage of spleen dampness and stagnation of water and grain and fluids."

This quotation fully describes the pathomechanism by which spleen qì fails to move, the fluids stagnate and form phlegm-rheum, and phlegm-rheum obstructs the spleen, transforming and engendering many types of transmuted patterns.

文献评述

《中藏经·论脾脏虚实寒热生死逆顺之法》："实者舌强直，不嗜食，呕逆，四肢缓。""太过则令人四肢沉重，语言謇涩。"脾实，是指脾为痰浊所困。痰气上逆，则呕吐、不欲食；痰浊阻于舌本，则舌强，言语不清；痰浊流于肢体，则四肢沉重。

《病机汇论•痰饮》："何痰饮之有哉？迨乎六气外侵，七情内乱，惑肥甘酒湿损伤脾胃，则气道壅滞，脉络不通，津液凝聚转为败浊，此为痰为饮之端也。"说明各种病因损伤于脾，脾不化津，生成痰饮。痰饮内停，阻塞气道经络，又可引起多种病变。

《张氏医通•痰饮》："先哲论，脾为生痰之源，肺为贮痰之器。又曰，治痰不理脾胃，非其治也。以脾土虚，则清者难升，浊者难降，留中滞膈，瘀而成痰。…在脾经者，名曰湿痰。脉缓面黄，肢体沉重，嗜卧不收，腹胀食滞，其痰滑而易出，二陈加枳术。"脾不升清，胃不降浊，湿停中焦，化生痰浊，痰浊困脾，则引起痰滑易出，腹胀肢重等症。

《不居集•痰饮》："脾胃为仓廪，所以纳谷。因脾弱不能运行，致血气失于滋养，故不周流气道，壅滞中焦，不能腐谷，遂停滞而为痰为饮。其变为寒为热，为喘为咳，为呕吐，为反胃，为肿满…不可尽状，是皆痰之变病。而其源则出于脾湿不流，水谷津液停滞之所致也。"充分阐述脾气不运，水津停滞而成痰饮，痰饮阻脾，化生多种变证的病机。

Summary of Phlegm-Turbidity Obstructing the Spleen
1. Phlegm-Turbidity Invading the Lung Cough and panting, oppression in the chest with copious phlegm that is slippery, disinhibited, and easy to expectorate.
2. Spleen Qì Failing to Move Glomus in the stomach duct and abdominal distention, torpid and reduced food intake, bland taste in the mouth, intestinal rumbling and diarrhea, fatigue and lack of strength, obesity.
痰浊阻脾
痰浊犯肺——咳嗽气喘，胸闷痰多，滑利易咯。
脾气失运——脘痞腹胀，纳呆食少，口淡无味，肠鸣腹泻，身倦乏力，形体肥胖。

1.4 Food and Drink Damaging the Spleen

Food and drink are the basic substances for the vital activities of the human body and provide a boost for its health. However, if they are provided in inappropriate amounts, they cause damage instead. For example, irregular eating, unclean food, or a predilection for strange foods can injure the stomach as well as the spleen.

As stated in the chapter, "Prevalence and Weakness of the Spleen and Stomach" in the *Pí Wèi Lùn* ("On the Spleen and Stomach"), "Dietary irregularities cause stomach disease...and when the stomach is diseased, the spleen has nothing to be endowed with." When food and drink damage the spleen, the most important result is its effect on spleen qì. When spleen qì is encumbered, movement and transformation functions are impaired, the movement of the spleen becomes difficult, food is not transformed, upbearing and downbearing is disturbed, and qì stagnates in the center burner. Therefore one observes such symptoms as oppression in the chest and glomus in the stomach duct, torpid intake and a bland taste in the mouth, abdominal distention and fullness, abdominal pain that refuses pressure, intestinal rumbling with diarrhea, sour-, putrid-, or foul-smelling feces, fatigued and cumbersome limbs, a thick and slimy tongue fur, and a slippery pulse.

The "Treatise on Food and Drink Damaging the Spleen" in the *Pí Wèi Lùn* ("On the Spleen and Stomach") also contains the following quotation: "The forty-ninth difficult issue states that taxation and fatigue from food and drink damage the spleen. It further states that when food and drink are doubled, the intestines and stomach are damaged, which results in intestinal afflux and hemorrhoids. Now regarding the spleen, it moves the fluids of the stomach, grinds the grain inside the stomach, and governs the five flavors. Damage to the stomach impairs the transformation of food and drink, prevents the mouth from tasting flavors, and causes fatigue and encumbrance of the four limbs, glomus and fullness of the heart and abdomen, shaking with desire to vomit and aversion to food, and occasional swill diarrhea or intestinal afflux. This illustrates the fact that when the stomach is damaged, the spleen is also damaged." The abdominal fullness with sloppy stool and encumbrance and fatigue of the four limbs mentioned here as a result of food damage indicate that the stomach disease has affected the spleen, that the spleen is now the main location of the disease, and that the emphasis is now on encumbered spleen qì failing to perform its movement and regulation functions. It is obvious that this is different from food and drink damaging the stomach.

This condition is treated by moving the spleen and moving qì, and by dispersing food and transforming stagnation. The recommended formula is *xiāng shā píng wèi sǎn* (Costusroot and Amomum Stomach-Calming Powder) from the *Yī Zōng Jīn Jiàn* ("Golden Mirror of Medicine"), a modified version of *píng wèi sǎn* (Stomach-Calming Powder).

Xiāng Shā Píng Wèi Sǎn 香砂平胃散
Costusroot and Amomum Stomach-Calming Powder

chén pí (陈皮 tangerine peel, Citri Reticulatae Pericarpium)
hòu pò (厚朴 official magnolia bark, Magnoliae Officinalis Cortex)
cāng zhú (苍术 atractylodes, Atractylodis Rhizoma)
gān cǎo (甘草 licorice, Glycyrrhizae Radix)
Plus:
shā rén (砂仁 amomum, Amomi Fructus)
xiāng fù zǐ (香附子 cyperus, Cyperi Rhizoma)
shān zhā (山楂 crataegus, Crataegi Fructus)
shén qū (神曲 medicated leaven, Massa Medicata Fermentata)
mài yá (麦芽 barley sprout, Hordei Fructus Germinatus)
zhǐ qiào (ké) (枳壳 bitter orange, Aurantii Fructus)
bái sháo yào (白芍药 white peony, Paeoniae Radix Alba)
shēng jiāng (生姜 fresh ginger, Zingiberis Rhizoma Recens)

饮食伤脾

饮食是人体生命活动的基本物质，有益于健康。稍有失宜，则反而为害。如饥饱失常，饮食不洁，偏嗜食物，既可损胃，又可伤脾。正如《脾胃论•脾胃胜衰》所云："饮食不节则胃病…胃既病，则脾无所禀受。"饮食伤脾，主要影响脾气，脾气困阻，运化失职，脾运艰难，化食无能，升降失司，气滞中焦，故见胸闷脘痞、纳呆口淡、腹胀腹满、腹痛拒按、肠鸣泻利、便下酸腐秽臭、四肢困倦、舌苔厚腻、脉滑等症。正如《脾胃论•饮食伤脾论》所云："<四十九难>曰：饮食劳倦则伤脾。又云：饮食自倍，肠胃乃伤，肠澼为痔。夫脾者行胃津液，磨胃中之谷，主五味也。胃既伤则饮食不化，口不知味，四肢困倦，心腹痞满，兀兀欲吐而恶食，或为飧泄，或为肠澼，此胃伤脾亦伤明矣。"这里言伤食引起腹满便溏，四肢困倦，是胃病及脾，病位应侧重于脾，为脾气受困，运化失司。与饮食伤胃，自然有别。治宜运脾行气，消食化滞。方选《医宗金鉴》香砂平胃散（平胃散加砂仁、香附、山楂、神曲、麦芽、枳壳、白芍、生姜。）

Literature Review of Food and Drink Damaging the Spleen

📖 *Zhēn Jiǔ Dà Chéng* ("Great Compendium of Acupuncture and Moxibustion"), "Song of the Foot Greater Yīn Spleen Channel"

"If people are merely intemperate in their eating or drinking or suffer from excessive taxation fatigue, this damages their spleen qì. Once the spleen and stomach are damaged, food and drink are not transformed, the mouth does not know flavors, the four limbs are cumbersome and fatigued, and the heart and abdomen suffer from glomus and fullness; this results in vomiting and diarrhea, as well as intestinal afflux (bloody stool due to intestinal stasis)."

This quotation describes the pathomechanism by which splenic transformation failure from food and drink-related damage to the spleen can lead to torpid intake, abdominal fullness, and diarrhea.

📖 *Dān Xī Xīn Fǎ Fù Yú* ("A Supplement to Dān-Xī's Experiential Therapy"), "Spleen and Stomach"

"When people are intemperate in their eating and drinking and lead an untimely way of life, they damage the spleen and stomach. When the stomach is damaged, it is unable to carry out intake. When the spleen is injured, it is unable to carry out transformation. When both the spleen and stomach are damaged, both intake and transformation are impaired, the original qì is weakened and the hundred evils can invade easily, causing such symptoms as bloating and oppression, glomus and accumulations, block and repulsion, counterflow vomiting, abdominal pain, and diarrhea."

This quotation further describes how food- and drink-related damage to the spleen and nontransformation of spleen qì can lead to bloating and oppression, abdominal pain, diarrhea, and other symptoms related to impaired splenic movement and transformation.

文献评述

《针灸大成•足太阴脾经歌》："人惟饮食不节，劳倦过甚，则脾气受伤矣。脾胃一伤，则饮食不化，口不知味，四肢困倦，心腹痞满，为吐泄，为肠澼。"阐述了饮食伤脾，脾失健运，可致纳呆、腹满、泄泻的病机。

《丹溪心法附余•脾胃》："人惟饮食不节，起居不时，损伤脾胃。胃损则不能纳，脾损则不能化，脾胃俱损，纳化皆难，元气斯弱，百邪易侵，而饱闷、痞积、关格、吐逆、腹痛、泄痢等症作矣。"进一步阐述饮食伤脾，脾气不化，可致饱闷、腹痛、泄痢等脾失健运的症状。

Summary of Food and Drink Damaging the Spleen
1. Stagnation of Stomach Qì Chest oppression and glomus in the stomach duct, torpid intake and bland taste in the mouth. 2. Impaired Splenic Movement and Transformation Abdominal distention and fullness, abdominal pain that refuses pressure, intestinal rumbling and diarrhea, sour, putrid, or foul smelling feces, encumbrance and fatigue of the four limbs.
饮食伤脾
胃气郁滞——胸闷脘痞，纳呆口淡。 脾失健运——腹胀腹满，腹痛拒按，肠鸣泻利，便下酸腐秽臭，四肢困倦。

1.5 Static Blood Accumulating in the Spleen

The spleen governs movement and transformation, and it also controls blood. Dietary irregularities or excessive taxation can damage the spleen and stomach, causing the breakdown of intake by the stomach and of movement and transformation by the spleen. This makes the spleen and stomach susceptible to qì stagnation. When spleen qì has been damaged for a long time, the spleen becomes vacuous and unable to contain blood. Blood spills to the outside of the channels and stagnates in the intestines, forming static blood. Once formed, static blood not only fails to carry out its ordinary function of nourishing, but also tends to interact with the juices inside the intestines, causing the fluids to stagnate there. They congeal and gather instead of dispersing, and form accumulations and gatherings.

The chapter, "The Source of Accumulations and Gatherings, Concretions and Conglomerations, Strings and Aggregations, and Glomus" in the *Zá Bìng Yuán Liú Xī Zhú* ("Incisive Light on the Source of Miscellaneous Disease"), explains:

"A sudden increase in food and drink causes intestinal fullness. An irregular way of life or excessive exertion of energy causes damage to the yáng network vessels. When the yáng network vessels are damaged, blood spills to the outside. When the yīn network vessels are damaged, blood spills internally. When blood spills internally, it causes bloody stool. When the network vessels of the intestines and stomach are damaged, blood spills to the outside of the intestines. When cold is present on the outside of the intestines, the juices contend with the blood, combine with it, and congeal into gatherings that are impossible to dissipate, leading to the formation of accumulations."

Static blood, as a pathogenic factor, collects in the stomach and intestines and can aggravate spleen qì encumbrance and stagnation. It influences the movement and transformation function of spleen qì, and manifests in symptoms such as concrete lumps below the heart, glomus blockage with pain, abdominal distention and fullness, fatigued limbs, vomiting and diarrhea, jaundice, and water swelling. This is referred to as spleen accumulation.

The chapter, "Accumulations and Gatherings" in the *Yī Biǎn* ("Lancing Stones of Medicine"), explains:

> "Spleen accumulation is called glomus qì. Located in the stomach duct, it is as big as an overturned plate and [manifests with] glomus blockage that cannot be moved, heart and back pain, reduced hunger and satiation upon looking, abdominal fullness with vomiting and diarrhea, and in chronic cases loss of use of the limbs, yellowing, failure of food and drink to be transformed into skin and flesh, swelling of the feet, and wasting of the flesh."

The symptom of yellowing is caused by congested earth and depressed wood impeding the free flow of gallbladder qì. The remaining symptoms are related to static blood accumulating in the spleen, spleen qì depression, qì stagnation and lack of free flow, and loss of movement and transformation.

In contemporary medicine, hepatosplenomegaly, liver cirrhosis and ascites, an enlarged drum-like abdomen, prominent green-blue veins on the abdomen, fine red lines in the face, neck and chest, and rock-like hardness of the liver and spleen are all related to spleen vacuity complicated by stagnation, internal damage from the seven affects, and vanquished earth and robbed wood. For example, the chapter, "Drum Distention" in the *Dān Xī Xīn Fǎ* ("Dān Xī's Heart-Approach"), states:

> "When the yīn of spleen earth is damaged, the office of transformation and transportation breaks down. Although the stomach receives grain, it is unable to move and transform it. Therefore, yáng naturally rises and yīn naturally falls, and heaven and earth fail to interact. The clear and the turbid mix and tunnels congest, heat transforms into dampness, and dampness and heat contend with each other, resulting in the formation of drum distention."

In this quotation, "the clear and the turbid mix and tunnels congest" refers to the process by which the movement and transformation of the spleen and stomach are disturbed, upbearing and downbearing break down, the clear and turbid fail to be separated, the qì dynamic becomes obstructed, the movement of blood becomes stagnant, and the channels, network vessels, and tunnels congest, resulting in qì stagnation, water collection, and the formation of drum distention. In this context, spleen vacuity leads to stasis and stasis encumbers the spleen, creating a vicious circle of mutual cause and effect. Therefore, the drum distention is prolonged and difficult to cure.

This condition is treated by harmonizing and rectifying the spleen and stomach, and by dispelling stasis and softening hardness. The recommended formula is either *gé xià zhú yū tāng* (Infradiaphragmatic Stasis-Expelling Decoction) from the *Yī Lín Gǎi Cuò* ("Correction of Errors in Medical Classics") or *biē jiǎ jiān wán* (Turtle Shell Decocted Pill) from the *Jīn Guì Yào Lüè* ("Essential Prescriptions of the Golden Coffer"), in combination with *liù jūn zǐ tāng* (Six Gentlemen Decoction).

Gé Xià Zhú Yú Tāng
膈下逐瘀汤 Infradiaphragmatic Stasis-Expelling Decoction

dāng guī (当归 Chinese angelica, Angelicae Sinensis Radix)

chuān xiōng (川芎 chuanxiong, Chuanxiong Rhizoma)

chì sháo yào (赤芍药 red peony, Paeoniae Radix Rubra)

táo rén (桃仁 peach kernel, Persicae Semen)

hóng huā (红花 carthamus, Carthami Flos)

mǔ dān pí (牡丹皮 moutan, Moutan Cortex)

wū yào (乌药 lindera, Linderae Radix)

yán hú suǒ (延胡索 corydalis, Corydalis Rhizoma)

wǔ líng zhī (五灵脂 squirrel's droppings, Trogopteri Faeces)

xiāng fù zǐ (香附子 cyperus, Cyperi Rhizoma)

zhǐ qiào (*ké*) (枳壳 bitter orange, Aurantii Fructus)

gān cǎo (甘草 licorice, Glycyrrhizae Radix)

Biē Jiǎ Jiān Wán 鳖甲煎丸
Turtle Shell Decocted Pill

zhì biē jiǎ (炙鳖甲 mix-fried turtle shell, Trionycis Carapax cum Liquido Frictus)

shè gān (射干 belamcanda, Belamcandae Rhizoma)

huáng qín (黄芩 scutellaria, Scutellariae Radix)

shǔ fù (鼠妇 wood louse, Armadillidium)

gān jiāng (干姜 dried ginger, Zingiberis Rhizoma)

dà huáng (大黄 rhubarb, Rhei Radix et Rhizoma)

guì zhī (桂枝 cinnamon twig, Cinnamomi Ramulus)

shí wéi (石韦 pyrrosia, Pyrrosiae Folium)

hòu pò (厚朴 officinal magnolia bark, Magnoliae Officinalis Cortex)

qū mài (瞿麦 dianthus, Dianthi Herba)

líng xiāo huā (凌霄花 campsis flower, Campsis Flos)

ē jiāo (阿胶 ass hide glue, Asini Corii Colla)

chái hú (柴胡 bupleurum, Bupleuri Radix)

qiāng láng (蜣螂 dung beetle, Catharsius)

sháo yào (芍药 peony, Paeoniae Radix)

mǔ dān pí (牡丹皮 moutan, Moutan Cortex)

zhè chóng (蟅虫 ground beetle, Eupolyphaga seu Steleophaga)

zhì fēng cháo (炙蜂巢 mix-fried hornet's nest, Vespae Nidus)

chì xiāo (赤硝 red niter, Nitrum Rubrum)

táo rén (桃仁 peach kernel, Persicae Semen)

rén shēn (人参 ginseng, Ginseng Radix)

bàn xià (半夏 pinellia, Pinelliae Rhizoma)

tíng lì zǐ (葶苈子 lepidium/descurainiae, Lepidii/Descurainiae Semen)

Liù Jūn Zǐ Tāng 六君子汤
Six Gentlemen Decoction

---

fú líng (茯苓 poria, Poria)

bái zhú (白术 white atractylodes, Atractylodis Macrocephalae Rhizoma)

rén shēn (人参 ginseng, Ginseng Radix)

zhì gān cǎo (炙甘草 mix-fried licorice, Glycyrrhizae Radix cum
    Liquido Fricta)

bàn xià (半夏 pinellia, Pinelliae Rhizoma)

chén pí (陈皮 tangerine peel, Citri Reticulatae Pericarpium)

瘀血积脾

脾主运化，又主统血。饮食不节，或劳倦过度，损伤脾胃，胃不主受纳，脾不司运化，脾胃容易气滞。日久伤及脾气，脾虚不能统摄血液，血溢脉外，停滞肠间，形成瘀血。瘀血既成，不仅失却正常的濡养作用，反而易与肠间汁沫、停滞津液相互作用，迫聚不散，形成积聚。如《杂病源流犀烛•积聚癥瘕痃癖痞源流》说："卒然多饮食则胀满，起居不节，用力过度则阳络脉伤，阳络伤则血外溢，阴络伤则血内溢，血内溢则后血，肠胃之络伤则血溢于肠外，肠外有寒，汁沫与血相搏，则并合凝聚不得散，而积成矣。"瘀血作为病理致病因素，停聚胃肠，又会加重脾气的困滞，影响脾气的运化，出现心下有形之包块，痞塞疼痛、腹胀腹满、四肢倦怠、呕吐腹泄、黄疸、水肿等症状，称为脾积。如《医碥•积聚》所说："脾积名痞气，在胃脘，大如覆盘，痞塞不通，心背痛，饥减饱见，腹满吐泄，久则四肢不收，发黄，饮食不为肌肤，足肿肉消。"除发黄是由土壅木郁，胆气不疏所为外，其余症状均系瘀血积脾，脾气郁滞，气滞不通和运化失职所致。现代医学中肝脾肿大，肝硬化腹水，腹大如鼓，腹壁青筋，面、颈、胸部丝状红缕，肝脾坚硬如石，皆为脾虚挟瘀，七情内伤，土败木贼使然。正如《丹溪心法•鼓胀》所云："脾土之阴受伤，转输之官失职，胃虽受谷，不能运化，故阳自升，阴自降，而成天地不交之否，清浊相混，坠道壅塞，热化为湿，湿热相搏，遂成鼓胀。"其中"清浊相混，坠道壅塞"就是脾胃运化失调，升降失司，清浊不分，气机阻滞，血行瘀阻，壅塞经络坠道，导致气滞、血瘀、水停，而成鼓胀。这里因脾虚致瘀，又因瘀困脾，互为因果，恶性循环，故鼓胀迁延难愈。治宜调理脾胃，祛瘀软坚。方选《医林改错》膈下逐瘀汤（当归、川芎、赤芍、桃仁、红花、丹皮、乌药、延胡索、五灵脂、香附、枳壳、甘草）或《金匮要略》鳖甲煎丸（炙鳖甲、射干、黄芩、鼠妇、干姜、大黄、桂枝、石苇、厚朴、瞿麦、紫葳、阿胶、柴胡、蜣螂、芍药、丹皮、地鳖虫、炙蜂巢、赤硝、桃仁、人参、半夏、葶苈），与六君子汤配合使用。

Literature Review of Static Blood Accumulating in the Spleen

📖 *Nàn Jīng* ("Classic of Difficult Issues"), "Fifty-Sixth Difficult Issue"

> "Spleen accumulation is called glomus qì. It is located below the stomach and is the size of a plate. If this condition is chronic and not cured, it causes the patient to suffer from loss of use of the limbs, jaundice, and food and drink failing to be transformed into skin and flesh."

Spleen accumulation is caused by a binding depression of spleen qì, leading to qì stagnation and blood stasis. The symptoms of abdominal distention and jaundice are related to congested earth and depressed wood.

文献评述

《难经•五十六难》："脾之积，名曰痞气，在胃下，大如盘。久不愈，令人四肢不收，发黄疸，饮食不为肌肤。"脾之积，是由脾气郁结，气滞血瘀所致。腹胀大、黄疸是土壅木郁。

Summary of Static Blood Accumulating in the Spleen
Static Blood Accumulating in the Spleen
Lumps below the heart, glomus blockage with pain, abdominal distention and fullness, fatigue of the four limbs, vomiting, diarrhea, jaundice, water swelling.
瘀血积脾
瘀血积脾——心下之包块，痞塞疼痛，腹胀腹满，四肢倦怠，呕吐，腹泄，黄疸，水肿。

To summarize, encumbrance of spleen qì by disease evils or pathological substances, such as emotions, cold-damp, phlegm-rheum, food and drink, or static blood leads to disorders of the spleen's movement and transformation, causing pathologies classed as spleen repletion. If the condition persists for a long time, it can also damage spleen qì, resulting in pathologic changes in the categories of spleen qì vacuity or spleen yáng vacuity. In terms of relationship with the other organs, breakdown in the free flow of the liver and binding depression of liver qì can arise from cold-damp encumbering the spleen, causing phlegm turbidity to obstruct the spleen. Static blood then accumulates in the spleen, congesting earth and depressing wood. Conversely, when emotional dissatisfaction causes binding depression of liver qì and liver qì invades the spleen, it can give rise to the pathologic change of disharmony between liver and spleen.

总之，脾气为情志、寒湿、痰饮、饮食、瘀血等病邪或病理产物所困，导致脾的运化失调，引起脾实一类的病机变化。病情日久，亦可损伤脾气，引起脾气虚、脾阳虚之类的病机变化。与其它脏腑的关系上，寒湿困脾，痰浊阻脾、瘀血积脾，土壅木郁，可致肝失疏泄，肝气郁结；反之，情志不遂，肝气郁结，肝气犯脾，均可形成肝脾失调的病机变化。

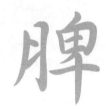

Chapter 2

Spleen Fire Exuberance
脾火亢盛

The spleen's yáng qì has the functions of warming, of stimulating, and of propelling the spleen's movement and transformation functions. If yáng qì becomes exuberant to the point of hyperactivity and superabundance, it can develop into the pathomechanism of spleen fire exuberance. A commonly seen cause is the contraction of evil from the six excesses, which depresses the spleen channel and transforms into fire. In the case of the contraction of dampness evil, it blocks and depresses central qì, and depressed dampness creates heat. Alternatively, the contraction of the evil of damp-heat causes damp-heat to decoct and phlegm-fire to be generated internally. Secondly, dietary irregularities and an internal accumulation of food, the long-term consumption of alcohol or a predilection for fatty and sweet foods impair the movement of the spleen. Alternatively, the excessive consumption of hot and spicy or stimulating foods impair the digestion of food, leading to heat brewing in the spleen channel, becoming depressed and transforming into fire. In addition, if excessive thought and preoccupation cause binding depression of the qì dynamic, this can also transform into fire, a situation referred to as "fire formation due to excess among the five minds." All of the above can lead to spleen fire exuberance. As is explained in the chapter on "The Seven Theories on Fire" in the *Yī Jiā Sì Yào* ("Physician's Four Essentials"), "In all cases of fire of the five minds... when thought and preoccupation have been excessive, fire will arise in the spleen."

In fact, spleen fire exuberance was already discussed amply as early as the *Nèi Jīng* ("Inner Canon"). The "Treatise on Needling Heat" in the *Sù Wèn* ("Plain Questions") states:

"Cases of spleen heat disease first [manifest in] head and cheek pain, a blue-green face, desire to vomit, and generalized heat. Heat struggle will then lead to lumbar pain with inability to bend forward or backward, abdominal fullness and diarrhea, and pain in the two sides of the jaw."

The "Treatise on Wilting" in the *Sù Wèn* ("Plain Questions") also states: "Spleen qì heat causes dryness of the stomach and thirst, numbness of the flesh, and flesh wilting." Subsequently, "Chapter on Jaundice" in the *Jīn Guì Yào Lǜe* ("Essential Prescriptions of the Golden Coffer"), contains the statement:

"This impediment is not a case of wind stroke. [The patient] will suffer from vexation in the four limbs, and the color of the spleen is invariably reflected in a yellow skin, which is caused by static heat moving there."

Regarding the pulse symptoms of spleen fire exuberance, the chapter, "Spleen Vacuity and Repletion" in the *Qiān Jīn Yào Fāng* ("A Thousand Gold Pieces Prescriptions"), further asserted:

"In cases of spleen repletion heat, the bar pulse in the left hand that is yīn and replete points to the foot greater yīn channel. The patient suffers from cold in the feet and heat in the lower legs, abdominal distention and fullness, vexation, and inability to lie down. This condition is referred to as spleen repletion heat."

This statement exerted a far-ranging influence on later generations, and the *Shèng Jì Zǒng Lù* ("Sages' Salvation Records") and *Jì Shēng Fāng* ("Yan's Lifesaving Formulas") both elaborated on it.

Lastly, the "Section on the Spleen" in the *Bǐ Huā Yī Jìng* ("Bihua's Medical Mirror") summarized the pathological manifestations of spleen fire exuberance comprehensively:

"As for the symptoms of spleen heat, the left bar pulse must be rapid, the tongue will be bitter, thin and yellow, and the lips red. Its symptoms include heat vomiting, drooling, throughflux diarrhea, diarrhea swells, red dysentery, abdominal pain, swelling and pain in the eyelids, liquor jaundice, dizziness, and yáng jaundice."

This laid the foundations for the pathomechanisms of spleen fire exuberance.

While the pathomechanisms of spleen fire exuberance are extremely complex, they can be summarized under two categories: The first one is pure spleen yáng exuberance forming repletion fire in the spleen channel. The other one is dampness and heat combining and binding spleen qì, forming the pathomechanism of damp-heat brewing in the spleen.

脾之阳气，具有温煦、激发、推动脾的运化功能。若阳气过盛，亢奋有余，则可发展形成脾火亢盛的病机。常见原因有感受六淫之邪，郁于脾经化火。如感受湿邪，阻郁中气，湿郁成热。或感受湿热之邪，湿热煎熬，痰火内生；其次饮食不节，食积内停，或长期饮酒，嗜食肥甘，损伤脾运；或过服辛辣刺激、不易消化食物，致脾经蕴热，郁而化火。此外，如思虑过度，气机郁结亦可化火，称为"五志化火"，均可引起脾火亢盛。正像《医家四要•火有七说》所说："凡有五志之火者...思虑过饱，则火起于脾。"

实际上早在《内经》时期已有关于脾火亢盛的不少论述。如《素问•刺热论》说："脾热病者，先头颊痛，颜青，欲呕，身热。热争则腰痛不可俯仰，腹满泄，两颔痛。"《素问•痿论》亦说："脾气热，则胃干而渴，肌肉不仁，发为肉痿。"《金匮要略•黄疸病篇》还有"痹非中风，四肢苦烦，脾色必黄，瘀热以行"的论述。《千金要方•脾虚实》对脾火亢盛的脉症作了进一步的肯定："脾实热，右手关上脉阴实者，足太阴经也。病苦足寒，胫热，腹胀满，烦扰，不得卧，名曰脾实热。"对后世产生深远影响。《圣济总录》、《济生方》均沿于此说。直到《笔花医镜•脾部》对脾火亢盛的病理表现作了全面概括："脾热之症，右关必数，舌苦薄而黄，唇赤，其症为热吐，为流涎，为洞泄，为泻渤，为赤痢，为腹痛，为目胞肿痛，为酒疸，为眩晕，为阳黄疸。"才奠定了脾火亢盛病机的基础。脾火亢盛的病机虽然十分复杂，但可概括于两类：一是单纯性的脾阳亢盛而形成脾经实火；另是湿与热合，胶结脾气，形成湿热蕴脾的病机。

2.1 Spleen Channel Repletion Fire

When spleen yáng is excessively hyperactive, it causes a superabundance of qì that amasses into fire. This can give rise to spleen fire. It is most often caused by food accumulation and enduring depression, by excessive consumption of acrid, hot-spicy, or stimulating foods, by fire formation due to excess among the five minds, or by the indiscriminant use of heating and supplementing therapies.

The spleen opens in the mouth, its bloom is in four whites of the lips (the lips and surrounding area), its channel connects to the root of the tongue and dissipates below the tongue, and it is associated with the eyelids. Therefore, when spleen fire blazes internally and the force of the fire follows the channels and flames upward, steaming the upper part of the body, you will observe such symptoms as parched lips and a dry tongue, mouth and tongue sores, a swollen tongue body, a painful, rigid, protruding, and hyperactive tongue, and goose mouth sores and dribbling. Qián Yǐ in his *Xiǎo Ér Yào Zhèng Zhí Jué* ("Key to Diagnosis and Treatment of Children's Diseases") focused exclusively on the use of *xiè huáng sǎn* (Yellow-Draining Powder) to clear spleen channel repletion fire and thereby treat spleen heat-related hyperactive tongue, mouth sores, bad breath, vexation thirst with rapid hungering, and dry mouth and lips, which are obvious signs of this condition. In the chapter, "Fire," in the *Yī Fāng Kǎo* ("Medical Remedies Researched"), Wú Kūn stated as follows in his comments on the use of *xiè huáng sǎn* (Yellow-Draining Powder):

> "The lips are the external indicator of the spleen. The mouth is the opening of the spleen. Therefore, when the lips and mouth are dry, we know that it is spleen fire."

The spleen governs movement and transformation. In the case of spleen channel repletion fire, exuberant fire accelerates movement, and food and grain are easily dispersed, thus causing large appetite with rapid hungering. The spleen governs the greater abdomen as well as the flesh and limbs. When spleen fire exuberates internally, it causes fire congestion, qì stagnation, and spleen qì encumbrance and blockage. Thus, one can observe distention and fullness in the greater abdomen and abdominal pain that refuses pressure. When fire heat scorches the fluids and the spleen fluids are unable to moisten the intestines, the result is constipation. Inability to moisten and nourish the flesh and limbs causes atrophy of the flesh and fatigued limbs that cannot be raised.

The chapter, "Fire Pathoconditions" in the *Zhèng Zhì Huì Bǔ* ("A Supplement to Patterns and Treatment"), states: "Abdominal distention and noise, bad breath, and swollen lips are [a sign of] spleen fire stirring." The chapter, "Spleen and Stomach" of the same text further explains: "You might observe large appetite and paradoxical emaciation of the limbs. This indicates a strong spleen and effulgent evil fire." Both these quotations demonstrate the objective existence of the pathomechanism of spleen channel repletion fire.

In addition, spleen fire exuberance can form splenic pure heat, which is most frequently caused by a predilection for fatty, sweet, or rich foods. The resulting counterflow ascent of spleen fire and turbid qì gives rise to a sweet and slimy ungratifying feeling in the mouth and fatness of the body. As stated in the chapter on "Splenic Pure Heat" in the *Shèng Jì Zǒng Lù* ("Sages' Salvation Records"):

> "When a patient suffers from a sweet taste, this indicates a spillage of the five flavors. It is called splenic pure heat. When food enters into yīn and promotes the growth of qì in yáng, it causes internal heat and center fullness in the person, resulting in exuberant yáng qì. Therefore, yáng alone causes splenic pure heat. Its sign is sweetness in the mouth. When it becomes chronic and is not treated, it turns into dispersion-thirst."

In short, spleen channel repletion fire can lead to many types of symptoms. The chapter, "Determining the Treatment of Spleen and Stomach

Vacuity and Repletion" in the *Jì Shēng Fāng* ("Yan's Lifesaving Formulas"), contains a detailed description:

> "As for repletion, repletion engenders heat, and heat causes vexation and oppression in the heart and chest, parched lips and dry mouth, generalized heat and pain in the cheeks, heaviness of the body and abdominal distention, a tendency toward hunger and tugging (cramping), and in severe cases, swelling and rigidity of the tongue root, sores inside the mouth, singing and music in one's dreams, fatigue and dropping of the limbs, and a replete tight pulse. These are the signs of repletion heat."

This is a comprehensive summary of the pathomechanism of spleen channel repletion fire.

This condition is treated by clearing and draining spleen fire. For mouth and tongue sores and dry and parched lips and mouth, the recommended formula is *xiè huáng sǎn* (Yellow-Draining Powder) from the *Xiǎo Ér Yào Zhèng Zhí Jué* ("Key to Diagnosis and Treatment of Children's Diseases"), or *xiè pí shēng má sǎn* (Spleen-Draining Cimicifuga Powder) from the *Tài Píng Shèng Huì Fāng* ("The Great Peace Sagacious Benevolence Formulary").

Xiè Huáng Sǎn 泻黄散 Yellow-Draining Powder
shí gāo (石膏 gypsum, Gypsum Fibrosum) *shān zhī zǐ* (山栀子 gardenia, Gardeniae Fructus) *huò xiāng yè* (藿香叶 patchouli leaf, Pogostemi Folium) *fáng fēng* (防风 saposhnikovia, Saposhnikoviae Radix) *gān cǎo* (甘草 licorice, Glycyrrhizae Radix)

Xiè Pí Shēng Má Sǎn 泻脾升麻散 Spleen-Draining Cimicifuga Powder
huáng lián (黄连 coptis, Coptidis Rhizoma) *huáng qín* (黄芩 scutellaria, Scutellariae Radix) *shuǐ niú jiǎo* (水牛角 water buffalo horn, Bubali Cornu) *shēng má* (升麻 cimicifuga, Cimicifugae Rhizoma) *mài mén dōng* (麦门冬 ophiopogon, Ophiopogonis Radix) *chái hú* (柴胡 bupleurum, Bupleuri Radix) *dà qīng yè* (大青叶 isatis leaf, Isatidis Folium) *fú shén* (茯神 root poria, Poria cum Pini Radice) *gān cǎo* (甘草 licorice, Glycyrrhizae Radix)

For a sore and swollen throat, vexation heat in the chest, and dry stool, the recommended formula is *xiè pí dà huáng sǎn* (Spleen-Draining

Rhubarb Powder) from the *Tài Píng Shèng Huì Fāng* ("Great Peace Sagacious Benevolence Formulary").

Xiè Pí Dà Huáng Sǎn 泻脾大黄散
Spleen-Draining Rhubarb Powder

dà huáng (大黄 rhubarb, Rhei Radix et Rhizoma)
huáng qín (黄芩 scutellaria, Scutellariae Radix)
mài mén dōng (麦门冬 ophiopogon, Ophiopogonis Radix)
chì fú líng (赤茯苓 red poria, Poria Rubra)
zhǐ qiào (*ké*) (枳壳 bitter orange, Aurantii Fructus)
chén pí (陈皮 tangerine peel, Citri Reticulatae Pericarpium)
bàn xià (半夏 pinellia, Pinelliae Rhizoma)
qián hú (前胡 peucedanum, Peucedani Radix)
gān cǎo (甘草 licorice, Glycyrrhizae Radix)

For conditions characterized mainly by abdominal distention and pain with constipation, the recommended formula is *má zǐ rén wán* (Cannabis Seed Pill) from the *Shāng Hán Lùn* ("On Cold Damage") to clear heat and drain the spleen, and to moisten the intestines and free the stool.

Má Zǐ Rén Wán 麻子仁丸
Cannabis Seed Pill

huǒ má rén (火麻仁 cannabis seed, Cannabis Semen)
dà huáng (大黄 rhubarb, Rhei Radix et Rhizoma)
hòu pò (厚朴 officinal magnolia bark, Magnoliae Officinalis Cortex)
zhǐ shí (枳实 unripe bitter orange, Aurantii Fructus Immaturus)
xìng rén (杏仁 apricot kernel, Armeniacae Semen)
sháo yào (芍药 peony, Paeoniae Radix)

For sweetness and sliminess in the mouth, the recommended formula is *qín lián wēn dǎn tāng* (Scutellaria and Coptis Gallbladder-Warming Decoction) with the addition of *huò xiāng* (Agastaches Herba) and *pèi lán* (Eupatorii Herba).

Qín Lián Wēn Dǎn Tāng 温胆汤
Scutellaria and Coptis Gallbladder-Warming Decoction

huáng qín (黄芩 scutellaria, Scutellariae Radix)
huáng lián (黄连 coptis, Coptidis Rhizoma)
chén pí (陈皮 tangerine peel, Citri Reticulatae Pericarpium)
bàn xià (半夏 pinellia, Pinelliae Rhizoma)
zhǐ shí (枳实 unripe bitter orange, Aurantii Fructus Immaturus)
zhú rú (竹茹 bamboo shavings, Bumbusae Caulis in Taenia)

shēng jiāng (生姜 fresh ginger, Zingiberis Rhizoma Recens)
dà zǎo (大枣 jujube, Jujubae Fructus)
gān cǎo (甘草 licorice, Glycyrrhizae Radix)
Plus:
huò xiāng (藿香 agastache, Agastaches Herba)
pèi lán (佩兰 eupatorium, Eupatorii Herba)

脾经实火

脾阳过度亢奋，气有余蓄积为火，可生脾火。多因食积久郁，或过食辛辣刺激，或五志化火，或滥用温补所生。脾开窍于口，其华在唇四白，脾之经脉连舌本，散舌下，眼胞属脾。故脾火内焰，火势循经上炎，熏蒸于上，则见唇焦舌燥、口舌生疮、舌体肿胀、舌强舌痛、吐舌弄舌、鹅口滞颐等症。钱乙《小儿药证直诀》专制泻黄散以清脾经实火，治疗脾热弄舌、口疮、口臭、烦渴易饥、口燥唇干即是明证。 吴崑 《医方考•火》在注释该方时说："唇者脾之外候，口者脾之窍，故唇干口燥，知脾火也。"

脾主运化，脾经实火，火盛运快，食谷易消，故善食而易饥。脾主大腹，又主肌肉四肢，脾火内盛，火壅气滞，脾气困塞，故可见大腹胀满、腹痛拒按。火热灼津，脾津不能润肠，则为便秘；不能濡养肌肉、四肢，则为肌肉萎缩，四肢倦怠不举。如《证治汇补•火症》说："腹胀有声，口臭唇肿，脾火动也。"《证诒汇补•脾胃》还说："或善食而四肢削瘦，此脾强而邪火旺也。"均论证脾经实火病机的客观存在。

此外，脾火亢盛，可成脾瘅。多因嗜食肥甘厚味，致使脾火浊气上逆而成，口中甜腻不爽，身体肥胖。如《圣济总录•脾瘅》云："有病口甘者，此五气之溢也，名曰脾瘅。夫食入于阴，长气于阳，令人内热而中满，则阳气盛矣。故单阳为瘅，其证口甘，久而弗治，转为消渴。"总之脾经实火可引起多种症状。《济生方•脾胃虚实论治》有段精辟的论述："及其实也，实则生热，热则心胸烦闷，唇焦口干，身热颊痛，体重腹胀，善饥善瘛（抽筋），甚则舌根肿强，口内生疮，梦见歌乐，四肢怠堕，脉来紧实者，是实热之候也。"是对脾经实火病机的全面概括。

治宜清泻脾火。口舌生疮，唇口干焦，方选《小儿药证直诀》泻黄散（石膏、山栀、藿香叶、防风、甘草），或《太平圣惠方》泻脾升麻散（黄连、黄芩、犀角屑、升麻、麦冬、柴胡、大青叶、茯神、甘草）。咽喉肿痛，胸中烦热，大便干燥，方选《太平圣惠方》泻脾大黄散（大黄、黄芩、麦冬、赤茯苓、枳壳、陈皮、半夏、前胡、甘草）。腹胀腹痛便秘为主，用《伤寒论》麻子仁丸，清热泻脾、润肠通便。口甘甜腻，用芩连温胆汤加藿香、佩兰。

Literature Review of Spleen Channel Repletion Fire

📖 *Líng Shū* ("Magic Pivot"), "Five Evils"

"When the evil is located in the spleen and stomach, the patient suffers from pain in the flesh. When yáng qì is superabundant and yīn qì is insufficient, there will be heat and large appetite."

This quotation describes the pathomechanism by which exuberant spleen channel repletion fire causes a large appetite due to overly accelerated decomposition, damage to the fluids from heat scorching, and loss of nourishment and pain in the flesh.

📖 *Zhū Bìng Yuán Hòu Lùn* ("Origin and Indicators of Disease"), "Symptoms of Spleen Disease"

"Spleen qì exuberance means a superabundance of the physical body, causing the patient to suffer from abdominal distention and fullness, inhibited urination, generalized heaviness, bitter hunger, wilting of the legs with inability to walk, tendency towards tugging (cramping) in the shins, and pain below the feet. These indicate spleen qì repletion that should be drained."

This quotation describes the pathomechanism of spleen fire exuberance with malfunctions in movement and transformation that can result in abdominal distention, generalized heaviness, wilting and limp legs, and foot pain.

📖 *Tài Píng Shèng Huì Fāng* ("Great Peace Sagacious Benevolence Formulary"), "Various Formulas for Treating Spleen Repletion by Draining the Spleen"

"Spleen repletion engenders heat, and heat causes an exuberance of yáng qì. When yáng qì is exuberant, it causes heart and chest vexation and heat, dry and parched lips and mouth, generalized heat, vexation, and pain, heaviness of the body with inability to turn sides, low voice, heart tension, a sore and inhibited throat, a swollen and rigid root of the tongue, sores inside the mouth, abdominal and rib-side distention and fullness, inability to rest and sleep, frequent appearance of singing and music in one's dreams, and a pulse that feels tight and replete. These are the signs of spleen repletion."

This quotation describes the pathomechanism by which yáng qì exuberance in the spleen generates spleen fire, and spleen fire harasses the upper part of the body, leading to heart and chest vexation and heat, dry and parched lips and mouth, mouth and tongue sores, a swollen and distended tongue body, fatigue of the limbs, and other symptoms.

📖 *Sù Wèn* ("Plain Questions"), "Treatise on Strange Diseases"

> "The Emperor said: 'In the case of a patient suffering from sweetness in the mouth, what is the name of this disease? How does one contract it?'

> Qí Bó said: 'This is a spillage of the five flavors. It is called splenic pure heat. The five flavors enter the mouth; they are stored in the stomach and the spleen moves their essential qì. When the fluids are in the spleen, a person will sense sweetness in the mouth. Because this is caused by fatty and fine [foods], this type of person must frequently consume sweet, fine, and fatty foods. Fat causes people to suffer from internal heat, while sweetness causes people to suffer from central fullness. Therefore, their qì spills upward, where it turns into dispersion-thirst.'"

This passage describes the pathomechanism by which an excessive diet of fatty and sweet foods forms internal heat, causing the fluids of the spleen to spill upward. This results in a sweet, slimy, and ungratifying sensation in the mouth.

文献评述

《灵枢•五邪》"邪在脾胃，则病肌肉痛。阳气有余，阴气不足，则热善饥。"阐述脾经实火亢盛，腐熟过快而善饥，热灼津伤，肌肉失养而疼痛的病机。

《诸病源候论•脾病候》："脾气盛，为形有余，则病腹胀满，溲不利，身重苦饥，足痿不行，腨（胫）善瘛（抽筋），脚下痛，是脾气之实也，宜泻之。"阐述脾火亢盛，运化失调，可引起腹胀、身重、足痿软、足痛的病机。

《太平圣惠方•治脾实泻脾诸方》："夫脾实则生热，热则阳气盛。阳气盛则心胸烦热，唇口干焦，身热烦疼，体重不能转侧，语声沉而心急，咽喉痛而不利，舌本肿强，口内生疮，腹胁胀满，不得安卧，梦多见歌乐，诊其脉紧实者，是脾实之候也。"论述脾的阳气亢盛，则生脾火，脾火上扰，可致心胸烦热、唇口干燥、口舌生疮、舌体肿胀、肢体倦怠等症的病机。

《素问•奇病论篇》："帝曰：有病口甘者，病名为何?何以得之?歧伯曰：此五气之溢也，名口脾瘅。夫五味入口，藏于胃，脾为之行其精气，津液在脾，故令人口甘也，此肥美之所发也，此人必数食甘美而多肥也。肥者令人内热，甘者令人中满，故其气上溢，转为消渴。"论述过食肥甘，化生内热，使脾津上溢，而引起口中甜腻不爽的病机。

Summary of Spleen Channel Repletion Fire

1. Internal Exuberance of Spleen Fire

   Parched lips and dry tongue, mouth and tongue sores, swollen and distended tongue body, stiff and painful tongue, protruding and hyperactive tongue, goose mouth sores and dribbling.

2. Fire Exuberance and Accelerated Movement

   Large appetite and rapid hungering.

3. Spleen Qì Encumbrance and Blockage

   Greater abdominal distention and fullness, abdominal pain that refuses pressure.

4. Fire Heat Scorching the Fluids

   Constipation.

5. Failure to Nourish the Flesh

   Atrophy of the flesh, fatigue of the four limbs and failure to raise them.

脾经实火

脾火内盛——唇焦舌燥，口舌生疮，舌体肿胀，舌强舌痛，吐舌弄舌，鹅口滞颐。

火盛运快——善食易饥。

脾气困塞——大腹胀满，腹痛拒按。

火热灼津——便秘。

不养肌肉——肌肉萎缩，四肢倦怠不举。

2.2 Damp-Heat Brewing in the Spleen

When dampness and heat combine and bind spleen qì, this is called damp-heat brewing in the spleen. The formation of damp-heat can be caused by the externally contracted evil of damp-heat, or it can be rooted in dampness evil, when dampness is depressed and transforms into heat. Alternatively, a predilection for hot and spicy or fat, sweet, and rich foods, or for drinking tea, liquor, or koumiss can brew into heat in the center to generate this condition. Or it can arise from a vacuity of spleen qì, causing a failure in the transformation of water-damp and the resulting transformation of the gathering dampness into heat.

Regardless of whether it is externally contracted or arises internally, it is always related closely to the strength or weakness of spleen qì in itself. Whenever people with a constitutional exuberance of center qì contract dampness evil or dampness arises internally on its own, damp-heat is engendered since heat is formed with yáng.

As explained in the "Treatise on Dampness" in the *Yī Guàn* ("Thorough Knowledge of Medicine"):

> "Dampness that is formed from greater yīn damp earth is not a condition that has entered from the outside. When yáng is exuberant, fire prevails and transforms into damp-heat."

The chapter, "Dampness" in the *Lín Zhèng Zhǐ Nán Yī Àn* ("A Clinical Guide with Case Histories") goes one step further:

> "When patients present with a somber red skin color and emaciation with solid flesh, their constitutional body is yáng. If they contract external dampness evil, it invariably tends to transform into heat. If they internally generate dampness evil, most often caused by sorghum or sweet liquors, they will invariably suffer from the pathoconditions of damp-heat or damp-fire."

These quotations stress the significance of constitutional factors in the formation of the pathomechanism of damp-heat.

Damp-heat brewing in the spleen can result in such pathomechanisms as the impairment of splenic movement and transformation, congested earth and depressed wood, and damp-heat brewing and steaming.

湿热蕴脾

湿与热合，胶结脾气，称为湿热蕴脾。湿热由生，可外感湿热之邪而致，亦可本为湿邪所中，湿郁化热而成；或嗜食辛热燥辣、肥甘厚腻、茶饮酒酪，蕴热于中而生；或由脾气虚弱，水湿不化，聚湿化热而发。无论外感还是内生湿热均与脾气自身的强弱有密切关系。凡中气素盛之人，感受湿邪，或湿自内生，从阳化热，皆生湿热。如《医贯•湿论》说：" 有太阴湿土所化之湿，不从外入者也。阳盛则火胜，化为湿热。"《临证指南医案•湿》则进一步指出："若其人色苍赤而瘦，肌肉坚结者，其体属阳。此外感湿邪，必易于化热；若内生湿邪，多因高粱酒醴，必患湿热，湿火之症。"充分强调体质因素在化生湿热病机中的重要意义。湿热蕴脾，可引起脾失健运，土壅木郁，湿热蕴蒸等病机变化。

2.2.1 Impairment of Splenic Movement and Transformation

The nature of damp-heat is sticky and clammy, like dense enshrouding mists. It manifests in conditions of depression and blockage; it brews and binds in the center burner, and blocks and obstructs the qì dynamic. This is bound to influence the upbearing and downbearing functions of the spleen and stomach, resulting in the pathological conditions of the spleen failing to upbear the clear, the stomach failing to downbear the turbid, and of qì stagnating in the center burner. The greater abdomen belongs to the spleen, and when the spleen fails to move and transform, qì stagnates in the stomach duct and abdomen where it also binds with the evil of damp-heat, becoming difficult to resolve. This causes persistent and irresolvable distention and fullness in the stomach duct and abdomen or localized dull pain that does not like pressure, or a sensation of fullness when pressure is applied.

As explained in the chapter, "Damp-Heat Abdominal Distention" in the *Zhèng Yīn Mài Zhì* ("Pathoconditions: Causes, Pulses, and Treatments"):

> "If the evil of damp-heat is contracted and enters through the intestines and stomach, cannot be discharged outward, and dampness becomes excessive, causing glomus blockage, the pathocondition of abdominal distention arises."

The bowel spleen and the viscus stomach are linked together in an intimate relationship with mutual influence, based on the "identical qì of damp earth". Spleen disease affects the stomach, causing failure of stomach qì to downbear, counterflow ascent of turbid qì, and impaired intake, resulting in the pathoconditions of aversion to food in general and oil in particular, and upflow nausea and vomiting.

When the spleen fails to perform its movement function and the evil of damp-heat flows downward and accumulates, it can strike and bind in the intestinal tract, impede the qì dynamic there, and cause the breakdown of the conveyance function of the large intestine. The result is pathoconditions like diarrhea, sloppy and ungratifying stools, scorching heat in the anus, yellow gruel-like stools with a foul smell, or dry and bound stools. When damp-heat pours down into the bladder and the qì transformation in the bladder breaks down, one might observe short voidings of reddish urine with distress and scorching heat, stagnation and roughness, and pain. When damp-heat brews in the spleen and spleen qì fails to upbear and is unable to distribute the fluids upward to supply the mouth, one can observe such pathoconditions as a dry mouth and thirst without large fluid intake.

In the *Shī Rè Bìng Piān* ("Treatise on Damp-Heat Disease"), Xuē Shēng-Bái stated:

> "Heat causes a failure to upbear the humors and subsequent thirst. Dampness causes an internal collection of fluids and subsequent failure to drink."

When damp-heat lying depressed and steaming prevents spleen qì from upbearing the clear to the head and damp-heat rises to cloud the clear orifices, it causes dizziness of the head and vision.

The "Treatise on Formulas for Damp-Heat" in the *Yī Lín Shéng Mò* ("Level Line Ink of the Forest of Medicine") states:

> "Damp-heat is caused by dampness engendering heat and is a disease of spleen-earth. …Its symptoms are dizziness of the head and general fatigue, lack of strength in the four limbs, unclear center qì, failure to ingest food and drink, yellow and turbid urine and sloppy stool and diarrhea …and in severe cases, heat effusion and aversion to cold and spontaneous periodic sweating with a soggy and rapid pulse."

From this statement, we can see that damp-heat brewing in the spleen and impairing splenic movement and transformation not only creates depression of spleen qì itself, but has further implications. These are the extremely complex pathomechanisms of spleen qì failing to upbear the clear, stomach qì failing to downbear, breakdown of the conveyance function of the large intestine and of the qì transformation of the bladder, and impediment of fluid transport.

This condition is treated by clearing heat and eliminating dampness, and by rectifying qì and moving the spleen. Conditions that are mainly characterized by glomus in the stomach duct with nausea and vomiting, and abdominal distention and fullness, are treated with *wáng shì lián pò yǐn* (Wang's Coptis and Official Magnolia Bark Beverage) from the *Huò Luàn Lǔn* ("On Cholera"), with the addition of *zhǐ ké* (*qiào*) (Aurantii Fructus), *mù xiāng* (Aucklandiae Radix), and *chén pí* (Citri Reticulatae Pericarpium).

Wáng Shì Lián Pò Yǐn 王氏连朴饮
Wang's Coptis and Officinal Magnolia Bark Beverage

huáng lián (黄连 coptis, Coptidis Rhizoma)
hòu pò (厚朴 officinal magnolia bark, Magnoliae Officinalis Cortex)
bàn xià (半夏 pinellia, Pinelliae Rhizoma)
shān zhī zǐ (山栀子 gardenia, Gardeniae Fructus)
dàn dòu chǐ (淡豆豉 fermented soybean, Sojae Semen Praeparatum)
lú gēn (芦根 phragmites, Phragmitis Rhizoma)
Plus:

zhǐ qiào (ké) (枳壳 bitter orange, Aurantii Fructus)
mù xiāng (木香 costusroot, Aucklandiae Radix)
chén pí (陈皮 tangerine peel, Citri Reticulatae Pericarpium)

Conditions that are mainly characterized by diarrhea and sloppy stool are treated with *gé gēn qín lián tāng* (Pueraria, Scutellaria, and Coptis Decoction) from the *Shāng Hán Lùn* ("On Cold Damage"), with the addition of *mù xiāng* (Aucklandiae Radix) and *bīng láng* (Arecae Semen).

Gé Gēn Qín Lián Tāng 葛根芩连汤
Pueraria, Scutellaria, and Coptis Decoction

gé gēn (葛根 pueraria, Puerariae Radix)
huáng qín (黄芩 scutellaria, Scutellariae Radix)
huáng lián (黄连 coptis, Coptidis Rhizoma)
gān cǎo (甘草 licorice, Glycyrrhizae Radix)
Plus:
mù xiāng (木香 costusroot, Aucklandiae Radix)
bīng láng (槟榔 areca, Arecae Semen)

Conditions that are mainly characterized by frequent urination with yellow or red urine are treated with *xìng rén huá shí tāng* (Apricot Kernel and Talcum Decoction) from the *Wēn Bìng Tiáo Bian* ("Systematized Identification of Warm Diseases").

Xìng Rén Huá Shí Tāng 杏仁滑石汤
Apricot Kernel and Talcum Decoction

xìng rén (杏仁 apricot kernel, Armeniacae Semen)
huá shí (滑石 talcum, Talcum)
tōng cǎo (通草 rice-paper plant pith, Tetrapanacis Medulla)
huáng qín (黄芩 scutellaria, Scutellariae Radix)
huáng lián (黄连 coptis, Coptidis Rhizoma)
yù jīn (郁金 curcuma, Curcumae Radix)
hòu pò (厚朴 officinal magnolia bark, Magnoliae Officinalis Cortex)
bàn xià (半夏 pinellia, Pinelliae Rhizoma)
chén pí (陈皮 tangerine peel, Citri Reticulatae Pericarpium)

脾失健运

湿热之性氤氲粘着，呈郁滞状态，蕴结中焦，阻碍气机，必然影响脾胃的升降功能，导致脾不升清，胃不降浊，气滞中焦的病理状态。大腹属脾，脾失健运，气滞脘腹，又与湿热之邪胶结难解，则为脘腹胀满、持续不解、或局部隐痛、不喜按压、或按之有充实

感 。如《症因脉治•湿热腹胀》说："湿热之邪，感入肠胃，不得外泄，湿淫太过，痞塞不通，则腹胀之症作矣。""脾与胃脏腑相连，""湿土同气"，关系密切，互为影响。脾病及胃，胃气不降，浊气上逆，不能受纳，则为厌食恶油、泛恶呕吐之症。

脾运失职，湿热之邪下流，积滞搏结肠道，阻碍肠道气机，大肠传导失司，可致腹泻、便溏不爽、肛门灼热 、便如黄糜、其气秽臭、或大便干结等症。湿热下注膀胱，膀胱气化失职，可见小便短赤、急迫灼热、滞涩疼痛。湿热蕴脾，脾气不升，不能输布津液上承于口，可见口干、渴不多饮等症。薛生白《湿热病篇》云："热则液不升而口渴，湿则饮内留而不引饮。"湿热郁蒸，脾气不能升清于头，湿热上蒙清窍，则为头晕目眩。正如《医林绳墨•湿热方论》所云："湿热者，因湿而生热也，脾土为病也。…其症头眩体倦，四肢乏力，中气不清，饮食不进，小便黄浊，大便溏泄…甚者发热恶寒，自汗时出，其脉濡而数。"由此可见，湿热蕴脾，脾失健运，不仅形成脾气自身的郁滞，还进一步影响脾气不能升清，胃气不能下降，大肠传导失司，膀胱气化失职，津液输布阻碍，病机十分复杂。

治宜清热除湿，理气运脾。若以脘痞呕恶、腹胀腹满为主者，选《霍乱论》王氏连朴饮（黄连、厚朴、半夏、焦山栀、豆豉、芦根）加枳壳、木香、陈皮。若以腹泄便溏为主，选《伤寒论》葛根芩连汤（葛根、黄芩、黄连、甘草）加木香、槟榔。若以小便频数、黄赤为主，选《温病条辨》杏仁滑石汤（杏仁、滑石、通草、黄芩、黄连、郁金、厚朴、半夏、橘皮）。

2.2.2 Earth Congestion and Wood Depression

When damp-heat brews and binds in the center burner, spleen qì is encumbered, damp-earth mounds and thickens, earth qì becomes congested, and wood, in turn, is depressed by it. Gallbladder qì fails to course freely and bile spills outward to the face, eyes, and skin instead of following the ordinary pathways, causing the eruption of jaundice. It can manifest as torpid intake, aversion to greasy foods, distention and fullness in the stomach duct and abdomen, and yellowing of the head, eyes, and skin of the whole body that is fresh and bright like the color of oranges. The movement of damp-heat into the skin causes itching, and the depression of gallbladder qì causes distention pain in the right rib-side.

The chapter, "Jaundice," in the *Yī Chún Shèng Yì* ("Refined and Surplus Meanings in Medicine") explains:

"It is said that a yellowing of the face and eyes with red and inhibited urination and calmness and somnolence means jaundice. This is related to an accumulation of dampness in the spleen, which causes fatigue and somnolence, and an accumulation of heat in the stomach, which causes yellowing and red urine."

The chapter, "Regular Jaundice," in the *Zhèng Yīn Mài Zhì* ("Patho-conditions: Causes, Pulses, and Treatments") also explains:

"The cause of regular jaundice is an accumulation of heat in the bowels and viscera, occurring simultaneously in the spleen and stomach. Con-tending with externally caused wind and dampness, it obstructs and de-presses the interstices, and damp-heat swelters, ferments, and creates yel-lowing."

While these two sources clearly indicate that damp-heat of the spleen and stomach causes the pathocondition of jaundice, they still fail to illustrate in detail how damp-heat brewing in the spleen results in the pathomecha-nism of bile spilling to the outside and creating yellowing. However, this can be deduced from an analysis on the basis of "restraining" shifts in five-phase theory: The gallbladder belongs to wood and the spleen be-longs to earth. When spleen qì is congested, earth qì is overly effulgent and instead of being coursed freely by gallbladder qì, rebels against it. Wood qì stagnation and blockage causes gallbladder qì depression, bile moves in counterflow, and jaundice is generated.

The chapter, "The Origin of Jaundice; Grain in the Gallbladder" in the *Sì Shèng Xīn Yuán* ("Four Sages' Original Heart"), explains:

"Old grain putrefies, congests, and entraps, obstructing spleen earth. Wood qì is entrapped and falls, and earth and wood become depressed and blocked, causing the disease of jaundice."

This offers an excellent summary and detailed description of the pathomechanism of congested earth and depressed wood.

This condition is treated by clearing heat and disinhibiting dampness, and by harmonizing the stomach and downbearing counterflow. The rec-ommended formula is *yīn chén hāo tāng* (Virgate Wormwood Decoction) from the *Shāng Hán Lùn* ("On Cold Damage"), with the addition of *huáng bǎi* (Phellodendri Cortex), *fú líng* (Poria), *bàn xià* (Pinelliae Rhi-zoma), *chén pí* (Citri Reticulatae Pericarpium), *zhǐ qiào (ké)* (Aurantii Fructus), *hòu pò* (Magnoliae Officinalis Cortex), *shān zhā* (Crataegi Fructus).

Yīn Chén Hāo Tāng 茵陈蒿汤
Virgate Wormwood Decoction

yīn chén hāo (茵陈蒿 virgate wormwood, Artemisiae Scopariae Herba)
shān zhī zǐ (山栀子 gardenia, Gardeniae Fructus)
dà huáng (大黄 rhubarb, Rhei Radix et Rhizoma)
Plus:

huáng bǎi (黄柏 phellodendron, Phellodendri Cortex)
fú líng (茯苓 poria, Poria)
bàn xià (半夏 pinellia, Pinelliae Rhizoma)
chén pí (陈皮 tangerine peel, Citri Reticulatae Pericarpium)
zhǐ qiào (*ké*) (枳壳 bitter orange, Aurantii Fructus)
hòu pò (厚朴 official magnolia bark, Magnoliae Officinalis Cortex)
shān zhā (山楂 crataegus, Crataegi Fructus)

土壅木郁

湿热蕴结中焦，脾气困阻、湿土阜厚，土气壅塞，木反被郁，胆气不疏，胆汁不循常道，外溢于面目肌肤，发为黄疸。可见纳呆厌油，脘腹胀满，头目全身皮肤发黄，鲜明如橘子色。湿热行于皮肤而作瘙痒，胆气郁滞而作右胁胀痛。《医醇剩义·黄疸》说："经曰：面目发黄，小溲赤涩，安静嗜卧者，黄疸也。此系脾有积湿，故倦怠嗜卧，胃有积热，故发黄溺赤。"《症因脉治·正黄疸》亦说："正黄疸之因，脏腑积热，并于脾胃之间，外因风湿相搏，闭郁腠理，湿热熏蒸，盦而成黄。"两处明确指出脾胃湿热形成黄疸之症，却未详细阐明湿热蕴脾引起胆汁外溢而成黄的病机，但可根据五行"相克"传变的理论分析而知。胆属木，脾属土，脾气壅塞，土气过旺，胆气不能疏土，反被土侮，木气滞塞，胆气郁滞，胆汁逆行，黄疸乃成。《四圣心源·黄疸根源·谷胆》说："陈腐壅遏，阻滞脾土，木气遏陷，土木郁塞，则病黄。"是对土壅木郁这一病机的高度概括和精辟阐述。

治宜清热利湿，和胃降逆。方选《伤寒论》茵陈蒿汤（茵陈、栀子、大黄）加黄柏、茯苓、半夏、陈皮、枳壳、厚朴、山楂。

2.2.3 Damp-Heat Lying Depressed and Steaming

The spleen governs the movement and transformation of water-damp and has the strongest affinity with dampness. Damp-heat tends to brew and bind in the center burner. Dampness encumbers heat and stops it, so they bind with each other. Dampness has a sticky and stagnating nature that traps heat and makes it deep-lying. Interior heat gradually becomes exuberant, resulting in unsurfaced generalized heat effusion. When dampness encumbers heat in the center, it brews heat inside the dampness, the power of heat forces it to the outside, and the steaming dampness becomes sweat. Heat follows sweat to be discharged, manifesting as fluctuating generalized heat effusion. When evil heat is trapped by dampness, it is not easy to outthrust since the sticky and slimy nature of dampness makes it difficult to expel and the force of the disease is not debilitated by sweating. Therefore one sees the pathocondition where the heat effusion is reduced during perspiration but relapses promptly.

The "Chapter on the Center Burner" in the *Zēng Bǔ Pìng Zhú Wēn Bìng Tiáo Bian* ("Supplemented Annotation to the Systematized Identification of Warm Diseases") explains:

> "The pulse is moderate with generalized pain, the tongue is pale yellow and slippery, there is thirst without large fluid intake or even no thirst at all, and heat effusion that is reduced during perspiration, but then flares up again."

Damp-heat depression and steaming in the spleen is one of the most fundamental and important pathomechanisms of damp-heat disease causing a generalized heat effusion that is continuous and difficult to resolve.

This condition is treated by clearing heat and disinhibiting dampness, and by diffusing the qì aspect. Recommended formulas include *huáng qín huá shí tāng* (Scutellaria and Talcum Decoction) from the *Wēn Bìng Tiáo Bian* ("Systematized Identification of Warm Diseases"), and *gān lù xiāo dú dān* (Sweet Dew Toxin-Dispersing Elixir) from the *Xù Míng Yī Lèi Àn* ("Supplement to the Classified Case Histories of Famous Physicians").

Huáng Qín Huá Shí Tāng 黄芩滑石汤 Scutellaria and Talcum Decoction
huáng qín (黄芩 scutellaria, Scutellariae Radix)
huá shí (滑石 talcum, Talcum)
fú líng pí (茯苓皮 poria skin, Poriae Cutis)
zhū líng (猪苓 polyporus, Polyporus)
tōng cǎo (通草 rice-paper plant pith, Tetrapanacis Medulla)
dà fù pí (大腹皮 areca husk, Arecae Pericarpium)
bái dòu kòu (白豆蔻 cardamom, Amomi Fructus Rotundus)

Gān Lù Xiāo Dú Dān 甘露消毒丹 Sweet Dew Toxin-Dispersing Elixir
bái dòu kòu (白豆蔻 cardamom, Amomi Fructus Rotundus)
huò xiāng (藿香 agastache, Agastaches Herba)
shí chāng pú (石菖蒲 acorus, Acori Tatarinowii Rhizoma)
bò hé (薄荷 mint, Menthae Herba)
lián qiáo (连翘 forsythia, Forsythiae Fructus)
shè gān (射干 belamcanda, Belamcandae Rhizoma)
chuān bèi mǔ (川贝母 Sichuan fritillaria, Fritillariae Cirrhosae Bulbus)

huáng qín (黄芩 scutellaria, Scutellariae Radix)
yīn chén hāo (茵陈蒿 virgate wormwood, Artemisiae Scopariae Herba)
huá shí (滑石 talcum, Talcum)
mù tōng (木通 trifoliate akebia, Akebiae Trifoliatae Caulis)

湿热郁蒸

脾主运化水湿，与湿的亲和力最强，湿热易蕴结中焦，湿困热停，相互胶结，湿性粘滞，遏热内伏，里热渐盛，则身热不扬；湿困热中，湿中蕴热，热势外迫，蒸湿为汗，热随汗泄，故见身热起伏；邪热为湿所遏，不易透达，湿性粘腻难去，病势不为汗衰，故见汗出热减，既而复热之症。如《增补评注温病条辨•中焦篇》说："脉缓身痛，舌淡黄而滑，渴不多饮，或竟不渴，汗出热减，继而复热。"湿热郁蒸于脾，是湿热病引起全身发热，缠绵难解的最基本、最重要的病机之一。

治宜清热利湿，宣通气分。方选《温病条辨》黄芩滑石汤（黄芩、滑石、茯苓皮、猪苓、通草、大腹皮、白蔻），或《续名医类案》甘露消毒丹（白蔻、藿香、石菖蒲、薄荷、连翘、射干、川贝母、黄芩、茵陈、滑石、木通）。

Literature Review of Damp-Heat Brewing in the Spleen

📖 *Yī Xué Zhèng Zhuàn* ("Orthodox Tradition of Medicine"), "Swelling and Distention"

"Again it is said that the various conditions of abdominal distention and enlargement are all associated with heat. When the spleen is vacuous and unable to restrain water, water seeps out and moves frenetically, causing puffy swelling throughout the body, face, eyes, and extremities. This is called water swelling. Alternatively, if the stomach is enlarged like a drum but the face, eyes, and four limbs are not swollen, it is called distention fullness or drum distention. Whenever the disease is a condition of damp-heat of spleen earth, the swelling is light, but the distention is severe."

This describes the pathomechanism by which damp-heat encumbers the spleen, causing a failure in the movement of the fluids so that water qì floods, which can lead to water swelling and drum distention.

📖 *Sù Wèn* ("Plain Questions"), "Treatise on Wind"

"Conditions of spleen wind manifest as profuse sweating with aversion to wind, generalized fatigue and falling, unwillingness to move the four

limbs, a faint and slightly yellow complexion that is the color of earth, no
pleasure in eating, and, when examining the area above the nose, a yellow coloration."

Zhāng Jǐng-Yuè commented:

"The reason for the generalized fatigue and unwillingness to use the
limbs is that the spleen governs the flesh and limbs. The faint and slightly
yellow complexion is the color of earth. The lack of appetite is due to the
fact that the spleen is diseased and unable to transform. The nose is the
king of the face and governs the response to the spleen and kidneys, thus
an examination of its color should indicate spleen earth."

This quotation points out that an encumbrance of the spleen by damp-
heat causes a breakdown of the movement and transformation functions.
This results in a lack of interest in food and drink, and in fatigue and lack
of strength in the limbs. When bile is distressed and forced to discharge
to the outside, it causes a yellowing of the facial complexion.

📖 *Zhèng Zhì Huì Bǔ* ("A Supplement to Patterns and Treatment"),
  "Jaundice"

"Jaundice is mostly related to greater yīn dampness earth and to an inability of the spleen to overcome dampness. When aggravated by fire heat,
this results in depression and yellowing. …Most often, it is caused by
food and drink taxation fatigue that has caused damage to spleen-earth.
Because of the failure in movement and transformation, damp-heat
amasses internally and, lacking a place from which to erupt and discharge, flows into the spleen and flesh and all over the limbs."

This describes the pathomechanism by which damp-heat encumbers the
spleen, causes the breakdown of movement and transformation, and
flows into the flesh and limbs, resulting in jaundice.

📖 *Zhāng Shì Yī Tōng* ("Zhang's Clear View of Medicine"), "Dampness"

"Damp-heat includes innumerable classifications, with such symptoms
as drum distention and water swelling, retching counterflow and acid
swallowing, jaundice and stagnant diarrhea, heaviness and pain of the
lumbus and legs, and foot qì impediment. They are all associated with
suffering from damp-heat."

Although damp-heat is not yet clearly located in the spleen in this quotation, an analysis on the basis of disease patterns shows that every one of
them is related to damp-heat encumbering the spleen and is caused by the
spleen's failure to move and transform.

📖 *Sì Shèng Xīn Yuán* ("Four Sages' Original Heart"), "Origin of Jaundice"

"Jaundice is caused by earth dampness and the subsequent contraction of
wind evil… When wind evil is contracted, defense qì becomes blocked
and enclosed and dampness excess cannot be thrust out. This causes the
damming and depression of spleen earth, the entrapment of liver wood,

dual fall of the liver and spleen, lack of dispersal of water and grains, and stasis turbidity of grain qì that transforms into heat. Stasis heat moves forward, flows downward into the bladder and causes blocked and inhibited urination and inhibited waterways. Stasis heat in the bladder lacks a path to discharge below, swelters, and oozes out, spreading throughout the whole body. This is how jaundice is formed."

This describes the pathomechanism by which damp earth and depressed wood cause the fall of liver and spleen qì, depressed dampness transforms into heat and impedes the bladder, and damp-heat lacks an exit road and swelters in the flesh, forming jaundice.

文献评述

《医学正传•肿胀》："又曰：诸腹胀大，皆属于热。夫脾虚不能制水，水渍妄行，故通身面目手足皆浮而肿，名曰水肿。或腹大如鼓，而面目四肢不肿者，名曰胀满，又名鼓胀。皆脾土湿热为病，肿轻而胀重也。"论述湿热困脾，水津失运，水气泛滥，可致水肿、鼓胀的病机。

《素问•风论篇》："脾风之状，多汗恶风，身体怠堕，四支（肢）不欲动，色薄微黄，不嗜食，诊在鼻上，其色黄。"张景岳注："身体怠惰四支不用者，脾主肌肉四肢也，色薄微黄，土之色也，不嗜食，脾病不能化也。鼻为面王，主应脾肾，故色诊当见于脾土。"指出脾为湿热所困，运化失职，则不思饮食、四肢倦怠乏力；迫逼胆汁外泄，则面色发黄。

《证治汇补•黄病》："黄疸多属太阴湿土，脾不能胜湿，复挟火热，则郁而生黄。…多因饮食劳倦，致伤脾土，不能运化，湿热内蓄，无由发泄，流于脾肉，遍于四肢。"论述湿热困脾，运化失司，流于肌肉四肢，引起黄疸的病机。

《张氏医通•湿》说："湿热证类最多，如鼓胀水肿，呕逆吞酸，黄疸滞下，腰腿重痛，脚气痹著等候，悉属湿热为患。"此处湿热，虽未明确定位于脾，但从所致病证进行分析，无不与湿热困脾相关，均由脾失健运所致。

《四圣心源•黄疸根源》："黄疸者，土湿而感风邪也。…一感风邪，卫气闭阖，湿淫不得外达，脾土堙郁，遏其肝木，肝脾双陷，水谷不消，谷气瘀浊，化而为热。瘀热前行，下流膀胱，小便闭涩，水道不利。膀胱瘀热，下无泄路，熏蒸淫泆（溢），传于周身，于是黄疸成焉。"阐述土湿木郁，肝脾气陷，湿郁化热，阻碍膀胱，湿热无出路，熏蒸于肌肤，形成黄疸的病机。

Summary of Damp-Heat Brewing in the Spleen

1. Impairment of Splenic Movement and Transformation

   Qì blockage in the stomach duct and abdomen: Persistent and ir-resolvable distention and fullness in the stomach duct and abdomen, perhaps with localized dull pain that does not like pressure or with a sensation of fullness when pressed.

   Impairment of downbearing by stomach qì: Aversion to food, in particular to greasy foods, upflow nausea and vomiting.

   Breakdown of conveyance: Diarrhea, sloppy and ungratifying stool, scorching heat in the anus, yellow gruel-like stool with foul smell, or dry and bound stools.

2. Earth Congestion and Wood Depression

   Breakdown of bladder function: Short voidings of reddish urine, scorching heat and pain in the urethra, urgency, and rough passage of urine.

   Failure of liquids to bear upward: Dry mouth, thirst without large fluid intake.

   Disharmony between spleen and stomach: Torpid intake and aversion to greasy foods, glomus in the stomach duct and abdominal distention.

   Bile spilling outward: Jaundice, yellowing of the skin, with a fresh and bright color like oranges.

   Damp-heat in the skin: Itching skin.

   Depression of gallbladder qì: Distention pain in the right rib-side.

3. Damp-Heat Depression and Steaming

   Dampness trapping heat, making it deep-lying: Unsurfaced generalized heat.

   Damp-heat adhering and binding: Heat effusion that is reduced with perspiration but relapses promptly.

湿热蕴脾

脾失健运

气滞脘腹——脘腹胀满，持续不解，或局部隐痛，不喜按压，或按之有充实感。

胃气不降——厌食恶油，泛恶呕吐。

传导失司——腹泻，便溏不爽，肛门灼热，便如黄糜，其气秽臭，或大便干结。

土壅木郁

膀胱失职——小便短赤，急迫灼热，滞涩疼痛。

津不上承—— 口干，渴不多饮。

脾胃失调——纳呆厌油，脘痞腹胀

胆汁外溢——黄疸，皮肤发黄，鲜明如橘子色。

湿热在皮——皮肤瘙痒。

胆气郁滞——右胁胀痛。

湿热郁蒸

湿遏热伏——身热不扬。

湿热胶结—— 汗出热减，既而复热。

When the pathomechanism of damp-heat brewing in the spleen due to repletion fire in the spleen channel develops further, it can lead to such pathomechanisms as spleen-stomach yīn vacuity, spleen-liver disharmony, and spleen-stomach damp-heat.

2.3 Spleen-Stomach Yīn Vacuity

An exuberance of spleen fire or a long-term retention of damp-heat that has transformed into heat can both damage yīn humor. First the damage affects spleen yīn, but then it spreads to stomach yīn, forming the pathomechanism of spleen-stomach yīn vacuity. One might observe manifestations like glomus in the stomach duct and abdominal distention, hunger with no desire to eat, emaciation and constipation, or a red tongue with scant fur. It is treated by enriching and nourishing spleen and stomach yīn. To nourish spleen yīn, sweet, calming, and moistening medicinals are used such as *shān yào* (Dioscoreae Rhizoma), *huáng jīng* (Polygonati Rhizoma), *qiàn shí* (Euryales Semen), *bái sháo* (Paeoniae Radix Alba), *fēng mì* (Mel) or *gān cǎo* (Glycyrrhizae Radix). To enrich stomach yīn, sweet, cold, cooling or moistening medicinals are used such as *shí hú* (Dendrobii Herba), *shā shēn* (Adenophorae seu Glehniae Radix), *shēng dì huáng* (Rehmanniae Radix Exsiccata), *lú gēn* (Phragmitis Rhizoma), *yù zhú* (Polygonati Odorati Rhizoma), or *mài dōng* (Ophiopogonis Radix). To supplement and nourish the yīn of spleen and stomach, both of these types of medicinals are used together.

脾胃阴虚

脾经实火、湿热蕴脾的病机进一步发展，可引起脾胃阴虚，脾肝不调，脾胃湿热等病机变化。

脾胃阴虚：脾火亢盛，或湿热久留化热，均可耗伤阴液，先伤及脾阴，然后波及胃阴，既而形成脾胃阴虚的病机。可见脘痞腹胀，饥不欲食，消瘦便秘，舌红苔少等表现。治宜滋养脾胃之阴。养脾阴，药选山药、黄精、芡实、白芍、蜂蜜、甘草等甘平濡润之品；滋胃阴，药选石斛、沙参、生地、芦根、玉竹、麦冬等甘寒凉润之剂。补养脾胃之阴，则宜两者兼用。

2.4 Spleen-Liver Disharmony

When damp-heat brews in the spleen, earth is effulgent and rebels against wood. The inability of the liver and gallbladder to course freely and the failure of the spleen's movement and transformation function constitute a mutually reinforcing cause and effect, forming the pathomechanism of spleen-liver disharmony. Since damp-heat in the spleen and stomach influence the liver and gallbladder, this means the simultaneous existence of spleen-stomach damp-heat and of liver-gallbladder damp-heat.

Although the former is the cause and the later the effect, it is habitually referred to as liver-gallbladder damp-heat. It results in aversion to food, in particular to greasy foods, torpid intake and abdominal distention, and in such symptoms as rib-side pain and bitter taste in the mouth, dizzy head, and jaundice. It is treated by coursing the liver and regulating the spleen, and by clearing and disinhibiting heat and dampness. The recommended formula is *dān zhī xiāo yáo sǎn* (Moutan and Gardenia Free Wanderer Powder) from the *Nǚ Kē Cuō Yào* ("Synopsis of Gynecology"), or a modification of *lóng dǎn xiè gān tāng* (Gentian Liver-Draining Decoction) from the *Yī Fāng Jí Jiě* ("Medical Formulas Gathered and Explained").

Dān Zhī Xiāo Yáo Sǎn 丹栀逍遥散 Moutan and Gardenia Free Wanderer Powder
chái hú (柴胡 bupleurum, Bupleuri Radix)
dāng guī (当归 Chinese angelica, Angelicae Sinensis Radix)
fú líng (茯苓 poria, Poria)
bái sháo yào (白芍药 white peony, Paeoniae Radix Alba)
bái zhú (白术 white atractylodes, Atractylodis Macrocephalae Rhizoma)
gān cǎo (甘草 licorice, Glycyrrhizae Radix)
bò hé (薄荷 mint, Menthae Herba)

mǔ dān pí (牡丹皮 moutan, Moutan Cortex)
shān zhī zǐ (山栀子 gardenia, Gardeniae Fructus)

Lóng Dǎn Xiè Gān Tāng 龙胆泻肝汤 Gentian Liver-Draining Decoction
lóng dǎn (龙胆 gentian, Gentianae Radix)
huáng qín (黄芩 scutellaria, Scutellariae Radix)
shān zhī zǐ (山栀子 gardenia, Gardeniae Fructus)
mù tōng (木通 trifoliate akebia, Akebiae Trifoliatae Caulis)
chē qián zǐ (车前子 plantago seed, Plantaginis Semen)
shēng dì huáng (生地黄 dried/fresh rehmannia, Rehmanniae Radix Exsiccata seu Recens)
dāng guī (当归 Chinese angelica, Angelicae Sinensis Radix)
zé xiè (泽泻 alisma, Alismatis Rhizoma)
chái hú (柴胡 bupleurum, Bupleuri Radix)
gān cǎo (甘草 licorice, Glycyrrhizae Radix)

脾肝不调

湿热蕴脾，土旺侮木，肝胆失疏与脾失健运互为因果，形成脾肝不调的病机。此乃脾胃湿热影响肝胆，是脾胃湿热与肝胆湿热并存。虽然前者为因，后者为果，但习惯上仍称为肝胆湿热。既有厌食恶油、纳呆腹胀，又见胁痛口苦、头眩、黄疸等症。治宜疏肝调脾，清利湿热。方选《女科撮要》丹栀逍遥散（逍遥散加丹皮、栀子），或用《医方集解》龙胆泻肝汤（龙胆草、黄芩、栀子、木通、车前子、生地、当归、泽泻、柴胡、甘草）加减。

2.5. Spleen-Stomach Damp-Heat

When damp-heat brews in the spleen and advances to invade the stomach, the spleen's failure to move and transform and the stomach's failure to harmonize and downbear influence each other, forming the pathomechanism of spleen-stomach dam-heat. Thus, one observes torpid intake and abdominal distention, diarrhea and sloppy stools, together with such manifestations as glomus in the stomach duct, nausea and retching, aversion to food, and belching. It is treated by harmonizing the spleen and stomach, and by clearing heat and disinhibiting dampness. The recommended formula is *lián pò yǐn* (Coptis and Officinal Magnolia Bark Beverage) from the *Huò Luàn Lùn* ("On Cholera").

> ### *Lián Pò Yǐn* 连朴饮
> #### Coptis and Officinal Magnolia Bark Beverage
>
> *huáng lián* (黄连 coptis, Coptidis Rhizoma)
> *hòu pò* (厚朴 officinal magnolia bark, Magnoliae Officinalis Cortex)
> *bàn xià* (半夏 pinellia, Pinelliae Rhizoma)
> *shí chāng pú* (石菖蒲 acorus, Acori Tatarinowii Rhizoma)
> *dàn dòu chǐ* (淡豆豉 fermented soybean, Sojae Semen Praeparatum)
> *shān zhī zǐ* (山栀子 gardenia, Gardeniae Fructus)
> *lú gēn* (芦根 phragmites, Phragmitis Rhizoma)

In addition, when damp-heat moves downward from the spleen and stomach into the large intestine, it can form the pathomechanism of damp-heat in the large intestine. One can observe symptoms like abdominal distention and pain, sloppy and ungratifying stool, or scorching heat in the anus. A chronic brewing of damp-heat influences the movement of qì and blood, causing qì stagnation and blood stasis. This can form such symptoms as concretions, conglomerations, accumulations, and gatherings.

脾胃湿热

湿热蕴脾，进而犯胃，脾失健运，胃失和降，相互影响，形成脾胃湿热的病机。既见纳呆腹胀、腹泻便溏，又见脘痞呕恶，厌食嗳气等表现。治宜调和脾胃，清热利湿。方选《霍乱论》连朴饮（黄连、厚朴、半夏、石菖蒲、淡豆豉、焦山栀、芦根）。

此外，湿热由脾胃下移大肠，可形成大肠湿热的病机，可见腹胀腹痛，便溏不爽，肛门灼热等症。湿热久蕴，影响气血运行，气滞血瘀，可形成癥瘕积聚等症。

脾

PART TWO

Pathomechanisms of Spleen Vacuity

脾虚的病机

脾

Spleen Vacuity
脾虚

The spleen and stomach are the source for blood and qì formation as well as the pivot for the upbearing and downbearing of the qì dynamic. Because they play such a significant role in the vital activities of the human body, physicians throughout the ages have referred to them as the "root of later heaven" (acquired constitution). In the course of vital activities and pathological processes, major damage to qì, blood, or fluids, or a disordered counterflow of the qì dynamic's upbearing and downbearing can influence spleen and stomach functions. Since this can result in vacuity detriment to the spleen and stomach, many diseases include the pathomechanism of spleen vacuity.

The "Treatise on Greater Yīn and Yáng Brightness" in the *Sù Wèn* ("Plain Questions") states: "When yáng pathways are replete, yīn pathways are vacuous." This expresses the important general observation that the spleen tends towards pathomechanisms of vacuity and the stomach towards pathomechanisms of repletion. The "Treatise on the Source of Diseases" in the *Yòu Kē Fā Huī* ("Elaboration on Pediatrics") states: "When the spleen and stomach are weakened by vacuity, the hundred diseases will arrive like a swarm of bees."

From the perspective of clinical practice, the pathomechanism of spleen vacuity is exceptionally common, aggravating all the other diseases. Many pathogenic factors, such as damage from the externally contracted six excesses, irregular food and drink, excessive taxation, prolonged thought and preoccupation, excessive vomiting and diarrhea, chronic diseases and disharmony, or lack of or improper treatment can all damage the spleen and cause the pathomechanism of spleen vacuity.

According to extant records from the silk manuscript *Zú Bì Shī Yī Mài Jiǔ Jīng* ("Moxibustion Canon of the Eleven Channels of the Limbs") from the Hàn tomb in Măwángduī, symptoms for the foot greater yīn vessel include such signs as abdominal pain, abdominal distention, and no pleasure in eating. This can be regarded as the earliest literary reference to the symptoms of spleen vacuity. The first formulations of the pathomechanism of spleen vacuity are found in the *Nèi Jīng* ("Inner Canon"). The "Chapter on the Original Spirit" in the *Líng Shū* ("Magic Pivot") states: "When spleen qì is vacuous, use of the limbs is lost and the five viscera are disquieted." The chapter, "Methods of Treating Visceral Qì in Accordance with the Seasons" in the *Sù Wèn* ("Plain Questions"), states: "Regarding spleen disease... vacuity is marked by abdominal fullness, rumbling intestines, swill diarrhea, and non-transformation of food."

Subsequent writers discussed the source of the pathomechanism of spleen disease. During the Hàn dynasty, Zhāng Zhòng-Jǐng stated, in the chapter on "Pulses, Patterns, and Treatments of Vomiting and Diarrhea Disorders" in the *Jīn Guì Yào Lüe* ("Essential Prescriptions of the Golden Coffer"): "When the instep yáng pulse is floating and rough, the floating indicates vacuity and the roughness, a damaged spleen. A damaged spleen fails to grind. Thus, eating in the morning causes vomiting in the evening; eating in the evening causes vomiting in the morning; and grain is habitually not transformed. This is called stomach reflux." This quote analyzes the pathomechanisms of spleen vacuity from the perspective of the pulse manifestation.

The chapter, "On the Methods for Treating Spleen Vacuity and Repletion, Cold and Heat, Life and Death, and Flow and Counterflow" in the *Zhōng Zàng Jīng* ("Central Treasury Canon"), states: "Spleen vacuity leads to an increase in aggregations, a susceptibility to acid swallowing, and incessant diarrhea." It also states: "Spleen vacuity leads to a failure of essential qì to overcome the loss of original qì, an inability to hold urine, and a pulse like running water." Being a relatively early text to discuss organ vacuity and repletion, it specifically mentioned spleen vacuity by name.

The Suí, Táng, and Sòng dynasties saw some developments in the pathomechanism of spleen vacuity. Both the *Zhū Bìng Yuán Hòu Lùn* ("Origin and Indicators of Disease") and the *Qiān Jīn Yào Fāng* ("A Thousand Gold Pieces Prescriptions") described the pathomechanism of spleen vacuity in accordance with the systematic classification of the five viscera. The chapter, "Vacuity, Repletion, and Abdominal Distention" in Qián Yǐ's *Xiǎo Ér Yào Zhèng Zhí Jué* ("Key to Diagnosis and Treatment of Children's Diseases"), states:

> "Small children can easily suffer from vacuity or repletion. When the spleen is vacuous, it cannot bear cold or warmth. When they ingest cold

foods, it generates cold; when they ingest warm foods, it generates heat. One should know this in order to avoid mistakes."

This quotation points out a special characteristic of the pathomechanism of spleen vacuity.

During the Jīn to Yuán period, the Yì-Shuǐ School achieved great results in researching the pathomechanism of spleen vacuity. Zhāng Yuán-Sù, the author of the *Zǎng Fù Biāo Běn Hán Rè Xū Shí Yòng Yào Shì* ("Medicinal Use for the Bowels and Viscera, Heat and Cold, Vacuity and Repletion"), introduced more systematic pattern identification for spleen and stomach diseases based on a classification into pathomechanisms of vacuity or repletion. In "Discussion of the Exuberance and Debilitation of the Spleen and Stomach" in the *Pí Wèi Lùn* ("On the Spleen and Stomach"), Lǐ Dōng-Yuán expressed the famous view of this pathomechanism:

"[On the basis of vacuity detriment to the spleen and stomach] the hundred diseases all arise from debilitation of the spleen and stomach."

Thereby, he comprehensively described the significance of the pathomechanism of spleen vacuity for diseases arising in the entire body. He established the basis for the "Spleen-Stomach Theory" and became the founder of the Earth-Supplementing School.

Following Lǐ Dōng-Yuán, every generation had outstanding physicians who researched spleen vacuity. Wáng Hǎo-Gǔ wrote the *Yīn Zhèng Lüè Lì* ("Examples of Yin Patterns"), inheriting the theories of Zhāng Yuán-Sù and Lǐ Dōng-Yuán. He began a "discussion on yīn patterns" and supplemented the shortcomings of Zhāng and Lǐ who, in their emphasis on spleen-stomach qì vacuity, had neglected the theory of spleen-stomach yáng vacuity.

During the Míng and Qīng periods, the pathomechanism of spleen vacuity was further developed and perfected. In the Míng period, Zhāng Jǐng-Yuè held the greatest esteem for the ideas of Lǐ Dōng-Yuán's spleen-stomach theory and produced an even more comprehensive description of the pathomechanisms in which spleen vacuity is related to the onset of disease in the five viscera. In the Qīng period, Wú Chéng began a discussion of spleen yīn vacuity in his *Bù Jū Jí* ("Non-limitation Collection"). Táng Róng-Chuān stated in the chapter, "What the Five Viscera Store; Spleen Stores Ideation" in the *Zhōng Xī Yī Huì Tōng Yī Jīng Jīng Yì* ("Combined Essences of Chinese and Western Medical Classics"): "When spleen yīn is insufficient, the ability to remember becomes impaired." This made the pathomechanism of spleen vacuity yet more substantial and complete.

For a long time, most practitioners of Chinese medicine thought that qì vacuity and yáng vacuity were the more common forms of spleen vacuity and mentioned yīn vacuity only rarely. But after extensive and in-depth research in more recent times, it is now believed that the pathomechanism of spleen yīn vacuity was first discussed in the Míng and Qīng periods and does in fact have real practical value in clinical application. Thus, its importance has gradually been recognized by everyone. The condition of spleen blood vacuity is rarely discussed to this day and still awaits further exploration.

脾胃为气血生化之源，又是气机升降之枢纽，在人体生命活动中具有极其重要的地位，被历代医家称为"后天之本"。在生命活动和疾病过程中，气、血、津液大量损耗，气机升降逆乱，均会影响脾胃功能，导致脾胃虚损的发生，故许多疾病中都包含着脾虚的病机。如《素问•太阴阳明论》说："阳道实，阴道虚"，对脾病多虚，胃病多实的病机趋向作了高度概括。《幼科发挥•原病论》说："脾胃虚弱，百病蜂起。"从临床实践出发，强调了诸多疾病中，脾虚病机尤为多见。多种病因，如外感六淫的损伤，饮食失调，劳倦过度，思虑日久，吐泻太过，病久失调，失治误治等均会伤脾而引起脾虚的病机。

据现存资料，马王堆汉墓帛书《足臂十一脉灸经》中，足太阴脉病候有腹痛、腹胀、不嗜食等病状，可以认为是脾虚症状的早期文字记录。脾虚病机的提法首见于《内经》。《灵枢•本神篇》："脾气虚，则四肢不用，五脏不安。"《素问•藏气法时论》："脾病者…虚则腹满，肠鸣，飧泄，食不化。"是后世讨论脾虚病机之滥觞。汉•张仲景《金匮要略•呕吐下利病脉证治》说："趺阳脉浮而涩，浮则为虚，涩则伤脾，脾伤则不磨，朝食暮吐，暮食朝吐，宿谷不化，名曰胃反。"从脉象分析了脾虚的病机变化。《中藏经•论脾脏虚实寒热生死逆顺之法》说："脾虚则多癖，喜吞酸，痢不已。"又说："脾虚则精气不胜元气之失，溺不能自持，其脉似水流。"较早讨论脏腑虚实，明确提出了脾虚的名称。隋唐宋代对脾虚的病机有所发展，《诸病源候论》，《千金要方》均按五脏系统归类，阐述脾虚病机。钱乙《小儿药证直诀•虚实腹胀》有："小儿易为虚实，脾虚不受寒温，服寒则生冷，服温则生热，当识此勿误也"之说，指出脾虚病机的特性。金元时代，易水学派对脾虚病机的研究取得巨大成就，张元素著《脏腑标本寒热虚实用药式》，根据虚实分类的病机对脾胃病进行比较系统的辨证。李东垣《脾胃论•脾胃盛衰论》从脾胃虚损出发，提出"百病皆由脾胃衰而生"的著名病机观点，全面阐述脾虚病机在全身发病中的重要意义，奠定了"脾胃学说"的基础，成为补土派的创始人。继东垣之后，研究脾虚的医家，代不乏贤。王好古著《阴证略例》，继承了张(元素)、李(东垣)的理论，提出"阴证论"，补充了张、李重视脾胃气虚，忽略脾胃阳虚理论之不足。明清时期，脾虚病机得到进一步发展和完善。明代•张景岳对东垣脾胃学说的思想推崇备致，并对脾虚与五脏发病关系的病机作了更为全面的论述。清代•吴澄在《不居集》中开创脾阴虚之说，唐容川《中西医汇通医精经义•五脏所藏•脾藏意》有"脾阴不足则记忆多忘"之言，从而使脾虚的病机更加充实和完善。长期以来，广大中医工作者认为脾虚以气虚和阳虚较为多见，较少提及阴虚。通过近代广泛深入的研究，认为脾阴虚的病机从明清开始已有论述，在临床上又有着实际的运用价值，逐渐受到大家的重视。关于脾的血虚，至今少见论述，有待深入发掘。

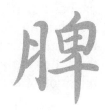

Chapter 1

Spleen Qì Vacuity

脾气虚

The *Huáng Dì Nèi Jīng* ("Yellow Emperor's Inner Canon") contains the earliest mention of the pathomechanism of spleen qì vacuity, providing a detailed and penetrating discussion. The chapter, "Methods of Treating Visceral Qì in Accordance with the Seasons" in the *Sù Wèn* ("Plain Questions") explains: "Regarding spleen disease, in vacuity there will be abdominal fullness, rumbling intestines, swill diarrhea, and non-transformation of food." This indicates that spleen qì vacuity can result in manifestations of all sorts of indigestion. The "Treatise on Comparative [Understanding of] Exuberance and Debilitation" in the *Sù Wèn* ("Plain Questions") also explains:

> "When spleen qì is vacuous, one will have dreams of insufficient food and drink. At the time when earth is dominant, one will have dreams of constructing walls and building houses."

These sources indicate that spleen qì vacuity can lead to a range of symptoms of the essence-spirit. The chapter, "Natural Lifespan" in the *Líng Shū* ("Magic Pivot"), states: "At the age of seventy, spleen qì is vacuous and the skin is desiccated." The "Discussion of the Root Spirit" in the same text also notes: "When spleen qì is vacuous, the use of the limbs is lost and the five viscera are disquieted." This quotation describes how spleen qì vacuity can result in generalized malnutrition.

Subsequently, the *Shāng Hán Lùn* ("On Cold Damage"), *Zhōng Zàng Jīng* ("Central Treasury Canon"), *Zhū Bìng Yuán Hòu Lùn* ("Origin and Indicators of Disease"), *Qiān Jīn Yào Fāng* ("A Thousand Gold Pieces Prescriptions"), and *Shèng Jì Zǒng Lù* ("Sages' Salvation Records") all elaborated substantially on this foundation. Lǐ Dōng-Yuán's *Pí Wèi Lùn* ("On the Spleen and Stomach") founded the Spleen-Stomach Theory on the basis of the idea that spleen qì vacuity causes debilitation of original qì, which in turn is the cause for the formation of disease. This laid the foundation for research on the pathomechanisms of spleen qì vacuity in the following generations. The "Discussion of the Exuberance and Debilitation of the Spleen and Stomach" in the *Pí Wèi Lùn* explains:

> "When spleen-stomach qì is vacuous, it causes inability to eat and emaciation, or reduced eating and obesity, and inability to lift the limbs in spite of obesity… When the spleen is vacuous, it results in emaciation."

There are many causes for spleen qì vacuity. For example, in the *Sù Wèn* ("Plain Questions"), we find passages such as: "When food and drink are doubled, the intestines and stomach are damaged" ("Treatise on Impediment"); "Food and drink taxation fatigue results in damage to the spleen" ("Treatise on Sickness"); "Thought damages the spleen" ("Treatise on the Movements of the Five Periods"); "When kidney heat spreads to the spleen, it passes into vacuity" ("On Qì Reversal"). All these disease causes can damage spleen qì. In addition, insufficient care in early childhood, debility in old age, constitutional insufficiency, enduring diarrhea and disinhibition, and lack of or improper treatment can also affect spleen qì. All these pathogenic factors cause spleen qì vacuity to be most common among the patterns of spleen vacuity. It is the most basic pathomechanism, but its manifestations are extremely complex. Broadly speaking, they can be divided into the aspects of spleen vacuity movement failure, spleen qì failing to upbear, failure of the spleen to control blood, and failure of spleen qì to provide luxuriance.

《黄帝内经》最早提出脾气虚的病机，并作了详细精辟的论述。如《素问•藏气法时论》说："脾病者...虚则腹满，肠鸣，飧泄，食不化。"指出脾气虚可引起消化不良的各种表现。《素问•方盛衰论》亦说："脾气虚，则梦饮食不足，得其时，则梦筑垣盖屋。"提示脾气虚，可引起一系列精神症状。《灵枢•天年》曰："七十岁，脾气虚，皮肤枯。"《灵枢•本神论》又说："脾气虚则四肢不用，五脏不安"，阐述了脾气虚可致全身营养不良。继后，《伤寒论》、《中藏经》、《诸病源候论》、《千金要方》、《圣济总录》都在此基础上作了大量的发挥。李东垣《脾胃论》基于脾气虚则元气衰，元气衰则疾病由此而生的思想，创立了脾胃学说，为后世研究脾气虚的病机奠定了基础。如《脾胃论•脾胃盛衰论》说："脾胃气虚，则不能食而瘦，或少食而肥，虽肥而四肢不举。...脾虚则肌肉瘦削。"导致脾气虚原因很多，如"饮食自倍，肠胃乃伤"（《素问•痹论》）；"饮食劳倦则伤脾"（《素问•本病论》）；"思伤脾"（《素问•五运行大论》）；"肾移热于脾，传为虚"（《素问•气厥论》）

等病因均可伤及脾气。此外，小儿喂养不良，成人年高体衰，先天禀赋不足，久泻久利，失治误治亦可引起。多种多样致病原因，使脾气虚在脾虚证中成为最常见、最基本的病机之一，表现十分复杂。概括起来可分为脾虚失运，脾气不升，脾不统血和脾气不荣等几个方面。

1.1   Spleen Vacuity Movement Failure

The spleen governs movement and transformation. It is able to digest grain and water, to absorb as well as convert and transport the essence of grain and water, and to participate in the digestion of food and drink. In addition, it is able to absorb water-humor, to distribute water-humor, and to regulate and balance the fluid metabolism in the human body. Spleen qì vacuity causes the breakdown of the movement and transformation functions. This results in two kinds of pathomechanisms: grain and water failing to move, and water-damp failing to transform.

脾虚失运

脾主运化，可消化水谷，吸收和转输水谷精微，参与饮食物的消化过程。又可吸收水液，输布水液，调节人体水液代谢平衡。脾气虚，运化功能失司，则有水谷失运、水湿不化两类病机变化。

1.1.1   Grain and Water Movement Failure

The spleen depends on the effulgence of spleen qì for the movement and transformation of grain and water. Only then can it assist the stomach in the digestion of grain and water, the absorption of nutritional substances, and their distribution throughout the entire body. In cases of spleen qì vacuity, grain and water cannot be digested, converted, and transported in a timely manner. They collect and stagnate below the heart, causing non-transformation of food, an exceedingly long absence of hunger, and torpid stomach intake. One tastes no flavors in the mouth and has no thought of food and drink, which manifests as the primary pathoconditions of torpid intake and reduced eating.

The chapter, "Spleen-Stomach Qì Vacuity and Inability to Eat and Drink" in the *Shèng Jì Zǒng Lù* ("Sages' Salvation Records"), states:

"It is said that grain and water enter the mouth and accumulate in the stomach, and that the spleen then disseminates their qì and moisture,

thereby enhancing the various organs. When the spleen viscus is insufficient and stomach qì is internally weakened, the person is unable to eat
and drink, and, even if eating, the food cannot be transformed."

This passage points out that the spleen transports and distributes the essence of grain and water for the stomach. When spleen qì is vacuous,
movement and transformation fail and food and drink are difficult to digest, causing absence of hunger for an exceeding length of time and reduced food intake.

The greater abdomen belongs to the spleen. When spleen qì is vacuous, it propels movement without force, preventing clear qì from upbearing and turbid qì from downbearing, and causing qì to stagnate in the
center. This results in abdominal distention. After meals, burden on the
spleen's movement function is increased, movement and transformation
are even more difficult, and qì stagnation is even more prominent. Thus
the distention and fullness is aggravated after meals.

The appearance of the stool is closely related to the spleen's ability to
move and transport grain and water. When spleen qì is vacuous, movement and transformation lack strength, grain and water are not transformed, damp qì stagnates and collects, and grain, water, and damp qì
flow downward into the intestines. As a result, the large intestine conveyance breaks down and water flows into the intestinal region, causing
dull pain in the center of the abdomen and faint rumbling in the intestines.
Grain and water are not transformed and instead pour down, and spleen
qì has difficulty controlling and containing them. This causes desire to
defecate after meals, thin sloppy stools, and nontransformation of whole
grains, which is recurrent and incessant. As stated in the chapter, "Methods of Treating Visceral Qì in Accordance with the Seasons" in the *Sù
Wèn* ("Plain Questions"), "Regarding spleen disease... in vacuity, there
will be abdominal fullness, rumbling intestines, swill diarrhea, and nontransformation of food." Swill diarrhea refers to stool that is thin and
contains residues of undigested food. Its most important pathomechanism
is exactly this one caused by spleen vacuity and nontransformation of
grain and water.

When spleen qì is vacuous and fails to propel movement, the conveyance and transformation of the large intestine is forceless, grain and water collect for a long time in the intestines, and liquids and humors are
absorbed extremely slowly, which can also cause constipation. This condition manifests in no bowel movement for several days, dry stools, or
sometimes an inability to defecate in spite of a desire to do so and exert-
ing great efforts to expel the stool, or expelling only a small amount of
stool, with sweating, shortness of breath, fatigued spirit, and lack of
strength after bowel movements.

Grain and water movement failure is treated by supplementing the center and boosting qì, and by fortifying the spleen and assisting movement. For conditions that are mainly characterized by torpid intake and reduced eating with abdominal distention, the recommended formula is *yì gōng sǎn* (Special Achievement Powder) from the *Xiǎo Ér Yào Zhèng Zhǐ Jué* ("Key to Diagnosis and Treatment of Children's Diseases") with additions:

Yì Gōng Sǎn 异功散
Special Achievement Powder
rén shēn (人参 ginseng, Ginseng Radix)
fú líng (茯苓 poria, Poria)
bái zhú (白术 white atractylodes, Atractylodis Macrocephalae Rhizoma)
gān cǎo (甘草 licorice, Glycyrrhizae Radix)
chén pí (陈皮 tangerine peel, Citri Reticulatae Pericarpium)
Plus:
mù xiāng (木香 costusroot, Aucklandiae Radix)
shā rén (砂仁 amomum, Amomi Fructus)

If the main symptoms are abdominal distention, abdominal pain, and sloppy stool, the recommended formula is *shēn líng bái zhú sǎn* (Ginseng, Poria, and White Atractylodes Powder) from the *Tài Píng Huì Mín Hé Jì Jú Fāng* ("Tài-Píng Imperial Grace Pharmacy Formulas"):

Shēn Líng Bái Zhú Sǎn 参苓白术散
Ginseng, Poria, and White Atractylodes Powder
rén shēn (人参 ginseng, Ginseng Radix)
fú líng (茯苓 poria, Poria)
bái zhú (白术 white atractylodes, Atractylodis Macrocephalae Rhizoma)
shān yào (山药 dioscorea, Dioscoreae Rhizoma)
biǎn dòu (扁豆 lablab, Lablab Semen Album)
lián zǐ ròu (莲子肉 lotus fruit, Nelumbinis Semen)
yì yǐ rén (薏苡仁 coix, Coicis Semen)
shā rén (砂仁 amomum, Amomi Fructus)
jié gěng (桔梗 platycodon, Platycodonis Radix)
gān cǎo (甘草 licorice, Glycyrrhizae Radix)

An alternate choice is *zī shēng wán* (Life-Promoting Pill) from the *Xiān Xǐng Zhāi Yī Xué Guǎng Bǐ Jì* ("Broad-Ranging Medical Notes from the Studio of Early Awaking") with modifications:

Zī Shēng Wán 资生丸
Life-Promoting Pill

rén shēn (人参 ginseng, Ginseng Radix)

fú líng (茯苓 poria, Poria)

bái zhú (白术 white atractylodes, Atractylodis Macrocephalae Rhizoma)

gān cǎo (甘草 licorice, Glycyrrhizae Radix)

shān yào (山药 dioscorea, Dioscoreae Rhizoma)

biǎn dòu (扁豆 lablab, Lablab Semen Album)

lián zǐ ròu (莲子肉 lotus fruit, Nelumbinis Semen)

yì yǐ rén (薏苡仁 coix, Coicis Semen)

shā rén (砂仁 amomum, Amomi Fructus)

jié gěng (桔梗 platycodon, Platycodonis Radix)

huò xiāng yè (藿香叶 patchouli leaf, Pogostemi Folium)

jú hóng (橘红 red tangerine peel, Citri Reticulatae Exocarpium Rubrum)

huáng lián (黄连 coptis, Coptidis Rhizoma)

zé xiè (泽泻 alisma, Alismatis Rhizoma)

qiàn shí (芡实 euryale, Euryales Semen)

jiāo shān zhā (焦山楂 scorch-fried crataegus, Crataegi Fructus Ustus)

chǎo mài yá (炒麦芽 stir-fried barley sprout, Hordei Fructus
    Germinatus Frictus)

bái dòu kòu (白豆蔻 cardamom, Amomi Fructus Rotundus)

For conditions mainly characterized by constipation and shortness of breath, the recommended formula is *huáng qí tāng* (Astragalus Decoction) from the *Jīn Guì Yì* ("Wings of the Golden Coffer") with additions:

Huáng Qí Tāng 黄芪汤
Astragalus Decoction

huáng qí (黄耆 astragalus, Astragali Radix)

chén pí (陈皮 tangerine peel, Citri Reticulatae Pericarpium)

huǒ má rén (火麻仁 cannabis seed, Cannabis Semen)

fēng mì (蜂蜜 honey, Mel)

Plus:

bái zhú (白术 white atractylodes, Atractylodis Macrocephalae Rhizoma)

rén shēn (人参 ginseng, Ginseng Radix)

shēng má (升麻 cimicifuga, Cimicifugae Rhizoma)

jié gěng (桔梗 platycodon, Platycodonis Radix)

zhǐ qiào (*ké*) (枳壳 bitter orange, Aurantii Fructus)

水谷失运

脾对水谷的运化，是依赖脾气的旺盛，才能助胃以消化水谷，吸收营养物质，输布全身。脾气虚弱，水谷不能按时消化、转输，停滞心下，食而不化，过时不饥，胃纳呆滞，故觉口中无味、不思饮食、出现纳呆食少的主症。如《圣济总录•脾胃气虚弱不能饮食》云："论曰：水谷入口，而聚于胃，脾则播其气泽，以埤（增加）诸脏腑而已。今脾脏不足，胃气内弱，故不能饮食，虽食亦不能化也。"指出脾为胃输布水谷精微，脾气虚，失于运化，饮食难消，故过时不饥，进食量少。

大腹属脾，脾气虚弱，推动无力，清气不升，浊气不降，气滞于中，则为腹胀。食后增加脾运负担，运化更难，气滞更为突出，故食后胀满益甚。大便的性状与脾的运化水谷功能密切相关。脾气虚弱，运化乏力，水谷不化，湿气滞留，水谷湿气下流肠中，导致大肠传导失司，水行肠间，则腹中隐痛，肠鸣幽幽；水谷不化而下注，脾气难于统摄，则食后欲便、大便溏薄、完谷不化、反复不止。如《素问•藏气法时论》所云："脾病者…虚则腹满，肠鸣，飧泄，食不化。"飧泄，即言大便稀薄，夹有不消化的食物残渣，主要病机就是脾虚不化水谷所致。

脾气虚弱，失于推动，大肠传化无力，水谷久停肠中，津液被缓缓吸收，又可引起便秘。表现为多日不便，大便干燥，或有时虽有便意，入厕努力排泄，仍不能排便，或排出少许大便，便后常兼汗出短气，神疲乏力等症状。

治宜补中益气，健脾助运。若以纳呆食少，腹胀为主，选《小儿药证直诀》异功散（人参、茯苓、白术、甘草、陈皮）加木香、砂仁。若以腹胀、腹痛、便溏为主，选《和剂局方》参苓白术散（人参、茯苓、白术、山药、扁豆、莲子肉、苡仁、砂仁、桔梗、甘草），或《先醒斋医学笔记》资生丸（人参、茯苓、白术、甘草、山药、扁豆、莲子肉、苡仁、砂仁、桔梗、藿香叶、橘红、黄连、泽泻、芡实、焦山楂、炒麦芽、白蔻）加减。若以便秘气短为主，选《金匮翼》黄芪汤（黄芪、陈皮、麻仁、白蜜）加白术、人参、升麻、桔梗、枳壳等药。

1.1.2   Water-Damp Failing to Transform

The spleen governs the movement and transformation of water-damp. When spleen qì is vacuous, it is unable to distribute or expel water-humor, and water-damp is not transformed. This can lead to pathomechanisms with such aspects as spleen vacuity with dampness collecting, spleen vacuity engendering phlegm, and spleen vacuity water swelling.

水湿不化

脾主运化水湿，脾气虚弱，不能输布、排泄水液，水湿不化，可引起脾虚湿停、脾虚生痰和脾虚水肿等方面的病机变化。

1.1.2.1 Spleen Vacuity with Dampness Collecting

When spleen qì is vacuous, it is unable to move and transform. Water-humor stagnates and converts into dampness, which collects in the center burner. Lodging water-damp can then in turn reversely encumber and harass spleen qì, bringing about qì stagnation in the stomach duct and abdomen. This causes glomus and oppression in the stomach duct and abdomen, and poor appetite.

In cases of qì vacuity with dampness collecting, damp qì scatters throughout the entire body and blocks channel qì; this results in a heavy and cumbersome head and body and aching pain in the limbs. When spleen qì is vacuous, the girdling vessel is insecure and damp turbidity flows downward. This can then result in such symptoms as continuously-flowing, clear-white, thin vaginal discharge.

As suggested by the expression "dampness engendered by spleen-earth" from the chapter on "Dampness Damage" in the *Yī Biǎn* ("Lancing Stones of Medicine"), this type of dampness disease "reaches everywhere, to the top and the bottom, to the center and the outside." "When it is in the center, it results in abdominal distention, glomus, and blockage." As a treatment for this pathomechanism, in which "dampness is engendered by pathological earth vacuity," this source proposes to use the method of "supplementing earth," with the intention of eliminating dampness by fortifying the spleen. It is thus an example of a concrete clinical application of the pathomechanism of spleen vacuity with dampness collecting.

This condition is treated by supplementing the center and nourishing qì, and by fortifying the spleen and eliminating dampness. Conditions that are mainly characterized by spleen vacuity with dampness collecting are best treated with *qī wèi bái zhú sǎn* (Seven-Ingredient White Atractylodes Powder) from the *Xiǎo Ér Yào Zhèng Zhí Jué* ("Key to Diagnosis and Treatment of Children's Diseases") with the addition of *yì yǐ rén* (Coicis Semen):

Qī Wèi Bái Zhú Sǎn 七味白朮散
Seven-Ingredient White Atractylodes Powder

rén shēn (人参 ginseng, Ginseng Radix)

fú líng (茯苓 poria, Poria)

bái zhú (白朮 white atractylodes, Atractylodis Macrocephalae Rhizoma)

gān cǎo (甘草 licorice, Glycyrrhizae Radix)

huò xiāng yè (藿香叶 patchouli leaf, Pogostemi Folium)

mù xiāng (木香 costusroot, Aucklandiae Radix)

gé gēn (葛根 pueraria, Puerariae Radix)

Plus:

yì yǐ rén (薏苡仁 coix, Coicis Semen)

For conditions that are mainly characterized by white discharge that is copious, clear, and thin, the recommended formula is *jiā wèi liù jūn zǐ tāng* (Six Gentlemen Decoction) from the *Zhōng Yī Fù Kē Zhì Liáo Xué* ("Therapeutics in Chinese Medical Gynecology") with modifications:

Jiā Wèi Liù Jūn Zǐ Tāng 加味六君子汤
Modified Six Gentlemen Decoction

rén shēn (人参 ginseng, Ginseng Radix)

fú líng (茯苓 poria, Poria)

bái zhú (白朮 white atractylodes, Atractylodis Macrocephalae Rhizoma)

gān cǎo (甘草 licorice, Glycyrrhizae Radix)

chén pí (陈皮 tangerine peel, Citri Reticulatae Pericarpium)

bàn xià (半夏 pinellia, Pinelliae Rhizoma)

cāng zhú (苍朮 atractylodes, Atractylodis Rhizoma)

shēng má (升麻 cimicifuga, Cimicifugae Rhizoma)

chái hú (柴胡 bupleurum, Bupleuri Radix)

shēng jiāng (生姜 fresh ginger, Zingiberis Rhizoma Recens)

脾虚湿停

脾气虚弱，不能运化，水液停滞，转化为湿，停留中焦。水湿滞留，反过来又会困扰脾气，导致脘腹气滞，引起脘腹痞闷、食欲不振。脾虚湿停，湿气散布周身，阻塞经气，则为头身困重、肢体酸痛。脾气虚，带脉不固，湿浊下流，又会引起带下绵绵、色白清稀等症状。如《医碥•伤湿》中有"脾土所生之湿"的提法，此类湿病，"上下中外，无处不到"。其"在中则腹胀痞塞。"针对这种"自病土虚生湿"的病机，提出用"补土"方法，通过健脾达到除湿的目标，是脾虚湿停病机在临床上的具体运用。

治宜补中养气，健脾除湿。若以脾虚湿停为主者，选《小儿药证直诀》七味白术散（人参、茯苓、白术、甘草、藿香叶、木香、葛根）加苡仁。若以白带量多清稀为主者，方选《中医妇科治疗学》加味六君子汤（人参、茯苓、白术、甘草、陈皮、半夏、苍术、升麻、柴胡、生姜）加减。

1.1.2.2 Spleen Vacuity Engendering Phlegm

When spleen qì is full and exuberant, its movement and transformation prevents internal dampness from collecting and prevents external dampness from invading, so phlegm-rheum does not arise. When spleen qì is vacuous and weak, water-damp fails to transform, gathering damp turns into rheum, and rheum transforms into phlegm, engendering pathogenic substances like phlegm-rheum. When phlegm-rheum is formed, it scurries along the channels in all directions. Flowing downward into the intestinal area, it gurgles faintly and generates rumbling intestines and diarrhea. Rising up and intimidating the heart, it impedes heart qì, causing stirring palpitations below the heart. Moving up into the lungs, it impairs the diffusion and downbearing of the lung, leading to shortness of breath, oppression in the chest, cough, and ejection of clear and thin phlegm.

As stated in the chapter on "Rheum Pathoconditions" in the *Zhèng Zhì Huì Bǔ* ("Combined Supplements to Patterns and Treatment"): "When patients with serious cases of spleen vacuity drink fluids, they sense it collecting and stagnating in the intestines, making the intestines rumble inside; in severe cases, it may even cause diarrhea." The chapter on "Phlegm-rheum" in the *Shǔ Zhōng Yī Cuàn* ("Sìchuān Medical Cullings") explains even more clearly: "Phlegm is precisely the essential humor of a person and is necessarily a product of the transformation of grain and water. It is entirely caused by vacuity of the center. Phlegm is identical with water. Its root is in the kidney and its tip in the spleen… As for it being in the spleen, when spleen vacuity causes the nontransformation of food and drink, it means that earth is failing to dam water." This elaborates in more detail on the pathomechanism of spleen vacuity engendering phlegm.

This condition is treated by supplementing the center and boosting qì, and by fortifying the spleen and transforming phlegm. The recommended formula is *xiāng shā liù jūn zǐ tāng* (Costusroot and Amomum Six Gentlemen Decoction) from the *Zhōng Guó Yī Xué Dà Cí Diǎn* ("Greater Dictionary of Chinese Medicine") with modifications:

Xiāng Shā Liù Jūn Zǐ Tāng 香砂六君子汤
Costusroot and Amomum Six Gentlemen Decoction

mù xiāng (木香 costusroot, Aucklandiae Radix)

shā rén (砂仁 amomum, Amomi Fructus)

bàn xià (半夏 pinellia, Pinelliae Rhizoma)

chén pí (陈皮 tangerine peel, Citri Reticulatae Pericarpium)

rén shēn (人参 ginseng, Ginseng Radix)

fú líng (茯苓 poria, Poria)

bái zhú (白术 white atractylodes, Atractylodis Macrocephalae Rhizoma)

 zhì gān cǎo (炙甘草 mix-fried licorice, Glycyrrhizae Radix cum Liquido Fricta)

脾虚生痰

脾气充盛，自能健运，内湿不停，外湿不侵，则痰饮不生。脾气虚弱，水湿不化，聚湿为饮，饮化为痰，产生痰饮等病理产物。痰饮生成，随经四窜，下流肠间，沥沥有声，而生肠鸣腹泻；上凌于心，阻碍心气，则为心下悸动；上行于肺，肺失宣降，则为气短、胸闷、咳嗽，吐痰清稀。如《证治汇补•饮症》云："更有脾虚之人，每遇饮后，即觉停滞肠中，肠鸣于内，甚或作泻。"《蜀中医纂•痰饮》更明确指出："痰即人之精液，无非水谷所化，悉由中虚而然。痰即水也，其本在肾，其标在脾。...在脾者，以脾虚饮食不化，土不制水也。"较为精辟地阐述了脾虚生痰的病机。

治宜补中益气，健脾化痰。方选《中国医学大辞典》香砂六君子汤（木香、砂仁、半夏、陈皮、人参、茯苓、白术、炙甘草）加减。

1.1.2.3 Spleen Vacuity Water Swelling

The spleen is located in the center burner and is the pivot of fluid metabolism. Above, it can transport liquids to the lung; below, it can move liquids to the kidney and bladder. Spleen qì is therefore of particular importance for the regularity of fluid metabolism. As stated in the "Separate Treatise on the Channels" in the *Sù Wèn* ("Plain Questions"):

> "Spleen qì dissipates essence. Above, it returns it to the lungs and regulates the waterways; below, it transports it to the bladder; thus it distributes water essence to all directions and makes it flow through all the five channels."

When spleen qi is vacuous, it is unable to move and transform fluids. Earth fails to dam water, and water qì floods over, percolates and pours into the channels and network vessels, steeps the organs, and floats and dissipates into the skin. This causes puffiness and swelling in the whole body, face, and eyes, with rather pronounced water swelling in the legs. When spleen qì fails to move, water-damp cannot be transported down to the bladder and its source of transformation is reduced, causing shortened or reduced urination. When water qì collects in the abdomen, it can lead to such symptoms as abdominal distention, torpid intake, and reduced eating.

As explained in the chapter on "Water Swelling" in the *Biǎn Què Xīn Shū* ("Heart Text of Biǎn Què"):

> "This pathocondition is due to spleen-stomach vacuity. It is caused by damage from eating or drinking cool substances, or by damage to spleen qì from ingesting attacking, restraining, or cooling drugs during sickness, so that it is unable to free the waterways. Therefore it flows into the four limbs and hundred bones, causing generalized puffy swelling, difficult urination, and diarrhea, making this disease most serious. Physicians of this age all use drugs that disinhibit water and dissipate the swelling, thereby hastening the patient's death."

This quotation emphasizes strongly that the cause for the pathomechanism of water swelling is found in water qì flooding due to spleen vacuity. If one stubbornly employs water-disinhibiting, swelling-dispersing, and freeing medicinals, this can accelerate the damage to spleen qì. It will not only fail to disinhibit water, but to the contrary aggravate the water swelling and worsen the patient's condition.

The "Section on Water Swelling" in the *Shèng Jì Zǒng Lù* ("Sages' Salvation Records") also explains:

> "The condition of water swelling is due to spleen and kidney qì vacuity so that it is unable to dam water and water qì moves frenetically, spilling into the skin."

This quotation again explains that spleen qì vacuity and breakdown of movement and transformation is one of the most important pathomechanisms to cause water swelling.

Spleen vacuity water swelling is treated by fortifying the spleen and boosting qì, and by disinhibiting water and dispersing swelling. The recommended formula is *liù jūn zǐ tāng* (Six Gentlemen Decoction) in combination with *wǔ líng sǎn* (Poria Five Powder) from the *Shāng Hán Lùn* ("On Cold Damage"):

Liù Jūn Zǐ Tāng 六君子汤
Six Gentlemen Decoction

bàn xià (半夏 pinellia, Pinelliae Rhizoma)
chén pí (陈皮 tangerine peel, Citri Reticulatae Pericarpium)

rén shēn (人参 ginseng, Ginseng Radix)

fú líng (茯苓 poria, Poria)

bái zhú (白术 white atractylodes, Atractylodis Macrocephalae Rhizoma)

zhì gān cǎo (炙甘草 mix-fried licorice, Glycyrrhizae Radix cum
Liquido Fricta)

Wǔ Líng Sǎn 五苓散 Poria Five Powder
zé xiè (泽泻 alisma, Alismatis Rhizoma) *zhū líng* (猪苓 polyporus, Polyporus) *bái zhú* (白术 white atractylodes, Atractylodis Macrocephalae Rhizoma) *fú líng* (茯苓 poria, Poria) *guì zhī* (桂枝 cinnamon twig, Cinnamomi Ramulus)

An alternative choice is *liù jūn zǐ tāng* (Six Gentlemen Decoction)
combined with *wǔ pí yǐn* (Five-Peel Beverage) from the *Zhōng Zàng Jīng*
("Central Treasury Canon") with modifications:

Wǔ Pí Yǐn 五皮饮 Five-Peel Beverage
jiāng pí (姜皮 ginger skin, Zingiberis Rhizomatis Cortex) *sāng bái pí* (桑白皮 mulberry root bark, Mori Cortex) *chén pí* (陈皮 tangerine peel, Citri Reticulatae Pericarpium) *dà fù pí* (大腹皮 areca husk, Arecae Pericarpium) *fú líng pí* (茯苓皮 poria skin, Poriae Cutis)

脾虚水肿

脾位于中焦，为水液代谢的枢纽，上可输津于肺，下可运津于肾与
膀胱，故脾气在水液代谢的调节中有特别重要的意义。正如《素问•
经脉别论》所云："脾气散精，上归于肺，通调水道，下输膀胱，水
精四布，五经并行。"脾气虚，不能运化水液，土不制水，水气泛
溢，渗注经络，浸渍脏腑，浮散肌肤，令人全身面目浮肿，下肢水
肿较为明显。脾气不运，水湿不能下输于膀胱，化源减少，则为尿
短尿少。水气停留于腹，可引起腹胀、纳呆食少等症状。如《扁鹊
心书•水肿》说："此症由脾胃虚弱，为饮食冷物所伤，或因病服攻
克凉药损伤脾气，致不能通行水道，故流入四肢百骸，令人遍身浮
肿，小便反涩，大便反泄，此病最重。世医皆用利水消肿之药，乃
速其毙也。"这里强调指出，引起水肿的病机是脾虚水气泛溢，如果
强施利水消肿通利之药，则会加速脾气的损伤，不仅不能利水，反

而加重水肿，增添病情。《圣济总录•水肿门》亦说：" 水肿之病，
以脾肾气虚，不能制水，水气妄行，溢于皮肤。"再次说明脾气虚，
运化失职是引起水肿的重要病机之一。

治宜健脾益气，利水消肿。方选六君子汤合《伤寒论》五苓散（泽
泻、猪苓、白术、茯苓、桂枝）。或以六君子汤合《中藏经》五皮
饮（生姜皮、桑白皮、陈皮、大腹皮、茯苓皮）加减。

Literature Review of Spleen Vacuity Movement Failure

📖 *Zhāng Shì Yī Tōng* ("Zhang's Clear View of Medicine"), "Damage from Food and Drink"

> "When patients suffer from no thought of food and drink, failure to digest food, and yet satiety after meals, it means that the spleen is vacuous and unable to move and transform."

This quotation points out the pathomechanism by which spleen qì vacuity and failure to move and transform, with nontransformation of food and drink so that they collect and stagnate in the center burner and impede the qì dynamic can lead to no thought of food and drink and yet bloating after eating.

📖 *Biàn Zhèng Lù* ("Records on Pattern Identification"), "Section on Center Fullness"

> "All conditions of center fullness are bound to have formed due to qì vacuity. If one fails to supplement spleen and stomach qì, how could the distention possibly be dissipated?"

The term center fullness indicates distention and fullness below the heart. It is mostly generated because of spleen qì vacuity, breakdown of movement and transformation, and qì stagnation in the center burner. Therefore it should be treated primarily by fortifying the spleen and boosting qì.

📖 *Jǐng Yuè Quán Shū* ("Jǐng-Yuè's Complete Compendium"), "Schema of Miscellaneous Patterns," "Diarrhea"

> "If dietary irregularities or a way of life not in accordance with the seasons have resulted in damage to the spleen and stomach, water will revolt, causing dampness, and grain will revolt, causing stagnation. Essential qì will be unable to transport and transform, causing it to downbear together with filth, and diarrhea will occur."

This quotation describes the pathomechanism by which damage to spleen qì and a breakdown of movement and transformation cause grain, water, and water-damp to flow downward, resulting in diarrhea.

📖 *Míng Yī Lèi Àn* ("Classified Case Histories of Famous Physicians"), "Case Histories of Wind Stroke"

> "Numbness in the forearm and limpness of the body means that the spleen is not functioning. Spontaneous discharge of phlegm-drool means that the spleen is unable to contain it. A deviated mouth and difficult speech mean that spleen qì is damaged."

This quotation points out the pathomechanism by which damage to spleen qì, formation of phlegm-rheum, and impediment of the channels and network vessels leads to drooling, deviated mouth and impeded speech, and numbness and fatigue of the limbs.

📖 *Yī Fāng Kǎo* ("Medical Remedies Researched"), "Section on Dampness"

> "When grain and water enter the stomach, there is bound to be dampness. If spleen-earth is effulgent, it is able to move and transform grain and water, return it to the lungs above, and make it reach the bladder below, without any damp qì collecting. It is only when the spleen is weak and unable to restrain dampness that it gathers and forms phlegm-rheum… When the spleen is fortified, it is sufficiently able to restrain dampness. When qì is disinhibited, the accumulated rheum will move spontaneously."

Spleen weakness refers to spleen qì vacuity so that it is unable to move and transform fluids. These collect and cause dampness, which transforms into rheum.

📖 *Yī Zōng Bì Dú* ("Indispensable Medical Reading"), "Phlegm-Rheum"

> "In cases of spleen-earth vacuity dampness, the clear is difficult to clear, and the turbid is difficult to downbear. They collect in the center and stagnate in the intestines, turning into phlegm. Therefore, for treating phlegm one should first supplement spleen. The spleen in turn will then normalize movement and transformation, and phlegm will transform on its own."

This quotation discusses why spleen qì vacuity and nontransformation of water-damp is an important pathomechanism that engenders dampness and phlegm.

📖 *Zhèng Zhì Huì Bǔ* ("Combined Supplements to Patterns and Treatment"), "Water Swelling"

> "All cases of damp swelling and fullness are related to the spleen. The spleen governs grain and water. When it is vacuous, movement breaks down, water-damp collects in the great channels and small network vessels, and they all become utterly turbid and putrid. Liquid and humor as well as blood all transform into water; therefore the face, eyes and four limbs are puffy and swollen."

This quotation points out that when spleen vacuity movement failure causes water-damp to collect and stagnate in the channels and network vessels, impeding the blood flow, it can take the shape of water swelling.

文献评述

《张氏医通•伤饮食》：”有不思饮食，食不克化，食后反饱，脾虚不能健运也。”指出脾气虚，失运健运，饮食不化，停滞中焦，阻碍气机，引起不思饮食、食后反饱作胀的病机。

《辨证录•中满门》：”盖中满之病，未有不因气虚而成者，不补脾胃之气，则胀从何而消。”中满是指心下胀满，多因脾气虚弱，运化失职，气滞中焦而成，故治疗应以健脾益气为主。

《景岳全书•杂证谟•泄泻》：”若饮食不节，起居不时，以致脾胃受伤，则水反为湿，谷反为滞，精华之气不能输化，乃至合污下降，而泻利作矣。”论述脾气受伤，运化失司，水谷水湿下流，引起腹泻下利的病机。

《名医类案•中风案》："臂麻体软，脾无用也。痰涎自出，脾不能摄也。口斜语涩，脾气伤也。”指出脾气损伤，化生痰饮，阻碍经络，引起流涎、口歪语謇、肢麻倦怠的病机。

《医方考•湿门》：”水谷入胃，无非湿也，脾土旺，则能运化水谷，上归于肺，下达膀胱，无湿气所留也。惟夫脾弱不能制湿，则积而成痰饮。…脾健则足以制湿，气利则积饮自行。”脾弱是脾气虚弱，不能运化水液，停聚为湿，转化为饮。

《医宗必读•痰饮》：”脾土虚湿，清者难清，浊者难降，留中滞肠，瘀而成痰。故治痰先补脾，脾复健运之常，而痰自化。”论述脾气虚，水湿不化，是生湿生痰的重要病机。

《证治汇补•水肿》：”诸湿肿满，皆属于脾。脾主水谷，虚而失运，水湿停留，大经小络，尽皆浊腐。津液与血，悉化为水，故面目四肢浮肿。”指出脾虚失运，水湿停滞经络，阻碍血行，可形成水肿。

Summary of Spleen Vacuity Movement Failure

1. Grain and Water Movement Failure

Torpid stomach intake: Lack of taste in the mouth, no thought of food and drink, torpid intake and reduced eating.

> *Qi stagnation in the center*: Abdominal distention, greatly increased fullness and swelling after eating.
>
> *Downward flow of damp turbidity*: Faintly rumbling intestines, thin sloppy stool, nontransformation of whole grains.
>
> *Forceless bowel movements*: Constipation, discharging a reduced amount of stool in spite of the desire to defecate and exerting great efforts to expel the stool, fatigued spirit and lack of strength after bowel movements.

2. Water-Damp Failing to Transform

Spleen vacuity with dampness collecting

> a) *Encumbrance and harassment of spleen qì*: Glomus and oppression of the stomach duct and abdomen, poor appetite, heaviness and encumbrance of the whole body, aching pain in the limbs.
>
> b) *Downward flow of damp turbidity*: Perpetual vaginal discharge that is white, clear, and thin.

Spleen vacuity engendering phlegm

> a) *Flowing down into the intestinal area*: Faint gurgling, rumbling intestines, diarrhea.
>
> b) *Rising up and intimidating the heart*: Stirring palpitations below the heart.
>
> c) *Rising up and steeping the lungs*: Shortness of breath and oppression in the chest, cough, ejection of clear and thin phlegm.

Spleen vacuity water swelling

> a) *Water qì invading upwards*: Puffiness and swelling in the entire body, face, and eyes.
>
> b) Reduced source of transformation: Scant urine.
>
> c) *Water qì collecting in the abdomen*: Abdominal distention, torpid intake and reduced eating.

脾虚失运
水谷不运——胃纳呆滞—口中无味，不思饮食，纳呆食少。
气滞于中—腹胀，食后胀满益甚。
湿浊下流—肠鸣幽幽，大便溏薄，完谷不化。
运便无力—便秘，虽有便意，入厕努力排泄， 便出量少，便后神疲乏力。
水湿不化——脾虚湿停—— 困扰脾气—脘腹痞闷，食欲不振， 周身困重，肢体酸痛。

湿浊下流—带下绵绵，色白清稀。

脾虚生痰——流于肠间—沥沥有声，肠鸣腹泻。

上凌于心—心下悸动。

上渍于肺—气短胸闷，咳嗽，吐痰清稀。

脾虚水肿——水气上犯—全身面目浮肿。

化源减少—尿少。

水气留腹—腹胀，纳呆食少。

1.2 Spleen Qì Fall

The spleen and stomach are the pivot of the qì dynamic's upbearing and downbearing in the human body. The chapter, "Some Questions on Medicine" in the *Yī Xué Zhèng Zhuàn* ("Orthodox Tradition of Medicine"), states: "The clear swiftly transforms into qì and relies on spleen qì to upbear it to the lung." The chapter, "On the Spleen and Stomach" in the *Lín Zhèng Zhǐ Nán Yī Àn* ("A Clinical Guide with Case Histories"), also states: "The spleen is supposed to upbear in order to fortify; the stomach is supposed to downbear in order to harmonize." Both explain that upbearing is the primary characteristic of spleen qì.

When spleen qì upbears the clear, it can not only transport the essence of grain and water up to the heart, lung, and head, face, ears and eyes, but it can also lift up the viscera inside and thereby preserve the stability of the location of the organs. If spleen qì is vacuous and unable to upbear the clear, it can develop into the pathomechanism of spleen qì fall.

The *Nèi Jīng* ("Inner Canon") mentions a disease called "drooping." The "Inquiry about Statements" in the *Líng Shū* ("Magic Pivot") explains:

> "When the stomach is not full, the various vessels are vacuous. When the various vessels are vacuous, the sinews are sluggish and fatigued. When the sinews are sluggish and fatigued, qì will be unable to return after vigorous sexual intercourse, causing the condition of drooping."

The Chinese character for drooping refers to a drooping appearance and a sluggish and forceless condition, due to flabbiness of the flesh and sinews. "When the stomach is not full" should include the pathomechanism of spleen vacuity and can be understood as insufficiency of spleen qì. In this condition, spleen qì fails to upbear the clear and is unable to move and transform the essence of grain and water to provide for the flesh and sinews. The sinews become flabby, which results in a sluggish, forceless, and drooping appearance.

This is the earliest description of the pathomechanism of spleen qì fall. The same text also explains: "When center qì is insufficient, there will be changes in the stool and urine and the intestines will hurt and rumble." The "Great Treatise on the Correspondences and Manifestations of Yīn and Yáng" in the *Sù Wèn* ("Plain Questions") also explains: "When clear qì is in the lower part of the body, it engenders swill diarrhea." This indicates even more clearly that when clear qì fails to upbear due to spleen vacuity movement failure and instead falls downward, it can lead to gastrointestinal dysfunctions and result in rumbling intestines and diarrhea.

Lǐ Dōng-Yuán explained in the chapter "On the Beginnings of Heat Stroke due to Food and Drink Taxation Fatigue" in the *Pí Wèi Lùn* ("On the Spleen and Stomach"): "When spleen and stomach qì flow downward, they prevent grain qì from upbearing and floating," describing in detail the pathomechanism of spleen qì fall resulting in internal damage and heat effusion. Lǐ Dōng-Yuán pioneered the use of *bǔ zhōng yì qì tāng* (Center-Supplementing Qì-Boosting Decoction) in accordance with the principle of "supplementing the center and upbearing yáng" and thereby established the foundation for the pathomechanism of spleen qì.

Xuē Yǐ mentioned the pathomechanism of spleen qì quite early. As he explained in his commentary on "Diarrhea" in the *Míng Yī Zá Zhù* ("Miscellaneous Works by Famous Physicians"), "When spleen qì fall occurs, one should use *bǔ zhōng yì qì tāng* (Center-Supplementing Qì-Boosting Decoction) to upbear and lift it." He also explained in the commentary on "Dysentery" in the same text: "When one is unable to cure center qì fall with inability to contain blood, one should use *bǔ zhōng yì qì tāng*."

While discussing the contributing factors of white turbidity pattern, Zhāng Jǐng-Yuè also mentioned the term "spleen qì fall." As he explained in the chapter, "Schema of Miscellaneous Patterns; White Turbidity" in the *Jǐng Yuè Quán Shū* ("Jǐng-Yuè's Complete Compendium"), "When white turbidity becomes chronic, it means spleen qì fall, failure of earth to restrain dampness, and lack of cleanliness in the waterways."

In the chapter "On the Spleen and Stomach" in the *Lín Zhèng Zhǐ Nán Yī Àn* ("A Clinical Guide with Case Histories"), Yè Tiān-shì emphasized even more strongly the significance of spleen qì fall at the onset of disease, based on the characteristic that "the spleen should upbear in order to fortify." He explained: "To summarize spleen and stomach disease, whether vacuity or repletion, cold or heat, dry or moist, they should certainly be distinguished carefully. The two terms "upbearing" and "downbearing" are particularly vital. When spleen qì fall consolidates a disease, even if it does not fall but merely fails to move and transform, it is still a disease." According to the progression of the pathomechanism, spleen qì fall can be divided into three levels of spleen qì failing to bear upward, center burner qì stagnation, and qì dynamic fall.

脾气下陷

脾胃为人体气机升降之枢纽。《医学正传•医学或问》曰："其清者倏焉而化为气，依脾气上升于肺。"《临证指南医案•脾胃门》也云："脾宜升则健，胃宜降则和。"均说明脾气的运动特点，是以上升为主。脾气升清，既可上输水谷精微于心、肺、头面耳目，又可升举内脏，维持脏腑位置的稳定。若脾气虚弱，不能升清，则可发展成为脾气下陷的病机。《内经》中有"弹"之病名。《灵枢•口问篇》说："胃不实则诸脉虚，诸脉虚则筋脉懈惰，筋脉懈惰则行阴（房室）用力，气不能复，故为弹。""弹"通"癉"，意为下垂貌，由于肌肉筋脉松弛而引起的懈惰无力状态。"胃不实"应包括脾虚的病机，可理解为脾气不足，失于升清，不能运化水谷精微供养肌肉筋脉，筋脉松弛而导致懈惰无力，下垂之貌，是对脾气下陷病机的最早描述。《灵枢•口问篇》说："中气不足，溲便为之变，肠为之苦鸣。"《素问•阴阳应象大论》又说："清气在下，则生飧泄"，更明确指出脾虚失运，清气不升，反而下陷可引起胃肠功能失调而导致肠鸣、腹泄。李东垣《脾胃论•饮食劳倦所伤始为热中论》说："脾胃之气下流，使谷气不得升浮"，较为精辟地阐述了脾气下陷引起内伤发热的病机。并根据"补其中而升其阳"的原则，首创补中益气汤，为脾气下陷的病机奠定了基础。薛已较早指出脾气下陷的病机。如他在注释《明医杂著•泄泻》时说："脾气下陷而致者，宜用补中益气汤升举之。"又在《明医杂著•痢疾》的注释中说："中气下陷不能摄血而不愈者，用补中益气汤。"张景岳在论述白浊证的成因中，也提出了"脾气下陷"的名称。如《景岳全书•杂证谟•白浊》说："白浊…其久也，则脾气下陷，土不制湿而水道不清。"叶天士《临证指南医案•脾胃门》根据"脾宜升则健"的特点，更强调脾气下陷在发病中的重要意义，他说："总之脾胃之病，虚实寒热，宜燥宜润，固当详辨。其于升降二字，尤为紧要。盖脾气下陷固病，即使不陷，而但不健运，已病矣。"脾气下陷，按其病机的发展过程可分为脾气不升、中焦气滞、气机下陷三个层次。

1.2.1 Spleen Qì Failing to Bear Upward

When spleen qì bears upward, the essence of grain and water bears upward along with clear yáng, thereby giving luxuriance to the heart, lung, and head, face, eyes, and ears and producing a marked moistening and nourishing effect. When spleen qì is vacuous, it is unable to upbear the clear. The essence of grain and water is unable to ascend and nourish the head and eyes, and clear yáng is unable to moisten the upper orifices. This manifests as dizziness and headache.

When spleen qì is unable to rise up to nourish the lung, lung qì becomes vacuous and unable to host qì and take charge of breathing, causing shortness of breath, shortage of qì, oppression in the chest, a low voice, and laziness to speak. When it is unable to rise up to nourish the heart, the heart spirit lacks governance, causing essence-spirit fatigue. When it is unable to rise up to nourish the ears, the clear orifices are without spirit, causing tinnitus and poor hearing.

The "Schema of Miscellaneous Patterns; Dizziness" in the *Jǐng Yuè Quán Shū* ("Jǐng-Yuè's Complete Compendium") explains:

> "When the cause of the original disease is qì vacuity, it means that clear qì is unable to bear upward, perhaps due to copious sweating and yáng collapse. It should be treated by upbearing yáng and supplementing qì."

Although qì vacuity is mentioned only in passing, it is common knowledge that the spleen is the source of engendering qì and that the spleen has the function of upbearing the clear. When spleen qì is vacuous and clear yáng fails to bear upward, the orifices in the head lose their nourishment, which is a notable cause for dizziness.

The chapter on "Dizziness" in the *Zhèng Zhì Huì Bǔ* ("Combined Supplements to Patterns and Treatment") suggests even more explicitly:

> "The spleen occupies the central region, upbears the soaring yáng of the heart and lung, and embanks the yīn of the kidney and liver. In cases of excessive taxation fatigue with copious sweating and yáng collapse, when original qì falls and clear yáng fails to upbear, dizziness arises owing to an insufficiency of center qì."

From this statement we can see that failure of the spleen to upbear the clear and insufficient nourishment of the clear orifices results in one of the most commonly seen pathomechanisms in the clinic, namely dizziness and flowery vision.

The chapter, "On the Passage and Transmutation of Vacuity and Repletion in the Spleen and Stomach" in the *Pí Wèi Lùn* ("On the Spleen and Stomach") states: "When stomach qì is vacuous, the ears, eyes, mouth, and nose are all diseased." What Lǐ Dōng-Yuán refers to as "stomach qì," in actuality also includes spleen qì. Thus it means that when spleen qì fails to upbear the clear, the head, face, and clear orifices are nourished improperly, which can result in the symptoms of dizziness, tinnitus, and poor hearing.

This condition is treated by fortifying the spleen and boosting qì, and by upbearing and supplementing clear yáng. The recommended formula is *bǔ zhōng yì qì tāng* (Center-Supplementing Qì-Boosting Decoction) from the *Pí Wèi Lùn* ("On the Spleen and Stomach"), with the addition of *màn jīng zǐ* (Viticis Fructus), *bái sháo* (Paeoniae Radix Alba), and *chuān xiōng* (Chuanxiong Rhizoma).

Bǔ Zhōng Yì Qì Tāng 补中益气汤 Center-Supplementing Qì-Boosting Decoction
huáng qí (黄耆 astragalus, Astragali Radix)
rén shēn (人参 ginseng, Ginseng Radix)
bái zhú (白朮 white atractylodes, Atractylodis Macrocephalae Rhizoma)
chái hú (柴胡 bupleurum, Bupleuri Radix)
shēng má (升麻 cimicifuga, Cimicifugae Rhizoma)
chén pí (陈皮 tangerine peel, Citri Reticulatae Pericarpium)
dāng guī (当归 Chinese angelica, Angelicae Sinensis Radix)
zhì gān cǎo (炙甘草 mix-fried licorice, Glycyrrhizae Radix cum Liquido Fricta)
Plus:
màn jīng zǐ (蔓荆子 vitex, Viticis Fructus)
bái sháo yào (白芍药 white peony, Paeoniae Radix Alba)
chuān xiōng (川芎 chuanxiong, Chuanxiong Rhizoma)

脾气不升

脾气上升，可使水谷精微随清阳之气上升，以荣心、肺、头面耳目，发挥其滋润营养作用。脾气虚弱，不能升清，水谷精微不能上养于头目，清阳不能濡润上窍，则见眩晕头痛；不能上养于肺，肺气虚不能主气司呼吸，则气短、少气、胸闷、声低懒言；不能上养于心，心神无主，则精神倦怠；不能上养于耳，清窍不灵，则耳鸣不聪。如《景岳全书•杂证谟•眩晕》说："原病之由，有气虚者，乃清气不能上升，或汗多亡阳而致，当升阳补气。"此处虽然概言气虚，但众所周知，脾为生气之源，脾又具有升清功能，脾气虚，清阳不升，头窍失养，是引起眩晕的重要原因。《证治汇补•眩晕》更明确提出："脾为中州，升腾心肺之阳，堤防肾肝之阴，若劳倦过度，汗多亡阳，元气下陷，清阳不升者，此眩晕出于中气不足也。"由此可见，脾不升清，清窍失养，是导致临床头昏眼花最常见的病机之一。《脾胃论•脾胃虚实传变论》："胃气一虚，耳、目、口、鼻，俱为之病。"东垣所指"胃气"，实际包括脾气在内。即言脾气失于升清，头面清窍失养，可引起头晕、耳鸣失聪等症状。

治宜健脾益气，升补清阳。用《脾胃论》补中益气汤（黄芪、人参、白术、柴胡、升麻、当归、炙甘草）加蔓荆子、白芍、川芎。

1.2.2   Center Burner Qì Stagnation

When spleen qì is vacuous, clear qì fails to upbear and instead stops and reverses its direction. Qì collecting in the center burner causes glomus blockage below the heart. Spleen qì stagnation in the center burner has a reciprocal influence on the spleen's failure to move and transform. This can aggravate the patient's condition even further, leading to such symptoms as glomus fullness below the heart and torpid stomach intake, which greatly worsen after meals.

The chapter, "Glomus Fullness" in the *Lèi Zhèng Zhì Cái* ("Systematized Patterns with Clear-Cut Treatments") states:

> When the spleen is unable to move qì to the lung and stomach so that it binds instead of dissipating, this causes glomus... In cases of enduring vacuity of center qì and nontransformation of the subtle essences, upbear the clear and downbear the turbid. Use *bǔ zhōng yì qì tāng* (Center-Supplementing Qì-Boosting Decoction) with the addition of *zhū líng* (Polyporus) and *zé xiè* (Alismatis Rhizoma). "

Zhāng Shì Yī Tōng ("Zhang's Clear View of Medicine") states:

> "*Shēng má* (Cimicifugae Rhizoma) and *chái hú* (Bupleuri Radix) upbear the clear from below the deepest ground; *fú líng* (Poria) and *zé xiè* (Alismatis Rhizoma) downbear the turbid from above the highest heaven. When they are mixed and negate each other, peace is created. In cases of spleen vacuity movement failure and vacuity glomus with reduced eating, warm and supplement the spleen as the origin. Use *sì jūn zǐ tāng* (Four Gentlemen Decoction) or *yì gōng sǎn* (Special Achievement Powder)."

This passage indicates that when spleen qì is unable to upbear and the qì dynamic is unable to move up to the lung and stomach and instead binds in the center burner, the glomus fullness pattern of stagnation and stoppage below the heart can arise.

This condition is treated by supplementing qì and moving the spleen, and by upbearing the clear and downbearing the turbid. The recommended formula is *bǔ zhōng yì qì tāng* (Center-Supplementing Qì-Boosting Decoction) from the *Pí Wèi Lùn* ("On the Spleen and Stomach"), with the addition of *zhū líng* (Polyporus) and *zé xiè* (Alismatis Rhizoma). An alternate choice is *liù jūn zǐ tāng* (Six Gentlemen Decoction) from the *Fù Rén Dà Quán Liáng Fāng* ("Compendium of Good

Remedies for Women") with the addition of *shēng má* (Cimicifugae Rhizoma) and *chái hú* (Bupleuri Radix).

Bǔ Zhōng Yì Qì Tāng 补中益气汤
Center-Supplementing Qì-Boosting Decoction [modified]

huáng qí (黄耆 astragalus, Astragali Radix)

rén shēn (人参 ginseng, Ginseng Radix)

bái zhú (白术 white atractylodes, Atractylodis Macrocephalae Rhizoma)

chái hú (柴胡 bupleurum, Bupleuri Radix)

shēng má (升麻 cimicifuga, Cimicifugae Rhizoma)

chén pí (陈皮 tangerine peel, Citri Reticulatae Pericarpium)

dāng guī (当归 Chinese angelica, Angelicae Sinensis Radix)

zhì gān cǎo (炙甘草 mix-fried licorice, Glycyrrhizae Radix cum Liquido Fricta)

Plus:

zhū líng (猪苓 polyporus, Polyporus)

zé xiè (泽泻 alisma, Alismatis Rhizoma)

Liù Jūn Zǐ Tāng 六君子汤
Six Gentlemen Decoction) [modified]

fú líng (茯苓 poria, Poria)

bái zhú (白术 white atractylodes, Atractylodis Macrocephalae Rhizoma)

rén shēn (人参 ginseng, Ginseng Radix)

zhì gān cǎo (炙甘草 mix-fried licorice, Glycyrrhizae Radix cum Liquido Fricta)

bàn xià (半夏 pinellia, Pinelliae Rhizoma)

chén pí (陈皮 tangerine peel, Citri Reticulatae Pericarpium)

Plus:

shēng má (升麻 cimicifuga, Cimicifugae Rhizoma)

chái hú (柴胡 bupleurum, Bupleuri Radix)

Alternatively, abdominal distention can arise when spleen qì is vacuous, fails to move and transform, and becomes unable to propel the movement of the qì dynamic, so that clear qì fails to upbear and turbid qì fails to downbear, causing qì to stagnate in the center. This type of abdominal distention has the special characteristics that the distention occurs even when hungry, that it is worst around midnight, and that it can be reduced with hiccup and flatus after meals or after pushing with gentle pressure. This is due to the fact that during times of hunger or in the middle of the night, there is no food and drink left to collect below the heart, and that this condition is caused entirely by spleen vacuity impairing movement and transformation, so that clear qì fails to upbear and qì stagnates in the center and cannot be dispersed or dissipated. This condition belongs to the category of vacuity distention and is called center vacuity qì stagnation.

The chapter, "Spleen Vacuity Abdominal Distention" in the *Zhèng Yīn Mài Zhì* ("Pathoconditions: Causes, Pulses, and Treatments"), explains:

> "The pathocondition of spleen vacuity abdominal distention is characterized by low food intake and general fatigue, spleen vacuity movement failure, uninhibited clear stool and urine, faint speech, and intermittently abating distention in the heart and abdomen that is relaxed in the morning and tense in the evening. This is the pathocondition of spleen vacuity abdominal distention."

Here, Qín Jǐng-Míng indicates that "intermittently abating distention that is relaxed in the morning and tense in the evening" is a particular sign of spleen vacuity abdominal distention. Its primary pathomechanism originates in lack of movement due to spleen vacuity, breakdown of upbearing and downbearing, and qì stagnation in the center.

This condition is treated by supplementing the spleen and upbearing the clear, and by moving qì and dissipating distention. The recommended formula is *xiāng shā liù jūn zǐ tāng* (Costusroot and Amomum Six Gentlemen Decoction) with the addition of *zhǐ qiào (ké)* (Aurantii Fructus), *hòu pò* (Magnoliae Officinalis Cortex), *wū yào* (Linderae Radix), *chái hú* (Bupleuri Radix), and *shēng má* (Cimicifugae Rhizoma).

Xiāng Shā Liù Jūn Zǐ Tāng 香砂六君子汤
Costusroot and Amomum Six Gentlemen Decoction [modified]

mù xiāng (木香 costusroot, Aucklandiae Radix)

shā rén (砂仁 amomum, Amomi Fructus)

fú líng (茯苓 poria, Poria)

bái zhú (白术 white atractylodes, Atractylodis Macrocephalae Rhizoma)

rén shēn (人参 ginseng, Ginseng Radix)

zhì gān cǎo (炙甘草 mix-fried licorice, Glycyrrhizae Radix cum Liquido Fricta)

bàn xià (半夏 pinellia, Pinelliae Rhizoma)

chén pí (陈皮 tangerine peel, Citri Reticulatae Pericarpium)

Plus:

zhǐ qiào (ké) (枳壳 bitter orange, Aurantii Fructus)

hòu pò (厚朴 official magnolia bark, Magnoliae Officinalis Cortex)
wū yào (乌药 lindera, Linderae Radix)
chái hú (柴胡 bupleurum, Bupleuri Radix)
shēng má (升麻 cimicifuga, Cimicifugae Rhizoma)

中焦气滞

脾气虚弱，清气不升，反而遏折，气停中焦，则为心下痞塞。脾气停滞中焦，与脾失健运互为影响，可使病情加剧，引起心下痞满、胃纳呆滞、食后尤甚等症状。如《类证治裁·痞满》云："<保命集>曰：脾不能行气于肺胃，结而不散，则为痞。…中气久虚，精微不化者，升清降浊。补中益气汤加猪苓、泽泻。<医通>曰：升、柴从九地之下而升其清，苓、泻从九天之上而降其浊，所以交否而为泰也。脾虚失运，食少虚痞者，温补脾元。四君子汤，异功散。"指出脾气不能上升，气机不能上行肺胃，停结于中焦，则会形成心下滞塞不通的痞满证。治宜补气运脾，升清降浊。方用《脾胃论》补中益气汤加猪苓、泽泻。或用《妇人大全良方》六君子汤加升麻、柴胡。

或因脾气虚弱，失于运化，不能推动气机运行，清气不升，浊气不降，气滞于中，发为腹胀。此类腹胀以饥时反胀、夜半胀甚，进食或推柔按压后，打呃矢气，胀满可减为特点。饥时或夜间，心下已无饮食停留，全因脾虚运化无力，清气不升，气滞于中，不能消散所致。此属虚胀，名曰中虚气滞。如《症因脉治·脾虚腹胀》说："脾虚腹胀之症：食少身倦，脾虚不运，二便清利，言语轻微，心腹时胀时退，朝宽暮急，此脾虚腹胀之症也。"这里秦景明指出"时胀时退，朝宽暮急"为脾虚腹胀的特征，其主要病机就是源于脾虚乏运，升降失司，气滞于中。治宜补脾升清，行气消胀。方选香砂六君子汤加枳壳、厚朴、台乌、柴胡、升麻。

1.2.3 Falling of the Qì Dynamic

When spleen qì is vacuous and unable to upbear the clear, uplifting is forceless and the qì dynamic sags into the lower body. This can cause the location of the internal organs to shift downward. When clear qì fails to bear upward and falls into the lower abdomen, it can lead to distention, fullness, and sagging distention and constraint in the lesser abdomen. When qì falls into the bladder, it can result in frequent desire to urinate. When qì falls into the essence gate, it can lead to such symptoms as seminal emission and premature ejaculation. The "Schema of Miscellaneous Patterns; Seminal Emission" in the *Jǐng Yuè Quán Shū* ("Jǐng-Yuè's Complete Compendium") states:

"As for the pattern of seminal emission ... when it coincides with taxation fatigue leading to emission, this means that sinew strength is impaired and that liver and spleen qì is weakened. Complete emissions that are caused by excessive pondering with the heart indicate an insufficiency of center qì and vacuity fall of the heart and spleen."

Although these two types have different disease causes, they both involve spleen qì fall and inability to contain essence, resulting in seminal emission and efflux diarrhea.

When the spleen fails to upbear the clear, it falls downward to the back and qì sags into the rectum. This can lead to a heavy and sagging sensation in the anus, frequent desire to defecate, bowel movements right after eating, unsuccessful straining with great effort during bowel movements, expelling rather small amounts of stool of dry or thin consistency, and perhaps shortness of breath and heart palpitations after defecating. Failure to contain qì as a result of spleen qì fall can lead to prolapse of the rectum. The chapter on "Symptom of Rectal Desertion" in the *Zhū Bìng Yuán Hòu Lùn* ("Origin and Indicators of Disease") explains:

"The anus is the indicator of the large intestine. When the large intestine is vacuous and cold and its qì surges downward, the anus will move outward."

The *Jǐng Yuè Quán Shū* ("Jǐng-Yuè's Complete Compendium"), "Schema of Miscellaneous Patterns; Prolapse of the Rectum" also explains:

"Spleen and kidney qì fall and desertion after enduring diarrhea and dysentery is caused either by center qì being vacuous and cold so that it cannot be contained and deserts, or by desertion due to taxation, overwork, vomiting, or diarrhea damaging the liver and spleen."

Although vacuity cold means yáng vacuity, it will invariably first damage spleen qì before causing spleen qì fall. Only when spleen qì fails to upbear the clear and preserve the normal location of the organs can it result in drooping and prolapse of the rectum.

When the qì dynamic falls and the organs shift downward as a result of the spleen failing to upbear the clear, this can manifest in drooping of the internal organs, such as prolapse of the stomach, prolapse of the liver, floating kidney, or uterine prolapse. The chapter, "Symptoms of Vaginal Protrusion and Desertion" in the *Zhū Bìng Yuán Hòu Lùn* ("Origin and Indicators of Disease") explains:

"Damage to the uterine network vessels, vacuity cold in the uterus, and downward surging of qì can cause vaginal protrusion. This is called desertion below. It can also be caused by desertion of the genitals due to straining and holding one's breath in childbirth."

The chapter, "Patterns and Treatment of Yīn Desertion" in the *Sān Yīn Jí Yī Bìng Zhèng Fāng Lùn* ("A Unified Treatise on Diseases, Patterns, and Remedies According to the Three Causes"), further explains:

> "Women who rush into labor tax themselves, straining, and choking excessively, [which leads to] vaginal desertion. If rectal desertion occurs or the vagina protrudes, this causes distress and painful swelling. Lifting heavy weights or sexual taxation can result in this condition, as well as continuous leaking of clear fluid and strangury."

Both these passages discuss how excessive taxation damage, injury to center qì, failure of the spleen to upbear the clear, and fall of the internal organs can lead to the various patterns of internal organ drooping such as uterine prolapse.

The spleen governs upbearing of the clear. When spleen qì is vacuous and clear qi fails to upbear, turbidity and dampness flow down. The clear is mixed with the turbid and percolates down into the intestinal region, which causes diarrhea. Owing to clear qì fall, the ripening transformation of food is disabled and grain and water flow continuously, often leading to enduring and incessant diarrhea and nontransformation of whole grains. As explained in the chapter, *Bǔ Zhōng Yǎng Qì Tāng* in the *Chéng Fāng Qiè Yòng* ("Effective Use of Set Formulas"):

> "When the spleen is vacuous and unable to upbear and lift, it causes more downbearing and less upbearing, leading to clear yáng fall, which results in diarrhea…When the diarrhea is not stopped, it means spleen qì fall."

The chapter, "Swill Diarrhea" in the *Jīn Guì Yì* ("Wings of the Golden Coffer"), explains:

> "Swill diarrhea means that the whole grains are not transformed… Again, when clear qì is in the lower body and engenders swill diarrhea, this is called yáng qì vacuity causing the fall."

Although this passage in general discusses yáng vacuity, it is in fact related to the inability of spleen qì to upbear the clear. In clinic, all cases of enduring diarrhea and frequent and increased defecation include the pathomechanism of spleen qì fall.

When due to spleen qì fall, essence is not transported and distributed normally and instead flows down into the bladder, one observes turbid urine, resembling rice water. The "Schema of Miscellaneous Patterns; Strangury-Turbidity" in the *Jǐng Yuè Quán Shū* ("Jǐng-Yuè's Complete Compendium") states:

> "White turbidity pattern means that turbidity is present in the urine. Its color is white like rice water… When this condition is enduring, it means that spleen qì fall has occurred, so earth is unable to contain dampness and the waterways are not cleared."

This type of white turbid urine is commonly seen in small children because they are most susceptible to spleen qì damage from dietary irregularities and to center qì fall, which cause the essence of grain and water to flow down into the bladder.

Sores in the front or back of the two yīn orifices can be caused by spleen qì fall. The reason for this is that sores can over time deplete qì and blood. As a result, spleen qì is easily damaged, clear yáng has difficulty upbearing, center qì falls, and turbidity and dampness pour down into the two yīn and become enmeshed with residual evil that has not been eliminated completely. This condition is lingering and difficult to treat. It leads to pudendal itching and pain and persistent ulcerating sores. The "Schema of Miscellaneous Patterns; Lower Body Gān Sore" in the *Jǐng Yuè Quán Shū* ("Jǐng-Yuè's Complete Compendium") states:

> "When lower body gān sores...coincide with fatigue at the end of day, they are caused by yáng qì vacuity and fall. [For treatment, use] *bǔ zhōng yì qì tāng* (Center-Supplementing Qì-Boosting Decoction)."

By supplementing the center, upbearing yáng, and revitalizing the qì dynamic, clear yáng is enabled to bear upward, turbid yīn is discharged outward, toxins are drawn out, and evil is dispelled. Thus, this chronic condition is treated. In short, the many chronic diseases of the area surrounding the two yīn are for the most part intimately linked to the pathomechanism of spleen qì fall.

Falling of the qì dynamic is treated by supplementing the center and boosting qì, and by upbearing yáng and lifting the fall. Conditions that are mainly characterized by heaviness and sagging in the lesser abdomen with frequent desire to defecate are best treated with *bǔ zhōng yì qì tāng* (Center-Supplementing Qì-Boosting Decoction) with the addition of *shān yào* (Dioscoreae Rhizoma), *wǔ wèi zǐ* (Schisandrae Fructus), and *yì zhì rén* (Alpiniae Oxyphyllae Fructus).

Bǔ Zhōng Yì Qì Tāng 补中益气汤 Center-Supplementing Qì-Boosting Decoction [modified]
huáng qí (黄耆 astragalus, Astragali Radix)
rén shēn (人参 ginseng, Ginseng Radix)
bái zhú (白术 white atractylodes, Atractylodis Macrocephalae Rhizoma)
chái hú (柴胡 bupleurum, Bupleuri Radix)
shēng má (升麻 cimicifuga, Cimicifugae Rhizoma)
chén pí (陈皮 tangerine peel, Citri Reticulatae Pericarpium)
dāng guī (当归 Chinese angelica, Angelicae Sinensis Radix)
zhì gān cǎo (炙甘草 mix-fried licorice, Glycyrrhizae Radix cum Liquido Fricta)

Plus:

shān yào (山药 dioscorea, Dioscoreae Rhizoma)

wǔ wèi zǐ (五味子 schisandra, Schisandrae Fructus)

yì zhì rén (益智仁 alpinia, Alpiniae Oxyphyllae Fructus)

Conditions that are mainly characterized by enduring diarrhea and disinhibition are treated with *bǔ zhōng yì qì tāng* (Center-Supplementing Qì-Boosting Decoction) without *dāng guī* (Angelicae Sinensis Radix), but with the addition of *hē zǐ* (Chebulae Fructus), *ròu dòu kòu* (Myristicae Semen), *wǔ wèi zǐ* (Schisandrae Fructus), and *wū méi* (Mume Fructus).

Bǔ Zhōng Yì Qì Tāng 补中益气汤
Center-Supplementing Qì-Boosting Decoction [modified]

huáng qí (黄耆 astragalus, Astragali Radix)

rén shēn (人参 ginseng, Ginseng Radix)

bái zhú (白术 white atractylodes, Atractylodis Macrocephalae Rhizoma)

chái hú (柴胡 bupleurum, Bupleuri Radix)

chén pí (陈皮 tangerine peel, Citri Reticulatae Pericarpium)

shēng má (升麻 cimicifuga, Cimicifugae Rhizoma)

zhì gān cǎo (炙甘草 mix-fried licorice, Glycyrrhizae Radix cum Liquido Fricta)

Plus:

hē zǐ (诃子 chebule, Chebulae Fructus)

ròu dòu kòu (肉豆蔻 nutmeg, Myristicae Semen)

wǔ wèi zǐ (五味子 schisandra, Schisandrae Fructus)

wū méi (乌梅 mume, Mume Fructus)

Conditions that are mainly characterized by rectal desertion and prolapse of the internal organs are treated with *bǔ zhōng yì qì tāng* (Center-Supplementing Qì-Boosting Decoction) with the addition of *cāng zhú* (Atractylodis Rhizoma), *bàn xià* (Pinelliae Rhizoma), *shā rén* (Amomi Fructus), *jié gěng* (Platycodonis Radix), and *zhǐ qiào (ké)* (Aurantii Fructus).

Bǔ Zhōng Yì Qì Tāng 补中益气汤
Center-Supplementing Qì-Boosting Decoction [modified]

huáng qí (黄耆 astragalus, Astragali Radix)

rén shēn (人参 ginseng, Ginseng Radix)

bái zhú (白术 white atractylodes, Atractylodis Macrocephalae Rhizoma)

chái hú (柴胡 bupleurum, Bupleuri Radix)

dāng guī (当归 Chinese angelica, Angelicae Sinensis Radix)

shēng má (升麻 cimicifuga, Cimicifugae Rhizoma)

chén pí (陈皮 tangerine peel, Citri Reticulatae Pericarpium)

zhì gān cǎo (炙甘草 mix-fried licorice, Glycyrrhizae Radix cum Liquido Fricta)

Plus:

cāng zhú (苍术 atractylodes, Atractylodis Rhizoma)

bàn xià (半夏 pinellia, Pinelliae Rhizoma)

shā rén (砂仁 amomum, Amomi Fructus)

jié gěng (桔梗 platycodon, Platycodonis Radix)

zhǐ qiào (*ké*) (枳壳 bitter orange, Aurantii Fructus)

Conditions that are mainly characterized by white turbidity in the urine, and genital sores and ulcerations are also treated with *bǔ zhōng yì qì tāng* (Center-Supplementing Qì-Boosting Decoction), but with the addition of *fú líng* (Poria), *qiàn shí* (Euryales Semen), and *shān yào* (Dioscoreae Rhizoma).

Bǔ Zhōng Yì Qì Tāng 补中益气汤
Center-Supplementing Qì-Boosting Decoction [modified]

huáng qí (黄耆 astragalus, Astragali Radix)

rén shēn (人参 ginseng, Ginseng Radix)

bái zhú (白术 white atractylodes, Atractylodis Macrocephalae Rhizoma)

chái hú (柴胡 bupleurum, Bupleuri Radix)

dāng guī (当归 Chinese angelica, Angelicae Sinensis Radix)

shēng má (升麻 cimicifuga, Cimicifugae Rhizoma)

chén pí (陈皮 tangerine peel, Citri Reticulatae Pericarpium)

zhì gān cǎo (炙甘草 mix-fried licorice, Glycyrrhizae Radix cum Liquido Fricta)

Plus:

fú líng (茯苓 poria, Poria)

qiàn shí (芡实 euryale, Euryales Semen)

shān yào (山药 dioscorea, Dioscoreae Rhizoma)

气机下陷

脾气虚弱，不能升清，升举无力，气机下坠，可使内脏位置下移。清气不升，陷于下腹，可引起小腹胀满、坠胀不舒。气坠膀胱，引起尿意频数；气坠精关，可致遗精早泄等症状。如《景岳全书•杂证谟•遗精》曰："遗精之证...有值劳倦即遗者，此筋力有不胜，肝脾之气弱也；有因用心思索过度彻遗者，此中气有不足，心脾之虚陷也。"两种不同病因，皆涉及脾气下陷，不能统摄精微，而致遗精滑泄。

脾不升清，下陷于后，气坠于肛，可引起肛门重坠、便意频数，食后即便，临厕虚挣努力，排便较少，便质可干可稀，或见便后气短心悸等症状。脾气下陷，气不收摄，可致脱肛。如《诸病源候论•脱肛候》说："肛门大肠候也，大肠虚冷，其气下冲者，肛门反出。"《景岳全书•杂证谟•脱肛》亦说："有因久泻久痢，脾肾气陷而脱者，有因中气虚寒不能收摄而脱者，有因劳役吐泻伤肝脾而脱者。"虽然虚寒、虚冷均为阳虚，但必须伤损脾气，才可导致脾气下陷。脾不升清，不能维持脏腑位置的恒定，方能引起直肠下垂而脱肛。

脾不升清，气机下陷，脏腑位置下移，可见胃下垂、肝下垂、肾下垂、子宫脱垂等内脏下垂的表现。如《诸病源候论•阴挺出下脱候》说："胞络伤损，子脏虚冷，气下冲则令阴挺出，谓之下脱。亦有因产用力偃气而阴下脱者。"《三因极一病证方论•阴脱证治》也说："妇人趣产，劳力努咽太过，致阴下脱，若脱肛状，及阴下挺出，逼迫肿痛。举重房劳，皆能发作，清水续续，小便淋露。"均阐述劳伤太过，损伤中气，脾不升清，脏器下陷，可引起诸如子宫脱垂之类的内脏下垂证候。

脾主升清，脾气虚弱，清气不升，浊湿下流，清浊交混，下渗肠间，则为腹泄。由于清气下陷，腐化无能，水谷长流，常致久泻不止，完谷不化。如《成方切用•补中养气汤》说："脾虚不能升举，则降多而升少，致清阳下陷则为泻痢 … 泻犹未止，是脾气下陷也。"《金匮翼•飧泄》说："飧泄，完谷不化也。…又清气在下，则生飧泄者，谓阳气虚则下陷。"这里虽然泛谈阳虚，实际主要与脾气不能升清有关。临床上，凡属久泻，或大便次数增多，大都包含脾气下陷的病机。

脾气下陷，精微不能正常输布，下流膀胱，则见小便混浊如米泔。如《景岳全书•杂证谟•淋浊》云："白浊证有浊在溺者，其色白如泔浆…及其久也，则有脾气下陷，土不制湿而水道不清者。"此类小便白浊，多见于小儿，是因饮食不节，脾气易伤，中气易陷，水谷精微下流膀胱所致。

前后二阴的疮疡，可由脾气下陷而致。是因疮疡日久，气血亏耗，脾气易伤，清阳难升，中气下陷，浊湿下注二阴，与未尽余邪胶结难解，病情缠绵难愈，引起外阴痒痛，疮疡溃烂难收。 如《景岳全书•杂证谟•下疳疮》云："下疳…日晡倦怠者，阳气虚而下陷也，补中益气汤。"补中升阳，干旋气机，清阳得升，浊阴外泄，托毒祛

邪，可疗顽疾。总之前后二阴的许多慢性疾病，多与脾气下陷的病
机有着密切的联系。

治宜补中益气，升阳举陷。若以少腹重坠、便意频数为主，用补中
益气汤加山药、五味子、益智仁。若以久泻久利为主，用补中益气
汤去当归加柯子、肉豆蔻、五味子、乌梅肉。若以脱肛、内脏下垂
为主，用补中益气汤加苍术、半夏、砂仁、桔梗、枳壳。若以小便
白浊、外阴疮疡溃烂为主，仍用补中益气汤加茯苓、芡实、山药。

Literature Review of Spleen Qì Fall

📖 *Pí Wèi Lùn* ("On the Spleen and Stomach"), "On Exuberance and Debility of the Spleen and Stomach"

> "When food and drink enter the stomach, they first move into the yáng pathways and cause yáng qì to upbear and float. Floating means that yáng qì scatters and fills the skin and hair. Upbearing means that it fills up the vertex. This makes the nine orifices free and disinhibited. If dietary irregularities have damaged a person's stomach qì so that it is unable to restrain and transform, to dissipate into the liver, to return to the heart, and to spill into the lung, taking in food will then cause clouding and veiling (clouded head and flowery vision) and desire to sleep. When lying down, the food is on one side of the body, and qì is temporarily soothed. This is the sign by which to recognize a movement failure of upbearing and effusing qì."

This quotation describes that when spleen qì upbears the clear and when yáng qì bears upward, the head obtains nourishment. If the spleen fails to upbear the clear and the clear orifices are deprived of nourishment, it causes clouded head and flowery vision.

📖 *Míng Yī Lèi Àn* ("Classified Case Histories of Famous Physicians"), "Case Histories of Wind Strike"

> "Dizziness and heaviness of the head and eyes is due to an inability of spleen qì to upbear."

This quotation expounds the pathomechanism of dizziness caused by failure of qì and blood to rise and nourish because spleen qì is unable to upbear.

📖 *Sù Wèn* ("Plain Questions"), "Chapter on Regulating the Channels"

> "Food and drink taxation fatigue damage the spleen and stomach. Both heat strike and cold strike are caused by spleen and stomach qì vacuity and a resulting inability to move and transform essence. This restrains grain and water, causing them to gather instead of dissipating, and to form distention and fullness."

When the spleen and stomach are vacuous and unable to move and transform the essence of grain and water, distention and fullness arise. This pathomechanism is caused by the inability of spleen qì to upbear the clear and by the inability of stomach qì to downbear the turbid, resulting in qì stagnation in the center burner.

📖 *Zá Bìng Yuán Liú Xī Zhú* ("Incisive Light on the Source of Miscellaneous Disease"), "The Source and Course of Swelling and Distention"

"Glomus fullness is a disease of the spleen. It is rooted in spleen qì vacuity, causing qì depression and inability to move, and glomus blockage and fullness below the heart."

This quotation describes how spleen qì vacuity, failure of clear qì to bear upward, failure of turbid qì to bear downward, and qì stagnation in the center burner results in the pathomechanism of glomus fullness.

📖 *Wēn Yì Lùn* ("On Warm Epidemics"), "On the Reckless Use of Qì-Breaking Medicinals"

"When epidemic toxin qì is passed on to the chest and stomach, it disinhibits the upbearing and downbearing of qì, resulting in distention and fullness. Actually, it is a case of visiting evil affecting root qì. Nevertheless, you only need to eliminate guest qì to make root qì upbear and downbear on its own and to immediately dissipate the distention and fullness."

Root qì refers to spleen and stomach qì. When evil qì damages root qì, the spleen and stomach are depleted, clear qì fails to upbear, and turbid qì fails to downbear. This can result in distention and fullness below the heart.

📖 *Xuē Shì Yī Àn* ("Case Histories of Master Xuē"), "Miscellaneous Works of Illustrious Physicians: Dream Emission and Seminal Efflux"

"Dān-Xī discussed how white turbidity is caused by the downward flow of turbid qì from the center of the stomach, which then percolates into the bladder. He said that no one is aware of this. Xuē notes that the junior steward Wáng Hán-Zhāi treated white turbidity with *bǔ zhōng yì qì tāng* (Center-Supplementing Qì-Boosting Decoction) with the addition of *fú líng* (Poria), *bàn xià* (Pinelliae Rhizoma), and double the amount of *bái zhú* (Atractylodis Macrocephalae Rhizoma)."

White turbidity that results from the downward flow of turbid qì from the center of the stomach to the bladder actually indicates a failure of the spleen to upbear the clear. It is caused by the downpour of the essence of grain and water. The fact that Dr. Xuē used *bǔ zhōng yì qì tāng* (Center-Supplementing Qì-Boosting Decoction) as a treatment with satisfying results provides ample proof that spleen qì fall can cause white turbidity.

📖 *Xuē Shì Yī Àn* ("Case Histories of Master Xuē"), "Miscellaneous Works of Illustrious Physicians: Urinary Incontinence" Xuē notes:

"It is said that failure of the bladder's retentive power causes enuresis and urinary incontinence, with very frequent and unconscious discharge... If urination is very frequent and perhaps exacerbated by taxation, it relates to spleen qì vacuity. Use *bǔ zhōng yì qì tāng* (Center-Supplementing Qì-Boosting Decoction) with the addition of *shān yào* (Dioscoreae Rhizoma) and *wǔ wèi zǐ* (Schisandrae Fructus)."

This quotation points out that frequent urination and urinary incontinence are not always caused by an insecurity of kidney qì, but can also result from spleen qì fall that causes qì to drop into the bladder.

📖 *Yī Zōng Jīn Jiàn* ("Golden Mirror of Medicine"), "Essential Secrets from the Heart in Gynecology: Various Patterns of the Anterior Yīn"

"Women's yīn protrusion can be caused by damage to the uterine network vessels, by excessive use of force during delivery, or by qì vacuity fall... In cases where something similar to a snake, fungus, or cock's comb protrudes from the vagina...when it is related to vacuity, it is invariably accompanied by heaviness, sagging, and clear urine. It should be treated with *bǔ zhōng yì qì tāng* (Center-Supplementing Qì-Boosting Decoction) with the addition of *qīng pí* (Citri Reticulatae Pericarpium Viride) and *zhī zǐ* (Gardeniae Fructus). Topically, apply *shé chuáng zǐ* (Cnidii Fructus) and *wū méi* (Mume Fructus) decocted in water to steam-wash it."

This passage describes how prolapse of the uterus can be caused by taxation-related damage to qì and spleen qì fall. It also discusses using a formula for supplementing the center and upbearing yáng to treat this condition. This in turn proves that spleen vacuity qì fall is an important pathomechanism that can lead to prolapse of the internal organs.

文献评述

《脾胃论•脾胃盛衰论》："饮食入胃，先行阳道，而阳气升浮也。浮者，阳气散满皮毛，升者，充塞头顶，则九窍通利也。若饮食不节，损其胃气，不能克化，散于肝，归于心，溢于肺，食入则昏冒（头昏眼花）欲睡，得卧则食在一边，气暂得舒，是知升发之气不行者此也。"论述脾气升清，阳气上升，可使头部得养。若脾不升清，清窍失养，则为头昏眼花。

《名医类案•中风案》："头目晕重，脾气不能升也。" 阐述脾气不能上升，气血不能上养，而致眩晕的病机。

《素问•调经篇》："因饮食劳倦，损伤脾胃。始受热中，末传寒中，皆由脾胃之气虚弱，不能运化精微，而制水谷聚而不散，而成胀满。"脾胃虚弱，不能运化水谷精微而成胀满，其病机就是因为脾气不能升清，胃气不能降浊，气滞中焦所致。

《杂病源流犀烛•肿胀源流》："痞满，脾病也，本由脾气虚，及气郁不能运行，心下痞塞填满。"论述脾气虚衰，清气不升，浊气不降，气滞中焦，而致痞满的病机。

《温疫论•妄投破气药论》："今疫毒之气，传于胸胃，以致升降之气不利，因而胀满，实为客邪累及本气，但得客气一除，本气自然升降，胀满立消。" 本气即脾胃之气，邪气伤及本气，脾胃亏损，清气不升，浊气不降，可致心下胀满。

《薛氏医案•明医杂著•梦遗滑精》"丹溪论白浊，为胃中浊气下流，渗入膀胱，而云无人知此也。薛按：少宰汪涵斋，白浊，用补中益气汤加茯苓、半夏，倍白术。"胃中浊气下流膀胱而引起白浊，实质上是指脾不升清，水谷精微下注所致，薛氏用补中益气汤治疗收到满意效果，充分论证脾气下陷可引起白浊。

《薛氏医案•明医杂著•小便不禁》："薛按：经云膀胱不约为遗溺，小便不禁，常常出而不觉也。...若小便频数，或劳而益甚，属脾气虚弱，用补中益气汤加山药、五味子。"指出小便频数或失禁，不仅多由肾气不固所致，也可由脾气下陷，气坠膀胱引起。

《医宗金鉴•妇科心法要诀•前阴诸证》："妇人阴挺，或因胞络损伤，或因分娩用力太过，或因气虚下陷...阴中突出一物如蛇，或如菌如鸡冠者...属虚者，必然重坠，小便清，宜补中益气汤加青皮、栀子，外用蛇床子、乌梅熬水薰洗之。"阐述子宫脱垂可因劳伤耗气，脾气下陷所致。并论述用补中升阳的方剂可治疗此疾，反证脾虚气陷是引起内脏下垂的重要病机。

Summary of Spleen Qì Fall

1. Spleen Qì Failing to Upbear

Improper nourishment of the head and eyes: Dizziness and headache.
Improper nourishment of the heart and lung: Shortness of breath and shortage of qì, low voice and laziness to speak, mental fatigue.
Improper nourishment of the ears: Tinnitus and poor hearing.

2. Center Burner Qì Stagnation

Spleen qì glomus blockage: Glomus and fullness below the heart, torpid stomach intake, abdominal distention and fullness that greatly worsens after meals.

Center burner qì depression: Distention even when hungry that is worst around midnight and can be reduced with hiccup and flatus after meals or after pushing with gentle pressure.

3. Qì Dynamic Fall

Qì falling into the lesser abdomen: Lower abdominal distention and fullness, intestinal prolapse, frequent desire to urinate, seminal emission.

Qì falling into the posterior yīn: Heaviness and prolapse of the anus, frequent desire to defecate, prolapse of the rectum.

Conveyance breakdown: Enduring and incessant diarrhea, nontransformation of whole grains.

Downpour of essence: Turbid urine resembling rice water.

Drooping of the internal organs: Sagging of the stomach or liver, floating kidney, or prolapse of the uterus.

Qì fall with downpouring of dampness: Genital sores that are persistent, ulcerating, and difficult to treat, pudendal itching and pain.

脾气下陷
脾气不升——头目失养——眩晕头痛。 心肺失养——气短少气，声低懒言，精神倦怠。
耳窍失养——耳鸣不聪。 中焦气滞——脾气痞塞——心下痞满，胃纳呆滞，腹部胀满，食后尤甚。 中焦气郁——饥时反胀，夜半胀甚，进食或推柔按压后，打呃矢气，胀满可减。 气机下陷——气陷少腹——下腹胀满，坠胀，尿意频数，遗精。
气陷后阴——肛门重坠，便意频数，脱肛。 传导失司——久泻不止，完谷不化。 精微下注——小便混浊如米泔。 内脏下垂——胃下垂，肝下垂，肾下垂，子宫脱垂。 气陷湿注——二阴疮疡，溃烂难收，外阴痒痛。

1.3 Spleen Failing to Control Blood

In its relationship to blood, spleen qì has a securing and containing effect and can thereby prevent and stanch the spillage of blood out of the vessels. "The Forty-Second Difficult Issue" in the *Nàn Jīng* ("Classic of Difficult Issues") explains: "The spleen governs the wrapping of the blood and warms the five viscera." This passage already includes the meaning that the spleen governs the control of blood.

The first instance of the phrase, "the spleen controls blood," is found in a commentary by Xuē Lì-Zhāi on the "Section on Regulating Menstruation; Introduction to Menstruation" of the *Fù Rén Dà Quán Liáng Fāng* ("Compendium of Good Remedies for Women"). Xuē stated: "Regarding the menses, the spleen controls blood and the liver stores blood." He further explained:

> "Blood constitutes the essential qì of grain and water. It harmonizes and regulates the five viscera, and moistens and matures the six bowels; in men, it transforms into semen; in women, it becomes breast milk above and becomes the sea of blood below. Thus, while the heart governs blood and the liver stores blood, it is also controlled by the spleen."

At the same time, Xuē further pointed out that spleen qì vacuity and a resultant failure of qì to control and contain the movement of blood can lead to various bleeding patterns. As he explained in his commentary on the chapter, "Dysentery" in the *Míng Yī Zá Zhù* ("Miscellaneous Works by Famous Physicians"): "When spleen qì is vacuous, it is unable to contain blood and return it to its origin." He also explained:

> "The qì in the spleen channel can be vacuous and therefore unable to contain blood… Generally speaking, blood pathoconditions are enduring and persistent. They are mostly caused by yáng qì vacuity with inability to engender blood, or by yáng qì vacuity with inability to contain blood."

He was thus the first author to propose the pathomechanism of spleen failing to control blood.

Following him, Gōng Tíng-Xián explained in the chapter, "Forgetfulness" in the *Shòu Shì Bǎo Yuán* ("Prolonging Life and Preserving the Origin"): "Thought and preoccupation damage the spleen so that it is unable to contain blood, causing blood to move frenetically."

The spleen's failure to control blood is actually a more advanced development of spleen qì vacuity and prominently reflects a disturbance of the controlling and containing function. When spleen qì fails to upbear, clear qì falls downward, weakening the securing and containing of blood in the lower part of the body. Therefore, the bleeding that results from this pathomechanism manifests mostly in the lower part of the body. It is common to observe symptoms of bleeding from the front and back of the two yīn, like bloody stool, bloody urine, profuse menstruation, or flooding and spotting. When spleen qì is unable to secure and contain, blood leaves the channels and spills into the skin, which can result in spontaneous bleeding of the flesh. If the blood in the upper body is not secured and contained, it can lead to bleeding from the head and face, such as blood ejection, expectoration of blood, and nosebleed.

The chapter, "On the Various Kinds of Bleeding" in the *Gǔ Jīn Míng Yī Huì Cuì* ("Combined Essence of Ancient and Modern Famous Physicians"), explains:

> "There are cases when thoughts are dissatisfying, depression damages the activity of fire, the spleen fails to control blood, and blood exits from the upper orifices. There are cases when one has labored excessively, taxation has damaged center qì, the spleen fails to control blood, and blood exits from the lower orifices."

Because it is due to spleen qì vacuity-related failure of the controlling and containing function and failure of the blood to stay in the channels, these types of bleeding conditions are generally accompanied by pronounced symptoms of qì vacuity like shortage of qì and lack of strength or fatigued spirit. The disease progressions are entangled and can relapse, with the bleeding starting and stopping over and over, mostly belonging to the category of chronic bleeding. Generally, the amount of blood lost is small, the color is pale white or dark purple, and the quality is clear and thin. Moreover, the spleen's failure to control blood is mostly caused by qì vacuity, but can also result from yáng vacuity causing failure to warm and contain.

As explained in the chapter, "Center Vacuity Blood Desertion" in the *Jīn Guì Yì* ("Wings of the Golden Coffer"):

> "The center consists of the spleen and stomach. The spleen controls blood. When it is vacuous, it is unable to contain blood. The spleen transforms blood. Spleen vacuity therefore causes an inability to move and transform. All these conditions are caused by the fact that the blood is ungoverned, causing desertion, falling, and frenetic movement. The color of the blood in these conditions is not very bright red, but either purple or black. This is caused by the vanquishing of yáng and manifests therefore mostly as patterns without heat, perhaps with nausea and vomiting. It should be treated with lǐ zhōng tāng (Center-Rectifying Decoction) to warm and supplement the spleen and stomach. When center qì has been rectified, the blood will return to the channels on its own."

The *Xuè Zhèng Lùn* ("On Blood Patterns") chapter, "Organ Pathomechanisms," also explains:

> "It is said that the spleen controls blood. The blood's upward and downward movement completely depends on the spleen. When spleen yáng is vacuous, it is unable to control the blood."

The two pathomechanisms of spleen yáng and spleen qì are not identical. However, because spleen yáng vacuity is an advanced development of spleen qì vacuity, spleen yáng vacuity with inability to control blood is in reality still a reflection of the pathomechanism of spleen qì vacuity and loss of the blood-controlling function.

This condition is treated by fortifying the spleen and supplementing the center, and by boosting qì and containing blood. The recommended formula is *guī pí tāng* (Spleen-Returning Decoction) from the *Chóng Dìng Yán Shì Jì Shēng Fāng* ("Revised Life-Saving Formulas of Master Yán").

Guī Pí Tāng 归脾汤 Spleen-Returning Decoction
huáng qí (黄耆 astragalus, Astragali Radix)
rén shēn (人参 ginseng, Ginseng Radix)
bái zhú (白术 white atractylodes, Atractylodis Macrocephalae Rhizoma)
fú líng (茯苓 poria, Poria)
dāng guī (当归 Chinese angelica, Angelicae Sinensis Radix)
lóng yǎn ròu (龙眼肉 longan flesh, Longan Arillus)
suān zǎo rén (酸枣仁 spiny jujube, Ziziphi Spinosi Semen)
yuǎn zhì (远志 polygala, Polygalae Radix)
mù xiāng (木香 costusroot, Aucklandiae Radix)
gān cǎo (甘草 licorice, Glycyrrhizae Radix)

For conditions that are mainly characterized by bloody stool and bloody urine, add *ē jiāo* (Asini Corii Colla), *dì yú* (Sanguisorbae Radix), and *mò hàn lián* (Ecliptae Herba).

For conditions that are mainly characterized by profuse menstruation and flooding and spotting blood precipitation, add *yì mǔ cǎo* (Leonuri Herba), *xù duàn* (Dipsaci Radix), and *wū méi* (Mume Fructus).

For conditions that are mainly characterized by spontaneous bleeding of the flesh, add *xiān hè cǎo* (Agrimoniae Herba), *pú huáng* (Typhae Pollen), *qiàn cǎo* (Rubiae Radix), and *zōng lǘ tàn* (Trachycarpi Petiolus Carbonisatus).

For conditions that are mainly characterized by blood ejection and nosebleed, add *cè bǎi yè* (Platycladi Cacumen), *ài yè* (Artemisiae Argyi Folium), *sān qī* (Notoginseng Radix), *bái jí* (Bletillae Rhizoma), and *hǎi piāo xiāo* (Sepiae Endoconcha).

脾不统血

脾气对血有固摄作用，可防止血液溢出脉外。《难经•四十二难》说："脾主裹血，温五脏。"其中已包含有脾主统血的意思。薛立斋在注解《妇人大全良方•调经门•月经序论》中首先提出"脾统血"的名称。他说："愚按经云脾统血，肝藏血。"又说："血者水谷之精气也，和调五脏，洒陈六腑，在男子则化为精，在妇人上为乳汁，下为血海。故虽心主血，肝藏血，亦皆统于脾。"同时薛氏还指出，脾气虚弱，气不能统摄血液运行可导致诸种出血病证。如在薛注《明医杂著•痢疾》中说："脾气虚弱，不能摄血归源。"又说："脾经气虚不能统血。""大凡血症久而不愈，多因阳气虚弱而不能生血，或因阳气虚而不能摄血。"首次提出了脾不统血的病机。其后龚廷贤在《寿世保元•健忘》中也说："思虑伤脾，不能摄血，致血妄行。"脾不统血实际上是脾气虚弱的进一步发展，突出地表现为统摄功能障碍。脾气不升，清气下陷，对下部血液固摄减弱，故本病机引起出血多见于人体的下部。常见便血、尿血、月经过多、或崩漏下血等前后二阴的出血症状。脾气不能固摄，血离经脉，泛溢于肌肤，亦可引起肌衄；如果对上部血液失于固摄，也可引起吐血、咯血、鼻衄等头面部出血症状。如《古今名医汇粹•诸血论》说："有思虑不遂，郁伤火动，脾不统血，而从上窍出者；有劳役过度，劳伤中气，脾不统血而从下窍也者。"由于是脾气虚弱，统摄无权，血不归经所致，故此类出血一般伴有明显的少气乏力，神疲倦怠等气虚症状。病程缠绵，反复发作，出出停停，多属于慢性失血范畴。一般出血量不多，颜色淡白或紫暗，血质清稀。此外，脾不统血多因气虚引起，也可由阳虚失于温煦和固摄所致。如《金匮翼•中虚脱血》说："中者，脾胃也。脾统血，脾虚不能摄血。脾化血，脾虚则不能运化。是皆血无所主，因而脱陷妄行。其血色不甚鲜红，或紫或黑，此阳败而然，故多无热证，而或见恶心呕吐，宜理中汤温补脾胃，中气得理，血自归经矣。"《血证论•脏腑病机》又说："经云：脾统血，血之运行上下，全赖于脾，脾阳虚则不能统血。"脾阳、脾气，二者病机不同，但因脾阳虚是脾气虚的进一步发展，故脾阳虚不能统血，实际上仍是脾气虚，统血无权病机的体现。

治宜健脾补中，益气摄血。方选《济生方》归脾汤（黄芪、人参、白术、茯苓、当归、龙眼肉、酸枣仁、远志、木香、甘草）。以便血、尿血为主，加阿胶、地榆、旱莲草；以月经过多、崩漏下血为主，加益母草、续断、乌梅；以肌衄为主，加仙鹤草、炒蒲黄、茜草根、棕榈炭；以吐血、鼻衄为主，加侧柏叶、艾叶、三七粉、白及、乌贼骨。

Literature Review of Spleen Failing to Control Blood

📖 *Jǐng Yuè Quán Shū* ("Jǐng-Yuè's Complete Compendium"), "Schema of Miscellaneous Patterns: Vacuity Detriment"

"Frequent tendency to vomiting and diarrhea due to taxation fatigue often manifests as blood ejection and bloody stool because of the spleen's failure to contain blood. They should be treated with *liù wèi huí yáng yǐn* (Six-Ingredient Yáng-Returning Beverage) with the addition of a large portion of *bái zhú* (Atractylodis Macrocephalae Rhizoma). Under no circumstances should one use cooling medicinals."

"In cases of bloody stool due to spleen and stomach qì vacuity, its color will not be very bright red, but either purple or black. This is caused by the vanquishing of yáng and manifests therefore mostly as patterns without heat, and as nausea and vomiting. The spleen should be able to control blood. When spleen qì is vacuous, blood cannot move and transform. All of these conditions are caused by the fact that the blood is ungoverned, causing desertion, fall, and frenetic movement."

This quotation discusses how spleen qì vacuity and inability to control and contain causes blood desertion and frenetic movement, which can lead to blood ejection, bloody stool, and other patterns of bleeding. It also describes in detail the special characteristic of blood loss that is caused by the spleen's failure to control blood.

📖 *Bù Jū Jí* ("Non-limitation Collection"), "Main Points of Blood Patterns"

"When excessive anxiety and thought injure the heart and spleen to the point that this results in blood ejection and expectoration of blood, the condition is generally not a fire pathocondition. It is common to observe shortness of breath, qì timidity, and a withered complexion, potentially with binding depression in the chest with inability to taste food, or no desire for food and drink in spite of the fact that the stomach is hungry, or fright and encumbrance of the spirit and ethereal soul with disquieted sleep. These are the result of center qì depletion and inability to contain."

This quotation points out that damage to the spleen from thought and preoccupation causes center qì depletion and inability to contain blood, which can result in all types of combined bleeding and qì vacuity manifestations.

文献评述

《景岳全书•杂证谟•虚损》：”若因劳倦而素易呕泻，多有脾不摄血，而为吐血下血者，宜用六味回阳饮大加白术主之，万不可用凉药。”又说：”脾胃气虚而大便下血者，其色不甚鲜红，或紫色、或黑色，此败阳而然，故多无热证，而见恶心呕吐。盖脾能统血，脾气虚则血不能运化，是皆血无所主，而脱陷妄行。"不仅论述脾气虚不能统摄，血脱妄行，可引起吐血、便血等出血之证，而且还详细描述脾不统血所致失血的特征。

《不居集·血证扼要》："忧思过度，损伤心脾，此致吐血、咯血者，其病多非火症。或常见气短、气怯、形色憔悴、或胸怀郁结，饮食无味，或腹虽作饥而不欲饮食，或神魂惊困而卧不安，是皆中气亏损，不能收摄所致。"指出思虑伤脾，中气亏损，不能摄血，可致各种出血兼气虚的表现。

Summary of Spleen Failing to Control Blood
1. Failure to Contain the Lower Body Bloody stool, bloody urine, profuse menstruation or flooding and spotting blood precipitation.
2. Flooding into the Skin Spontaneous bleeding of the flesh.
3. Failure to Contain the Upper Body Blood ejection, expectoration of blood, nosebleed.
脾不统血
不摄于下——便血，尿血，月经过多，或崩漏下血。
泛于肌肤——肌衄。
不摄于上——吐血，咯血，鼻衄。

1.4 Spleen Qì Failing to Provide Luxuriance

The spleen governs movement and transformation, absorbs the essence of grain and water, forms the fluids of qì and blood, and nourishes and moistens the whole body. Therefore it is said that the spleen and stomach are the root of later heaven (acquired constitution) and the source of blood and qì formation. When spleen qì vacuity results in nontransformation of essence and in nonformation of qì and blood, this can lead to pathomechanisms of improper nourishment in the whole body. When spleen qì fails to provide luxuriance, one can differentiate between improper nourishment of the body and improper nourishment of the offices and orifices.

脾气不荣

脾主运化，吸收水谷精微，化生气血津液，营养滋润全身，故有脾胃为后天为本，气血生化之源之说。脾气虚弱，精微不化，气血不生，则会引起全身失养的病机。脾气不荣有形体、官窍失养之别。

1.4.1 Improper Nourishment of the Body

The spleen governs movement and transformation, absorbs the essence of grain and water, and can form qì and blood, thereby filling out the flesh and nourishing the whole body. When spleen qì is vacuous, it is unable to form qì and blood and to nourish the flesh. As the flesh is nourished improperly, its function is reduced. Therefore, one observes symptoms such as emaciation, atrophy of the flesh, and in severe cases, limp wilting and loss of use. The "Treatise on Abnormal Spleen Pulse" in the *Qiān Jīn Yào Fāng* ("A Thousand Gold Pieces Prescriptions") explains that spleen qì vacuity "causes emaciation of the whole body." Moreover, the chapter on "Spleen and Stomach Qì Vacuity and Marked Emaciation of the Flesh and Body" in the *Shèng Jì Zǒng Lù* ("Sages' Salvation Records") explains:

> "If the spleen and stomach are vacuous and unable to move and transform grain and water, qì and blood are consumed and unable to irrigate the body. Therefore, the flesh is not bountiful and is markedly emaciated."

This explains that emaciation of the flesh, atrophy, limpness, and loss of use are also closely related to the pathomechanism of spleen vacuity with improper nourishment.

The spleen governs the four limbs. When the spleen fails to upbear the clear and clear yáng is unable to dissipate into the limbs, their function is reduced. As a result, you can observe symptoms like limpness of the limbs and body, inability to raise the limbs, paralysis and insensitivity, a forceless walk, and numbness in the fingers. The "Treatise on Greater Yīn and Yáng Brightness" in the *Sù Wèn* ("Plain Questions") points out:

> "Why is it that spleen disease causes the limbs to lose their function?
>
> Qí Bó said: 'The limbs are all endowed with qì by the stomach, but [stomach qì] is unable to reach to the end of the channels [on its own]. It is only because of the spleen that [the limbs] can receive their endowment. When the spleen is diseased and is unable to move the fluids for the stomach, the limbs fail to receive their endowment of grain and water qì. Their qì is debilitated day by day, the path of the vessels is inhibited, the sinews and bones, muscles and flesh all lack the foundation from which they are formed, and therefore they lose their function."

The "Treatise on Abnormal Spleen Pulse" in the *Qiān Jīn Yào Fāng* ("A Thousand Gold Pieces Prescriptions") also explains:

> "When spleen qi is vacuous, the limbs lose their function... In the case of vacuity...the limbs cannot be raised and the body is heavy like a mountain."

The "Treatise on the Prevalence and Debilitation of the Spleen and Stomach" in the *Pí Wèi Lùn* ("On the Spleen and Stomach") advances this further:

> "Dual vacuity of spleen and stomach leads to inability to eat and emaciation or to low food intake with fatness, and to inability to raise the limbs in spite of being fat."

These quotations provide abundant arguments that spleen qi failing to upbear the clear for the stomach, inability to distribute the essence of grain and water to the four directions, and improper nourishment of the limbs is an important pathomechanism leading to limpness and numbness of the limbs.

When spleen qì is vacuous, it is unable to form the fluids of qì and blood and to nourish and moisten the skin. Thus, the liquids are reduced and fail to enrich, and blood is depleted and loses luxuriance. This results in symptoms like dry skin, scaling, elastic flaking, desiccated hair, and in extreme cases encrusted skin. The "Treatise on the Natural Life-Span" in the *Líng Shū* ("Magic Pivot") explains: "At the age of seventy, spleen qì is vacuous and the skin desiccated." The "Treatise on Disease and Non-Reception of Qì in the Organs and Channels in Stomach Vacuity" in the *Pí Wèi Lùn* ("On the Spleen and Stomach") states:

> "When the stomach is vacuous, [the rest of the body] fails to receive qì and therefore becomes vacuous also. The fluids fail to moisten, the mouth and throat feel dry during sleep, and the skin and hair are lusterless."

This further indicates how the spleen's failure to move fluids for the stomach, resulting in a reduction of liquids and failure to moisten, causes desiccation of the skin and hair.

Improper nourishment of the body is treated by supplementing the spleen and boosting qì, and by fortifying movement and upbearing the clear. Conditions that are mainly characterized by emaciation and withered skin, and limpness and numbness of the limbs, are treated with *tiáo zhōng yì qì tāng* (Center-Regulating Qì-Boosting Decoction) from the *Pí Wèi Lùn* ("On the Spleen and Stomach").

Tiáo Zhōng Yì Qì Tāng 调中益气汤
Center-Regulating Qì-Boosting Decoction

huáng qí (黄耆 astragalus, Astragali Radix)

rén shēn (人参 ginseng, Ginseng Radix)

cāng zhú (苍朮 atractylodes, Atractylodis Rhizoma)

chái hú (柴胡 bupleurum, Bupleuri Radix)

shēng má (升麻 cimicifuga, Cimicifugae Rhizoma)

chén pí (陈皮 tangerine peel, Citri Reticulatae Pericarpium)

mù xiāng (木香 costusroot, Aucklandiae Radix)

gān cǎo (甘草 licorice, Glycyrrhizae Radix)

Plus:

jī xuè téng (鸡血藤 spatholobus, Spatholobi Caulis)

Conditions that are mainly characterized by dry, scaling, and encrusted skin are treated with *bǔ zhōng yì qì tāng* (Center-Supplementing Qì-Boosting Decoction) with the addition of *shēng dì huáng* (Rehmanniae Radix Exsiccata), *hé shǒu wū* (Polygoni Multiflori Radix), *táo rén* (Persicae Semen), *tiān dōng* (Asparagi Radix), and *mài dōng* (Ophiopogonis Radix).

Bǔ Zhōng Yì Qì Tāng 补中益气汤
Center-Supplementing Qì-Boosting Decoction [modified]

huáng qí (黄耆 astragalus, Astragali Radix)

rén shēn (人参 ginseng, Ginseng Radix)

bái zhú (白朮 white atractylodes, Atractylodis Macrocephalae Rhizoma)

chái hú (柴胡 bupleurum, Bupleuri Radix)

chén pí (陈皮 tangerine peel, Citri Reticulatae Pericarpium)

shēng má (升麻 cimicifuga, Cimicifugae Rhizoma)

dāng guī (当归 Chinese angelica, Angelicae Sinensis Radix)

zhì gān cǎo (炙甘草 mix-fried licorice, Glycyrrhizae Radix cum
    Liquido Fricta)

Plus:

shēng dì huáng (生地黄 dried/fresh rehmannia, Rehmanniae Radix
    Exsiccata seu Recens)

hé shǒu wū (何首乌 flowery knotweed, Polygoni Multiflori Radix)

táo rén (桃仁 peach kernel, Persicae Semen)

tiān mén dōng (天门冬 asparagus, Asparagi Radix)

mài mén dōng (麦门冬 ophiopogon, Ophiopogonis Radix)

形体失养

脾主运化，吸收水谷精微，能化生气血，以充养肌肉，营养全身。脾气虚弱，不能化生气血，营养肌肉，肌肉失养，及功能衰退，则见形体消瘦、肌肉萎缩、甚则痿弱不用等症状。如《千金要方•脾脏病脉论》说：脾气"虚则举体消瘦。"又如《圣济总录•脾胃气虚肌体羸瘦》说："若脾胃虚弱，不能运化水谷，则气血减耗，无以灌溉形体，故肌肉不丰而羸瘦也。"说明肌肉消瘦、萎缩及痿软不用亦与脾虚失养的病机有密切关系。

脾主四肢，脾不升清，清阳不能散布四肢，四肢功能减退，可见肢体软弱、四肢不举、麻痹不仁、行走无力、十指麻木等症状。正如《素问•太阴阳明论》指出："脾病而四肢不用，何也？岐伯曰：四肢皆禀气于胃，而不得至经，必因于脾，乃得禀也。今脾病不能为胃行其津液，四肢不得禀水谷气，气日以衰，脉道不利，筋骨肌肉皆无以生，故不用焉。"又如《千金要方•脾脏病脉论》说："脾气虚，则四肢不用。"又说："虚则…四肢不举，身重如山。"《脾胃论•脾胃胜衰论》还进一步指出："脾胃俱虚，则不能食而瘦；或食少而肥，虽肥而四肢不举。" 充分论证脾气不能为胃升清，水谷精微不能四布，四肢失养是引起肢软肢麻的重要病机。

脾气虚弱，不能化生气血津液，营养滋润皮肤，津少失滋，血亏失荣，则见皮肤干燥、脱屑、弹性下降、毛发枯槁、甚至肌肤甲错等症状。正如《灵枢•天年论》所说："七十岁，脾气虚，皮肤枯。"《脾胃论•胃虚脏腑经络皆无所受气而俱病论》云："胃虚则无所受气而亦虚，津液不濡，睡觉口燥咽干而皮毛不泽也。"进一步指出脾不为胃行其津液，津少失濡，则皮肤、毛发枯燥。

治宜补脾益气，健运升清。以消瘦肌萎，肢软肢麻为主，用《脾胃论》调中益气汤（黄芪、人参、苍术、柴胡、升麻、橘皮、木香、甘草）加鸡血藤。以皮肤干燥、脱屑、肌肤甲错为主者，仍选补中益气汤加生地、首乌、桃仁、天冬、麦冬。

1.4.2 Improper Nourishment of the Offices and Orifices

The "Great Treatise on the Correspondences and Manifestations of Yīn and Yáng" in the *Sù Wèn* ("Plain Questions") points out: "Grain qì flows into the spleen… The six channels are streams, the intestines and stomach are seas, and the nine orifices are qì that flows like water." This quotation explains that the nine orifices and the spleen and stomach are closely related in terms of their physiological functions. The reason for this is that the nine orifices are governed by the five viscera and that the grain and water essence of the five viscera originate in the spleen and stomach. When spleen qì vacuity prevents the essence of grain and water from forming the essential qì of the five viscera and from supplying the nine orifices, the offices [sensory organs] and orifices are nourished improperly, causing pathological changes.

"The Jade Swivel Treatise on True Viscera Pulses" in the *Sù Wèn* ("Plain Questions") contains the following statement: "When the spleen fails to reach, this causes stoppage in a person's nine orifices." The "General Treatise on Vacuity and Repletion" of the same text states even more clearly: "Headache, tinnitus, and inhibition of the nine orifices arises from the intestines and stomach."

Formed by the spleen and stomach, qì and blood dissipate essence into the liver and flow through the channels to provide luxuriance to the eyes. When the eyes receive nourishment, they are bright. If spleen qì is vacuous and qì and blood are unable to rise and nourish the eyes, one can observe symptoms like dizziness and flowery vision, fatigued eyesight, blurred vision, drooping eyelids, food intake without taste, sloppy stool, pale tongue, and a moderate, weak, and forceless pulse.

The "Section on the Seven Orifices; Comprehensive Treatise on Eye Disorders" in the *Zhāng Shì Yī Tōng* ("Zhang's Clear View of Medicine") states:

> "The essential qì of the five viscera and six bowels is all endowed by spleen-earth and from there rises to pass into the eyes, which are the gathering place of blood. Therefore, spleen vacuity means that the essential qì of the five viscera loses its charge and is unable to return to the eyes."

Lǐ Dōng-Yuán states in the chapter on "Eye Disease" in the *Yī Xué Zhèng Zhuàn* ("Orthodox Tradition of Medicine"):

> "For this reason, the blood and qì of the five viscera, six bowels, twelve channels, and 365 network vessels is all received from spleen-earth and rise up to pass into the eyes, making them bright… Vexing situations, dietary irregularities, or excessive labor make the spleen and stomach vacuous… The spleen is the head of all yīn and the eyes are the gathering place of the blood vessels. Therefore, spleen vacuity causes a breakdown of the essential qì of the five viscera so that they are unable to return and brighten the eyes."

These quotations point out that the manifold pathomechanisms of eye diseases are often related to spleen vacuity and essential qì insufficiency, failure of clear yáng to upbear, and improper nourishment of the eyes.

The ears are the orifices of the kidney and are in charge of hearing. Thus, the *Nèi Jīng* ("Inner Canon") states, "Kidney qì flows to the ears. When the kidney is harmonious, one is able to hear the five notes." The kidney is the root of earlier heaven, but in reality depends on the nourishment of later heaven by the spleen and stomach. If the spleen and stomach are vacuous, qì and blood lack the source of their formation. Alternatively, when spleen qì is vacuous, kidney essence will invariably become depleted and the ear orifices undernourished, which can lead to tinnitus and deafness.

"Inquiry about Statements" in the *Líng Shū* ("Magic Pivot") states:

"What causes qì to make a person's ears ring? The ears are the gathering place of the ancestral vessels. Therefore, when the stomach is empty, the ancestral vessels are vacuous, which in turn causes them to flow downward. Since a part of the vessels is exhausted, this causes tinnitus."

The stomach governs intake and absorption, ripening and rotting, and normal downbearing. Stomach qì does not by itself possess the ability to transport the essence of grain and water upward. Therefore, a vacuity of the ancestral vessels is actually a failure of the spleen to upbear the clear. When it is unable to transport the fluids upward from the stomach, the ear orifices are nourished improperly, resulting in tinnitus.

The "Section on Ear Patterns" in the *Gǔ Jīn Yī Tǒng Dà Quán* ("Complete Compendium of Medical Works, Ancient and Modern") discusses the use of *yì qì cōng míng tāng* (Qì-Boosting Sharp and Bright Decoction) as primary treatment for deafness due to taxation and overwork. It explains:

"Dietary irregularities or physical taxation and overwork lead to an insufficiency of the spleen and stomach. This makes a person susceptible to suffering from internal obstruction and deafness. Taking this [medicine] will more than double a person's mental strength, boost original qì naturally, lighten and fortify the body, and brighten the ears and eyes."

This passage points out that spleen and stomach vacuity and improper nourishment of qì and blood can lead to impaired hearing and in severe cases, deafness.

The lung opens at the nose, and the lung channel is connected to the stomach and intestines channels. The foot yáng brightness stomach vessel begins at the nose, and the channels of the spleen and stomach are therefore also linked to the nose orifice. Moreover, spleen-earth nourishes lung-metal and the spleen and stomach carry out movement and transformation. This makes lung qì abundant and frees and disinhibits the nose. If spleen vacuity prevents clear qì from rising and penetrating to the nose, this results in nasal congestion, runny nose with clear snivel, and loss of the sense of smell.

The "Section on the Seven Orifices; Nose" in the *Zhāng Shì Yī Tōng* ("Zhang's Clear View of Medicine") explains:

"It is said that ancestral qì runs into the nose to form the sense of smell. Now, ancestral qì is the qì that is formed inside the stomach. If hunger or satiety or overwork have damaged a person's spleen and stomach, construction and movement qì is unable to bear up and evil blocks the holes and orifices. Thus the nose is inhibited and unable to detect fetor or fragrance."

Commenting on the chapter on "Nasal Congestion" in the *Míng Yī Zá Zhù* ("Miscellaneous Works by Famous Physicians"), Xuē Jǐ explained:

"Regarding the former pathocondition, if damage from hunger, satiety, or overwork prevents the qì that is formed in the spleen and stomach from rising up and allows evil to harm the empty orifices, the result is inhibition and inability to detect fragrance or fetor. You should nourish the spleen and stomach to cause yáng qì to upbear and penetrate to the nose."

The ancients not only described in detail the relationship between inhibited nasal orifices and the spleen and stomach, but also stressed the importance of supplementing and nourishing spleen qì for treating nasal diseases. This contributed enormously to the pathomechanism and methods for treating nose conditions.

The mouth is the orifice of the spleen, as is reflected in the expression from the *Líng Shū* ("Magic Pivot"), "Outward Manifestations and Diseases Caused by the Five Viscera": "The mouth and lips are the office of the spleen." "Treatise on the Engenderment of the Five Viscera" in the *Sù Wèn* ("Plain Questions") also states: "The spleen... its luxuriance is in the tongue." This quotation indicates that the spleen and mouth are closely linked in terms of physiology. When spleen qì is vacuous and unable to rise and provide luxuriance, the mouth and tongue are improperly nourished. This can lead to such symptoms as bland taste in the mouth, erosion of the oral cavity, drooling from the corners of the mouth, and a limp tongue. As stated in the chapter, "Channels" in the *Líng Shū* ("Magic Pivot"):

"Foot greater yīn qì expiry results in a failure of the vessels to provide luxuriance to the flesh. Failure of the vessels to provide luxuriance causes limpness of the flesh. Limpness of the flesh causes a limp tongue."

This quotation points out that spleen qì vacuity and inability to rise and nourish the tongue body can result in a limp tongue.

The chapter, "Phlegm-drool" in the *Yòu Kē Shì Mí* ("Explanation of Pediatric Mysteries") explains:

"Profuse drooling in young children also arises because spleen qì is insufficient and unable to distribute fluids to the four directions. If you fail to treat the root by supplementing and boosting center qì before you dispel phlegm-drool, you will be forced to eliminate it incessantly and the disease will eventually turn into vacuity desertion, because phlegm-drool, while being the pathogenic fluid, is also attached to original qì."

This passage not only indicates clearly that spleen qì vacuity and inability to receive and contain can lead to drooling from the corners of the mouth in young children, but it also emphasizes the need to employ methods for supplementing the center and fortifying the spleen to advance the treatment.

The chapter, "On the Source and Course of Mouth, Tongue, Lip, and Teeth Diseases" in the *Zá Bìng Yuán Liú Xī Zhú* ("Incisive Light on the Source of Miscellaneous Disease"), explains:

"Oral putrescence is caused by eroding mouth sores… When center burner qì is insufficient, vacuity fire rises up to flood into the mouth, causing putrescence."

This passage indicates that while oral putrescence is in the majority of cases caused by repletion fire, it can also be due to vacuity of spleen qì, unable to rise and nourish, causing vacuity yáng to harass the upper body so that the tongue ulcerates and forms sores. For oral cavity diseases that are enduring and incessant with recurring ulcerations, it recommends the treatment principle of supplementing the center and fortifying the spleen.

Improper nourishment of the offices and orifices is treated by supplementing the center and fortifying the spleen, and by upbearing yáng and boosting qì. For dizziness and flowery vision, fatigued eyesight, blurred vision, and drooping eyelids, the recommended formula is *bǔ zhōng yì qì tāng* (Center-Supplementing Qì-Boosting Decoction) from the *Pí Wèi Lùn* ("On the Spleen and Stomach").

Bǔ Zhōng Yì Qì Tāng 补中益气汤
Center-Supplementing Qì-Boosting Decoction

huáng qí (黄耆 astragalus, Astragali Radix)

rén shēn (人参 ginseng, Ginseng Radix)

bái zhú (白术 white atractylodes, Atractylodis Macrocephalae Rhizoma)

chái hú (柴胡 bupleurum, Bupleuri Radix)

chén pí (陈皮 tangerine peel, Citri Reticulatae Pericarpium)

shēng má (升麻 cimicifuga, Cimicifugae Rhizoma)

dāng guī (当归 Chinese angelica, Angelicae Sinensis Radix)

zhì gān cǎo (炙甘草 mix-fried licorice, Glycyrrhizae Radix cum Liquido Fricta)

For tinnitus and deafness, it is *bǔ zhōng yì qì tāng* (Center-Supplementing Qì-Boosting Decoction) with a heavy emphasis on *rén shēn* (Ginseng Radix) and *huáng qí* (Astragali Radix). An alternative is *yì qì cōng míng tāng* (Qì-Boosting Sharp and Bright Decoction) from the *Gǔ Jīn Yī Tǒng Dà Quán* ("Complete Compendium of Medical Works, Ancient and Modern").

Yì Qì Cōng Míng Tāng 益气聪明汤
Qì-Boosting Sharp and Bright Decoction

rén shēn (人参 ginseng, Ginseng Radix)
huáng qí (黄耆 astragalus, Astragali Radix)
gé gēn (葛根 pueraria, Puerariae Radix)
shēng má (升麻 cimicifuga, Cimicifugae Rhizoma)
màn jīng zǐ (蔓荆子 vitex, Viticis Fructus)
bái sháo yào (白芍药 white peony, Paeoniae Radix Alba)
huáng bǎi (黄柏 phellodendron, Phellodendri Cortex)
gān cǎo (甘草 licorice, Glycyrrhizae Radix)

For nasal congestion and runny nose, *sì jūn zǐ tāng* (Four Gentlemen Decoction) is used with the addition of *chái hú* (Bupleuri Radix), *shēng má* (Cimicifugae Rhizoma), *xīn yí* (Magnoliae Flos), and *cāng ěr zǐ* (Xanthii Fructus).

Sì Jūn Zǐ Tāng 四君子汤
Four Gentlemen Decoction

rén shēn (人参 ginseng, Ginseng Radix)
fú líng (茯苓 poria, Poria)
bái zhú (白术 white atractylodes, Atractylodis Macrocephalae Rhizoma)
zhì gān cǎo (炙甘草 mix-fried licorice, Glycyrrhizae Radix cum
    Liquido Fricta)
Plus:
chái hú (柴胡 bupleurum, Bupleuri Radix)
shēng má (升麻 cimicifuga, Cimicifugae Rhizoma)
xīn yí (辛夷 magnolia flower, Magnoliae Flos)
cāng ěr zǐ (苍耳子 xanthium, Xanthii Fructus)

For a bland taste in the mouth, *shēn líng bái zhú sǎn* (Ginseng, Poria, and White Atractylodes Powder) or *xiāng shā liù jūn zǐ tāng* (Costusroot and Amomum Six Gentlemen Decoction) are used (these formulas are referenced in previous sections).

For a limp tongue and drooling from the corners of the mouth, *bǔ zhōng yì qì tāng* (Center-Supplementing Qì-Boosting Decoction) with the addition of *fú líng* (Poria) and *zé xiè* (Alismatis Rhizoma) is used.

For oral putrescence, *bǔ zhōng yì qì tāng* (Center-Supplementing Qì-Boosting Decoction) or *huáng qí jiàn zhōng tāng* (Astragalus Center-Fortifying Decoction) can be used.

Huáng Qí Jiàn Zhōng Tāng 黄芪建中汤 Astragalus Center-Fortifying Decoction
huáng qí (黄芪 astragalus, Astragali Radix) *guì zhī* (桂枝 cinnamon twig, Cinnamomi Ramulus) *bái sháo yào* (白芍药 white peony, Paeoniae Radix Alba) *shēng jiāng* (生姜 fresh ginger, Zingiberis Rhizoma Recens) *dà zǎo* (大枣 jujube, Jujubae Fructus) *zhì gān cǎo* (炙甘草 mix-fried licorice, Glycyrrhizae Radix cum   Liquido Fricta) *yí táng* (饴糖 malt sugar, Maltosum)

官窍失养

《素问•阴阳应象大论》指出："谷气通于脾…六经为川，肠胃为海，九窍为水注之气。"说明九窍与脾胃在生理功能上有密切的关系。这是因为九窍为五脏所主，五脏的水谷精微源于脾胃，脾气虚弱，水谷精微不能化生五脏之精气而供养九窍，官窍失养，则会发生病变。如《素问•玉机真藏论》有脾"其不及，则令人九窍不通"的论述。《素问•通评虚实论》更明确指出："头痛耳鸣，九窍不利，是肠胃所生也。"

脾胃所化生的气血，散精于肝，通过经脉上荣于目，目得其养则明矣。若脾气虚弱，气血不能上养于目，可见引起头昏眼花、视力疲劳、视力模糊、眼睑下垂、纳食乏味，便溏，舌淡，脉缓弱无力等症状。如《张氏医通•七窍门•目疾统论》："夫五脏六腑之精气，皆禀受于脾土，而上贯于目，目者血之宗也。故脾虚则五脏之精气皆失所司，不能归于目。"《医学正传•目病》"东垣曰：是以五脏、六腑、十二经脉、三百六十五络，其血气皆受于脾土，而上贯于目而为之明。…因事烦扰，饮食失节，劳役过度，致脾胃虚弱。…夫脾者诸阴之首，目者血脉之宗也，故脾虚则五脏之精气皆失所司，不能归明于目矣。"指出眼部多种疾病的病机多与脾虚精气不足，清阳不升，目失所养有关。

耳为肾之窍，司听觉，故《内经》曰："肾气通于耳，肾和则能闻五音矣。"肾为先天之本，实有赖后天脾胃的涵养，若脾胃虚弱，气血生化乏源，或脾气虚，清阳不升，肾精必亏，耳窍失养，可致耳鸣耳聋。如《灵枢•口问篇》云："人之耳鸣者，何气使然？耳者，宗脉之所聚也，故胃中空虚则宗脉虚，虚则下溜，脉有所竭者，故耳鸣。"胃主受纳、腐熟，以下降为顺，胃气本身不具备上输水谷精微的功能，所以宗脉虚，实际上是脾不升清，不能为胃上输津微，耳窍失养，从而引起耳鸣。《古今医统大全•耳证门》论述劳役耳聋，用益气聪明汤主治时说："饮食不节，劳役形体，脾胃不足，得受内障耳聋之患。服此令人精神过倍，元气自益，轻身健体，耳目聪明。"指出脾胃虚弱，气血失养，可致听力下降，甚至耳聋。

肺开窍于鼻，肺之经脉与胃肠之经脉相通，足阳明胃经的经脉起于鼻，故脾胃之经脉亦与鼻窍相连。又脾土养肺金，脾胃健运，则肺气充沛，鼻窍通利。若脾虚弱，清气不能上通鼻窍，则鼻塞不通，鼻流清涕、嗅觉失灵。如《张氏医通•七窍门•鼻》说："经云：其宗气走于鼻而为臭，夫宗气者，胃中生发之气也，若因饥饱劳役，损其脾胃，则营运之气不能上升，邪塞孔窍，故鼻不利而不闻香臭也。"薛己对《明医杂著•鼻塞》作补注时说："前症若因饥饱劳役所伤，脾胃发生之气不能上升，邪害空窍，故不利而不闻香臭者，宜养脾胃，使阳气上升而鼻窍通。"前贤不仅精辟阐述了鼻窍不利与脾胃的关系，并强调补养脾气，可治疗鼻病，大大丰富了治疗鼻疾的病机和方法。

口为脾之窍，《灵枢•五阅五使篇》称"口唇者，脾之官也。"《素问•五脏生成篇》又曰"脾…其荣舌也。"指出脾与口在生理上有密切联系。脾气虚，不能上荣，口舌失养，可引起口淡无味、口腔糜烂、口角流涎、舌萎软等症状。如《灵枢•经脉篇》云："足太阴气绝者，则脉不荣肌肉，脉不荣则肌肉软，肌肉软则舌萎。"指出脾气虚，不能上养舌本，可致舌萎软。《幼科释谜•痰涎》说："小儿多涎，亦由脾气不足，不能四布津液而成。若不治其本，补益中气，而徒去祛其痰涎，痰涎虽病液，亦元气所附，去之不已，遂成虚脱。"不仅明确指出脾气虚不能收摄，可致小儿口角流涎，而且强调要用补中健脾的方法进行治疗。《杂病源流犀烛•口舌唇齿病源流》说："口糜者，口疮糜烂也。…中焦气不足，虚火上泛亦口糜。"提出口糜虽然因实火而致者居多，但也可因脾气虚弱，不能上养，虚阳上扰而口舌溃烂生疮。为久病不已，反复溃烂的口腔疾病提出补中健脾的治疗法则。

治宜补中健脾，升阳益气。头昏眼花、视力疲劳、视力模糊、眼睑下垂，用《脾胃论》补中益气汤。耳鸣耳聋，选补中益气汤重用参、芪，或用《古今医统大全》益气聪明汤（人参、黄芪、葛根、升麻、蔓荆子、白芍、黄柏、甘草）。鼻塞流涕，用四君子汤加柴胡、升麻、辛夷、苍耳。口淡无味，用参苓白术散或香砂六君子汤。舌萎、口角流涎，用补中益气汤加茯苓、泽泻。口糜用补中益气汤或黄芪建中汤。

Literature Review of Spleen Qì Failing to Provide Luxuriance

📖 *Zhōng Zàng Jīng* ("Central Treasury Canon"), "On Flesh Impediment"

> "The spleen is the root of the flesh. When spleen qì has been lost, the flesh is not luxurious and the skin is not smooth and lustrous. As a result, the interstices are loose and the various evils of wind-cold and summer-heat-damp can easily enter. This will cause enduring impediment in the flesh."

This passage describes that, because the spleen governs flesh, spleen vacuity and improper nourishment result in the pathomechanism of luster-less skin and limp flesh.

📖 *Pí Wèi Lùn* ("On the Spleen and Stomach"), "Treatise on Exuberance and Debilitation of the Spleen and Stomach"

> "Dual vacuity of the spleen and stomach causes inability to eat and emaciation. Spleen vacuity results in whittling of the flesh, meaning emaciation and feebleness."

This quotation describes that vacuity of the spleen and stomach and improper nourishment of the flesh results in the pathomechanism of emaciation and cumbersome fatigue.

📖 *Yī Zōng Bì Dú* ("Indispensable Medical Reading"), "Wilting"

> "Yáng brightness vacuity causes blood and qì to be scanty and unable to moisten and nourish the ancestral sinews, which slacken as a result. Slack ancestral sinews mean that the girdling vessel is unable to contract and pull, causing wilting and loss of function in the feet."

Yáng brightness vacuity generally indicates spleen and stomach vacuity. This is because when the stomach is unable to absorb and the spleen is unable to move, they cannot form the essence of grain and water and properly nourish the flesh and ancestral sinews. This causes atrophy of the flesh, limpness of the sinews and vessels, and inability to walk.

📖 *Tài Píng Shèng Huì Fāng* ("Great Peace Sagacious Benevolence Formulary"), "Treatise on the Spleen"

"The spleen receives the essence of grain and water, transforms it into qì and blood, and uses it to nourish the bowels and viscera and fill the skin. If its qì is not luxuriant, it is unable to assist the stomach in moving its fluids and nourishing the entire body. This results in heaviness, sluggishness and fatigue of the body, and inability to raise the limbs…This is a symptom of spleen vacuity."

This quotation describes the pathomechanism by which spleen qì is vacuous and unable to upbear the clear, the essence of food and grain is unable to provide nourishment for the whole body, and the limbs become limp and forceless as a result.

📖 *Zhèng Yīn Mài Zhì* ("Pathoconditions: Causes, Pulses, and Treatments"), "Internal Damage and Inability to Raise the Four Limbs"

"Moreover, the hands and feet are endowed with qì by spleen-earth. Deficiency causes spleen qì depletion and in turn, inability to raise the limbs."

This quotation describes the pathomechanism by which spleen qì is depleted, the limbs are improperly nourished, and the hands and feet become limp and forceless.

📖 *Qiān Jīn Yào Fāng* ("A Thousand Gold Pieces Prescriptions"), "Extreme of the Flesh"

"When consummate yīn suffers a disease, it causes impediment of the flesh. When the flesh impediment does not stop but is complicated by a contraction of evil, this lodges internally in the spleen, and the body itches all over like mice are running around on it."

The spleen is the viscus of consummate yin. When spleen vacuity causes the skin to be improperly nourished and this is complicated by a contraction of external evil that runs into the interstices, it can cause itchy skin.

📖 *Míng Yī Lèi Àn* ("Classified Case Histories of Famous Physicians"), "Case Histories of Wind Strike"

"Itching and white scaling mean an inability of spleen qì to provide luxuriance."

This quotation describes the pathomechanism by which a failure of spleen qì to upbear prevents qì and blood from nourishing the upper body or being distributed to the outside, resulting in itching and scaling of the skin.

📖 *Pí Wèi Lùn* ("On the Spleen and Stomach"), "On Nine Orifices Stoppage Due to Spleen and Stomach Vacuity"

"The spleen constitutes consummate yīn and is rooted in the earth. When there is tangible earth that fills up the source of the nine orifices below, it makes them unable to rise and penetrate to heaven. Thus it is said that disharmony of the five viscera results in stoppage in the nine orifices."

This quotation describes the pathomechanism by which spleen qì vacuity and qì shortage causes a failure to generate essence, and an insufficiency of essence causes blood depletion, insufficiency of qì and blood, improper nourishment of the five viscera, and loss of luxuriance in the offices and orifices, resulting in various types of pathological manifestations.

📖 *Pí Wèi Lùn* ("On the Spleen and Stomach"), "Treatise on Diseases from Stomach Vacuity: the Large Intestine, Small Intestine, and Five Viscera are All Ascribed to the Stomach"

"The *Nèi Jīng* ("Inner Canon") states that tinnitus, deafness, and inhibition of the nine orifices are caused by the intestines and stomach. This is because these symptoms are due to stomach weakness and inability to nourish the hand greater yáng small intestine and hand yáng brightness large intestine channels. In other words, they are contracted because of stomach weakness."

The stomach governs intake and absorption, ripening and rotting; the spleen governs movement and transformation, and upbearing of the clear. The stomach weakness mentioned here refers to difficulty forming the essence of grain and water. This is bound to include spleen vacuity with inability to upbear the clear and improper nourishment of the offices (sensory organs) and orifices, leading to the symptoms of tinnitus, deafness, and inhibition of the nine orifices.

📖 *Zhāng Shì Yī Tōng* ("Zhang's Clear View of Medicine"), "Section on the Seven Orifices: Closed Eyes"

"The foot greater yīn sinew makes up the upper eyelid rim; the foot yáng brightness sinew makes up the lower eyelid rim… When true yáng is unable to rise and bear upward, it causes liking for warmth and fear of brightness. [Treat it with] *bǔ zhōng yì qì tāng* (Center-Supplementing Qì-Boosting Decoction)."

Based on the method of using *bǔ zhōng yì qì tāng* (Center-Supplementing Qì-Boosting Decoction), we can in turn deduce that the pathomechanism of closed eyes is caused by spleen qì vacuity and failure of clear yáng to bear upward.

📖 *Xuē Shì Yī Àn* ("Case Histories of Master Xuē"), "Food and Drink Taxation Fatigue, Depletion Injury, Original Qì Vacuity, and Similar Symptoms"

> "A scholar presented with tightness and dryness in both eyes and inability to gaze up at the end of the day. This is a case of original qì fall. I used *bǔ zhōng yì qì tāng* (Center-Supplementing Qì-Boosting Decoction) with the addition of *rén shēn* (Ginseng Radix) and *huáng qí* (Astragali Radix). He recovered after several preparations."

Dry eyes and inability to gaze up are both caused by a failure of the spleen to upbear the clear and improper nourishment of the eyes. Therefore, Dr. Xuē obtained satisfactory treatment results by employing *bǔ zhōng yì qì tāng* (Center-Supplementing Qì-Boosting Decoction).

📖 *Zhāng Shì Yī Tōng* ("Zhang's Clear View of Medicine"), "The Nose"

> "Modern doctors use *xīn yí* (Magnoliae Flos) to treat nasal congestion and loss of sense of smell. They use it indiscriminately regardless of whether it is a new or enduring, hot or cold condition. Little do they know that yáng qì of the lung and stomach may be vacuous and unable to penetrate up to the chest, which causes turbid yīn qì to rise and interfere, occupy the location of clear yáng, and block it. Therefore it is appropriate to use the acrid and warming fragrance of *xīn yí* (Magnoliae Flos) to penetrate and free."

In lung and stomach yáng vacuity, the downbearing action of stomach qì constitutes the normal flow and is necessary to enable spleen qì to fulfill its upbearing and diffusing function. Moreover, it is only through the upbearing and diffusing action of lung and spleen qì that they can fulfill their function of diffusing and penetrating to the nose.

文献评述

《中藏经·论肉痹》："脾者肉之本，脾气已失，则肉不荣，肌肤不滑泽，则腠理疏，凡风寒暑湿之邪易为入，故久不治为肉痹也。"论述脾主肌肉，脾虚失养，引起肌肤不泽，肌肉萎软的病机。

《脾胃论·脾胃盛衰论》："脾胃俱虚，则不能食而瘦；脾虚则肌肉削，即食□也。"论述脾胃虚弱，肌肉失养，引起形体消瘦、困倦的病机。

《医宗必读·痿》亦说："阳明虚则血气少，不能润养宗筋，故弛纵，宗筋纵则带脉不能收引，故足痿不用。"阳明虚，泛指脾胃虚弱，是胃不能纳，脾不能运，水谷精微不能化生，肌肉与宗筋失养，故肌肉萎缩，筋脉萎软，不能行走。

《太平圣惠方·脾脏论》："夫脾受水谷之精，化为气血，养于脏腑，充于肌肤。若其气不荣，则不能与胃行其津液，周养身形。致体重懈惰，四肢不举…则是脾虚不足之候也。"论述脾气虚弱，不能升清，水谷精微不能营养形体，而四肢软弱无力的病机。

《症因脉治·内伤四肢不举》："手足又禀气于脾土，不及，则脾气亏损，四肢亦不举。"论述脾气亏损，四肢失养，手足软弱无力的病机。

《千金要方·肉极》："至阴遇病为肌痹，肌痹不已，复感于邪，内舍于脾，体痒淫淫，如鼠走其身上。"脾为至阴之脏，脾虚肌肤失养，复感外邪，行走于皮里，可致皮肤瘙痒。

《名医类案·中风案》："痒起白屑，脾气不能营也。"阐述脾气不能上升，气血不能上养，不能外布，而致皮肤瘙痒脱屑的病机。

《脾胃论·脾胃虚则九窍不通论》说："脾为至阴，本乎地也。有形之土，下填九窍之源，使不能上通于天，故曰五脏不和，则九窍不通。"阐明脾气虚弱，气少则精微不生，精微不足则血亏，气血不足五脏失养，官窍失荣，而引起各种病理表现的病机。

《脾胃论·大肠小肠五脏皆属于胃，胃虚则俱病论》："《内经》云耳鸣、耳聋、九窍不利，肠胃之所生也，此胃弱不能滋养手太阳小肠，手阳明大肠，故有此症，然亦只从胃弱而得之。"胃主受纳、腐熟，脾主运化、升清。此处胃弱仅水谷精微难于化生，必然包括脾虚不能升清，官窍失养，才能引起耳鸣、耳聋、九窍不利等症状。

《张氏医通·七窍门·目闭不开》："足太阳之筋，为目上纲，足阳明之筋，为目下纲。…真阳不能上升者，则喜暖怕亮，补中益气汤。"从使用补中益气的方法，反证目闭不能开的病机是因脾气虚弱，清阳不能升举所致。

《薛氏医案·饮食劳倦亏损元气虚等症》："一儒者，日晡两目紧涩，不能瞻视，此元气下陷，用补中益气汤加参、芪。数剂而愈。"目涩、不能瞻视，是指目睛干涩，不能上视，均由脾不升清，目睛失养所致，故用补中益气汤治疗而收到满意疗效。

《张氏医通·鼻》："近世以辛黄仁治鼻塞不闻香臭，无问新久寒热，一概用之。殊不知肺胃阳气虚衰，不能上透于脑，致浊阴之气上干，清阳之位而窒塞者，故宜辛黄之辛温香窜以通达之。"肺胃阳虚，其中胃气以下降为顺，脾气才具有向上升宣的功能，藉肺脾之气向上升宣，才能发挥宣通鼻窍的作用。

Summary of Spleen Qì Failing to Provide Luxuriance

1. Improper Nourishment of the Body

Improper nourishment of the flesh: Emaciation, atrophy of the flesh, in severe cases wilting.

Improper nourishment of the limbs: Limpness of the limbs, inability to raise the limbs, paralysis and insensitivity, forceless walk, numbness in the fingers.

Improper nourishment of the skin: Dry skin, scaling, elastic flaking, desiccated hair, encrusted skin.

2. Improper Nourishment of the Offices and Orifices

Improper nourishment of the eyes: Dizziness and flowery vision, fatigued eyesight, drooping eyelids.

Improper nourishment of the ears: Tinnitus and deafness, impaired hearing.

Improper nourishment of the nose: Runny nose with clear snivel, loss of sense of smell.

Improper nourishment of the mouth: Bland taste in the mouth and no sense of taste, mouth sores and drooling, limp tongue.

脾气不荣

形体失养——肌肉失养——形体消瘦，肌肉萎缩，甚则痿弱。

四肢失养——肢体软弱，四肢不举，麻痹不仁，行走无力，十指麻木。

皮肤失养——皮肤干燥，脱屑，弹性下降，毛发枯槁，肌肤甲错。

官窍失养——目睛失养——头昏眼花，视力疲劳，眼睑下垂。

耳窍失养——耳鸣耳聋，听力下降。

鼻窍失养——鼻流清涕，嗅觉失灵。

口舌失养——口淡乏味，口疮流涎，舌萎软。

1.5 Qì Vacuity Heat Effusion

When spleen qì is vacuous, clear yáng fails to upbear and yáng qì floats astray into the fleshy exterior. There it becomes depressed and causes heat effusion, resulting in the pathomechanism of spleen vacuity heat effusion. This type of heat effusion is characterized by heat that is of moderate strength, erupts intermittently, and is aggravated by taxation, inability to endure wind-cold, yáng qì that intermittently becomes floating and stretched during times of fatigue, heat effusion that is reduced by sweating, and potentially occasional high fever that persists without abating. Accompanying symptoms are a pale white facial complexion, dizziness and flowery vision, shortness of breath and laziness to speak, fatigued spirit and lack of strength, a pale tongue body, and a vacuous and weak pulse.

The chapter, "On the Beginnings of Heat Stroke from Food and Drink Taxation Fatigue" in the *Pí Wèi Lùn* ("On the Spleen and Stomach") states:

> "Therefore, when a spleen pattern is first contracted, it results in elevated qì and panting, generalized heat and vexation, a surging and large pulse and headache, perhaps with incessant thirst, inability to bear wind-cold on the skin, and aversion to cold and heat effusion… When spleen and stomach qì flow downward, grain qì is unable to float up. When this lack of movement occurs in the spring, the body lacks yáng to protect its construction and defense, so that it becomes unable to endure wind-cold. This results in aversion to cold and heat effusion. All this is caused by an insufficiency of spleen and stomach qì."

Lǐ Dōng-Yuán thus suggested that spleen vacuity heat effusion is caused by taxation fatigue consuming qì, by damaged spleen qì, and by center qì fall. Therefore he used *bǔ zhōng yì qì tāng* (Center-Supplementing Qì-Boosting Decoction) in his treatments, since it fortifies the spleen, boosts qì, and upbears yáng with its sweetness and warmth. Thus he established the principle of "eliminating heat with warmth and sweetness." This source shows an application that corresponds to the pathomechanism of spleen vacuity heat effusion in clinic.

Qì vacuity heat effusion is treated by fortifying the spleen and boosting qì, just as in the above quotation "to eliminate great heat with warmth and sweetness." The recommended formula is *bǔ zhōng yì qì tāng* (Center-Supplementing Qì-Boosting Decoction) with modifications.

气虚发热

脾气虚弱，清阳不升，阳气浮越肌表，郁而发热，则为脾虚发热的病机。此类发热，热势不高、时作时止、遇劳则甚、不任风寒，当劳累时阳气浮张，阵阵而作，汗出热减；或偶有高热，持续不退。兼面色淡白，头晕眼花，气短懒言，神疲乏力，舌质淡，脉虚弱等症状。《脾胃论•饮食劳倦始为热中论》云："故脾证始得，则气高而喘，身热而烦，其脉洪大而头痛，或渴不止，其皮肤不任风寒而生寒热。…脾胃之气下流，使谷气不得升浮，是春生之令不行，则

无阳以护其荣卫，则不任风寒，乃生寒热，此皆脾胃之气不足所致
也。"李东垣认为脾虚发热是劳倦耗气，脾气损伤，中气下陷所致。
故用甘温健脾，益气升阳的补中益气汤治疗，创造"甘温除热 "的大
法，是脾虚发热病机应运于临床的典范。治宜健脾益气，正所谓甘
温除大热。方选补中益气汤加减。

Literature Review of Qì Vacuity Heat Effusion

📖 *Sù Wèn* ("Plain Questions"), "Treatise on Regulating the Channels"

> "Owing to the presence of taxation fatigue, bodily qì is reduced, grain qì
> is not exuberant, the upper burner does not move, the lower stomach duct
> is stopped, stomach qì becomes hot, and hot qì fumes inside the chest,
> causing internal heat."

This is a description of the pathomechanism by which Lǐ Dōng-Yuán's
"debilitation of the spleen and stomach and insufficiency of original qì"
results in qì vacuity heat effusion.

📖 *Zhèng Zhì Zhǔn Shéng* ("Level-Line of Pattern Identification and
Treatment"), "Miscellaneous Diseases: Onset of Disease"

> "Food and drink taxation fatigue internally damages original qì. This re-
> sults in center yáng fall and internally arising vacuity heat. Therefore, Lǐ
> Dōng-Yuán developed the theory of supplementing the center and boost-
> ing qì and used such sweet and warm medicinals as *rén shēn* (Ginseng
> Radix) and *huáng qí* (Astragali Radix) to greatly supplement qì and lift
> its fall. This is a case of using qì [-boosting] medicinals to supplement an
> insufficiency of qì."

This quotation describes how food and drink taxation fatigue causes internal damage to spleen qì and center qì fall, which can then engender
vacuity heat and subsequently qì vacuity heat effusion. Therefore, the
author applies the method of boosting qì with sweetness and warmth to
eliminate great heat.

📖 *Yī Biǎn* ("Lancing Stones of Medicine"), "Heat Effusion"

> "Center qì can become debilitated and unable to move, either because
> qì is dissipated as a result of taxation fatigue, because qì is bound as a
> result of thought and preoccupation, or because qì is famished as a re-
> sult of hunger. This causes it to stagnate in the center or fall down-
> ward, which in turn results in depression and formation of heat. The
> symptoms of this condition are laziness, fatigue and somnolence,
> panting on moving, fatigued and cumbersome limbs, occasional so-
> liloquy, inability to distinguish between head and tail, fever at mid-
> night that either goes into temporary remission at daybreak or never

breaks day or night, or clamoring followed by fever at sunrise, remission when the weather is cloudy and damp, vexing heat in the five hearts, and in severe cases a burning sensation in the flesh, sinews, and bones. This is what Lǐ Dōng-Yuán refers to as yáng vacuity heat effusion."

This quotation describes the pathomechanism and clinical manifestations of qì vacuity heat effusion. It is due to internal damage from taxation fatigue, injury to spleen qì, depression of the qì dynamic, downward fall, failure of clear yáng to bear upward, and yáng floating into the fleshy exterior.

文献评述

《素问·调经论》：”有所劳倦，形气衰少，谷气不盛，上焦不行，下脘不通，胃气热、热气熏胸中，故内热。”这是李东垣”脾胃虚衰、元气不足”而引起气虚发热的病机论述。

《证治准绳·杂病·发病》说：”饮食劳倦为内伤元气，此则中阳下陷，内生虚热，故东垣发补中益气之论，用人参、黄芪等甘温之药，大补其气而提其下陷，此用补气药以补气之不足也。”论述饮食劳倦，内伤脾气，中气下陷，可生虚热，此乃气虚发热，故用甘温益气之法，消除大热。

《医碥·发热》：”或劳倦气散，或思虑气结，或饥饿气馁，中气因而衰微，不能运行。或滞于中，或陷于下，而郁滞成热。证见怠懒嗜卧，行动喘乏，四肢困倦，或时自言自语，不知首尾，夜分即热，天明暂缓，或昼夜不解，或日出气喧则热，天阴应凉则缓，五心烦热，甚则肌肉筋骨如烧，此东垣所谓阳虚发热也。”论述劳倦内伤，脾气受损，气机郁滞、下陷，清阳不升，阳浮肌表，引起气虚发热的病机和临床表现。

Summary of Qì Vacuity Heat Effusion
Qì Vacuity Heat Effusion
Heat of moderate strength that is reduced with sweating, erupts intermittently, and is aggravated by taxation; inability to endure wind-cold; occasional high heat effusion that persists without abating.
气虚发热
热势不高，汗出热减，时作时止，遇劳则甚，不任风寒。偶有高热，持续不退。

Conclusion

In conclusion, the pathomechanisms of spleen qì vacuity are extremely complex. They can be differentiated by two important aspects.

The Influence on the Root Viscera

When spleen qì vacuity has persisted for a long time, yáng qì is debilitated and vacuity cold arises internally. This can develop into spleen yáng vacuity. When spleen qì vacuity prevents it from forming yīn humor, it can develop into spleen yīn vacuity or dual vacuity of qì and yīn in the spleen. When spleen qì vacuity prevents it from moving the fluids, dampness obstructs the center burner, which can result in spleen vacuity damp obstruction. When spleen qì vacuity prevents it from promoting the movement of the qì dynamic, qì stagnates in the center burner, which can result in the pathomechanism of center vacuity qì stagnation.

The Relationship to the Other Viscera

The "Chapter on Greater Yīn and Yáng Brightness" in the *Sù Wèn* ("Plain Questions") explains: "The five viscera and six bowels are all endowed with qì by the stomach." This indicates that the other four viscera (liver, heart, lung, and kidney) all depend on nourishment from the spleen and stomach and are closely related to the spleen and stomach. An advanced development of the pathomechanism of spleen qì vacuity can result in pathomechanisms like qì vacuity of the spleen and stomach, dual vacuity of the heart and spleen, qì vacuity of the spleen and lung, liver depression and spleen vacuity, and qì vacuity of the spleen and kidney.

Qì Vacuity of the spleen and stomach

The spleen and stomach are both located in the center burner. When spleen qì is vacuous, it most easily leads to stomach qì depletion, causing the pathomechanism of qì vacuity in the spleen and stomach. In clinic, this is the most commonly seen development. It manifests in symptoms of simultaneous vacuity of the spleen and stomach, like glomus in the stomach duct, abdominal distention, no thought of food and drink, nausea and vomiting, and sloppy stool. It is treated by supplementing the center and boosting qì, and by regulating and harmonizing the spleen and stomach.

Recommended formulas include modifications of *sì jūn zǐ tāng* (Four Gentlemen Decoction) and *yì gōng sǎn* (Special Achievement Powder) from the *Xiǎo Ér Yào Zhèng Zhí Jué* ("Key to Diagnosis and Treatment of Children's Diseases"), or *liù jūn zǐ tāng* (Six Gentlemen Decoction) from the *Fù Rén Dà Quán Liáng Fāng* ("Compendium of Good Remedies for Women").

Sì Jūn Zǐ Tāng 四君子汤
Four Gentlemen Decoction

rén shēn (人参 ginseng, Ginseng Radix)

fú líng (茯苓 poria, Poria)

bái zhú (白术 white atractylodes, Atractylodis Macrocephalae Rhizoma)

zhì gān cǎo (炙甘草 mix-fried licorice, Glycyrrhizae Radix cum
Liquido Fricta)

Yì Gōng Sǎn 异功散
Special Achievement Powder

rén shēn (人参 ginseng, Ginseng Radix)

fú líng (茯苓 poria, Poria)

bái zhú (白术 white atractylodes, Atractylodis Macrocephalae Rhizoma)

gān cǎo (甘草 licorice, Glycyrrhizae Radix)

chén pí (陈皮 tangerine peel, Citri Reticulatae Pericarpium)

Liù Jūn Zǐ Tāng 六君子汤
Six Gentlemen Decoction

fú líng (茯苓 poria, Poria)

bái zhú (白术 white atractylodes, Atractylodis Macrocephalae Rhizoma)

rén shēn (人参 ginseng, Ginseng Radix)

zhì gān cǎo (炙甘草 mix-fried licorice, Glycyrrhizae Radix cum
Liquido Fricta)

bàn xià (半夏 pinellia, Pinelliae Rhizoma)

chén pí (陈皮 tangerine peel, Citri Reticulatae Pericarpium)

Dual vacuity of the heart and spleen

The heart governs blood. When spleen qì is vacuous, it is unable to form heart blood. This can evolve into the pathomechanisms of heart blood vacuity and dual vacuity of the heart and spleen. In this case, one can observe torpid intake with reduced eating, abdominal distention, and sloppy stool, together with symptoms like heart palpitations, insomnia, profuse dreaming, and forgetfulness. It is treated by supplementing the spleen and boosting qì, and by nourishing the heart and quieting the spirit. The recommended formula is *guī pí tāng* (Spleen-Returning Decoction) from the *Chóng Dìng Yán Shì Jì Shēng Fāng* ("Revised Life-Saving Formulas of Master Yán") with modifications.

Guī Pí Tāng 归脾汤
Spleen-Returning Decoction

huáng qí (黄耆 astragalus, Astragali Radix)

rén shēn (人参 ginseng, Ginseng Radix)

bái zhú (白术 white atractylodes, Atractylodis Macrocephalae Rhizoma)

fú líng (茯苓 poria, Poria)

dāng guī (当归 Chinese angelica, Angelicae Sinensis Radix)

lóng yǎn ròu (龙眼肉 longan flesh, Longan Arillus)

suān zǎo rén (酸枣仁 spiny jujube, Ziziphi Spinosi Semen)

yuǎn zhì (远志 polygala, Polygalae Radix)

mù xiāng (木香 costusroot, Aucklandiae Radix)

gān cǎo (甘草 licorice, Glycyrrhizae Radix)

Qì vacuity of the spleen and lung: The spleen and lung stand in a mother-child relationship and are mutually engendering. When spleen qì is vacuous, earth is unable to engender metal. This can evolve into the pathomechanism of lung qì vacuity. As stated in the "Treatise on Exuberance and Debility of the Spleen and Stomach" in the *Pí Wèi Lùn* ("On the Spleen and Stomach"), "When lung-metal contracts evil, this results from a vacuity of the spleen and stomach, so that they are unable to engender the lung, causing the contraction of disease. Thus, there is coughing, shortness of breath, qì ascent, inability of the skin and hair to resist cold, reduced essence-spirit and thirst, and melancholy and unhappy emotions."

In a more advanced development, spleen qì vacuity and lung qì vacuity are seen simultaneously, thus forming the pathomechanism of qì vacuity of the spleen and lung. In that case, one will observe symptoms like torpid intake and reduced eating, abdominal distention, and sloppy stool, together with coughing and forceless panting, shortness of breath, and low voice. This condition is treated by fortifying the spleen and boosting qì, and by supplementing earth and engendering metal. The recommended formula is *liù jūn zǐ tāng* (Six Gentlemen Decoction) in combination with *bǔ fèi tāng* (Lung-Supplementing Decoction) from the *Yǒng Lèi Qián Fāng* with modifications.

Bǔ Fèi Tāng 补肺汤
Lung-Supplementing Decoction

rén shēn (人参 ginseng, Ginseng Radix)

huáng qí (黄耆 astragalus, Astragali Radix)

sāng bái pí (桑白皮 mulberry root bark, Mori Cortex)

zǐ wǎn (紫菀 aster, Asteris Radix)

shú dì huáng (熟地黄 cooked rehmannia, Rehmanniae Radix Praeparata)

wǔ wèi zǐ (五味子 schisandra, Schisandrae Fructus)

Liver depression and spleen vacuity: The spleen governs movement and transformation, and the liver governs blood storage and free coursing. When spleen qì is vacuous, it is unable to form blood and nourish the substance of the liver. This can result in insufficiency of liver blood, constraint of the liver system, and breakdown of free coursing, forming the pathomechanism of liver depression and spleen vacuity. In this case, one will observe torpid intake, abdominal distention, and sloppy stool, together with symptoms like dizziness and flowery vision, distention and pain in the chest and rib-sides, and constrained emotions. This condition is treated by coursing the liver and opening the depression, and by fortifying the spleen and boosting qì. The recommended formula is a modified version of *chái sháo liù jūn zǐ tāng* (Bupleurum and Peony Six Gentlemen Decoction) from the *Tài Píng Huì Mín Hé Jì Jú Fāng* ("Tài-Píng Imperial Grace Pharmacy Formulas").

Chái Sháo Liù Jūn Zǐ Tāng 柴芍六君子汤
Bupleurum and Peony Six Gentlemen Decoction

fú líng (茯苓 poria, Poria)

bái zhú (白术 white atractylodes, Atractylodis Macrocephalae Rhizoma)

rén shēn (人参 ginseng, Ginseng Radix)

zhì gān cǎo (炙甘草 mix-fried licorice, Glycyrrhizae Radix cum Liquido Fricta)

bàn xià (半夏 pinellia, Pinelliae Rhizoma)

chén pí (陈皮 tangerine peel, Citri Reticulatae Pericarpium)

chái hú (柴胡 bupleurum, Bupleuri Radix)

bái sháo yào (白芍药 white peony, Paeoniae Radix Alba)

Qì vacuity of the spleen and kidney: The kidney stores earlier heaven essential qì. The kidney must also receive a supplemental provision of later heaven essential qì, which is formed by the spleen and stomach, to be able to exercise its physiological functions. When spleen qì is vacuous, it is unable to form essential qì and nourish earlier heaven. This can result in depletion of the kidney's essential qì, emerging as the pathomechanism of qì vacuity of the spleen and kidney. In this case, one will see torpid intake, abdominal distention, diarrhea, and sloppy stool together with symptoms of impaired kidney functions like limp aching lumbus and knees, dizziness, and tinnitus. This condition is treated by supplementing and boosting the spleen and kidney. The recommended formula is a modification of *liù jūn zǐ tāng* (Six Gentlemen Decoction) in combination with *jīn guì shèn qì wán* (Golden Coffer Kidney Qì Pill).

Jīn Guì Shèn Qì Wán 金匮肾气丸
Golden Coffer Kidney Qì Pill

shú dì huáng (熟地黄 cooked rehmannia, Rehmanniae Radix Praeparata)
shān yào (山药 dioscorea, Dioscoreae Rhizoma)
mǔ dān pí (牡丹皮 moutan, Moutan Cortex)
fú líng (茯苓 poria, Poria)
zé xiè (泽泻 alisma, Alismatis Rhizoma)
shān zhū yú (山茱萸 cornus, Corni Fructus)
fù zǐ (附子 aconite, Aconiti Radix Lateralis Praeparata)
ròu guì (肉桂 cinnamon bark, Cinnamomi Cortex)

The spleen and stomach hold the center [within the five phases] and enable movement to the four sides. When spleen qì is vacuous, it can lead to improper nourishment in the other four viscera. This can result in many types of combined pathomechanisms of the viscera and bowels.

总之

脾气虚的病机发展十分复杂，主要有两个方面：

其一、对本脏的影响。脾气虚日久，阳气虚衰，虚寒内生，可发展为脾阳虚；脾气虚，不能化生阴液，可发展形成脾阴虚或脾的气阴两虚；脾气虚，不能运化水液，湿阻中焦，可引起脾虚湿阻；脾气虚，不能推动气机运行，气滞中焦，可引起中虚气滞的病机。

其二、与它脏的关系。《素问•太阴阳明篇》说："五脏六腑皆禀气于胃"，指出肝、心、肺、肾其它四脏皆依靠脾胃的滋养，与脾胃有密切的关系。脾气虚的病机进一步发展可引起脾胃气虚，心脾两虚，脾肺气虚，肝郁脾虚，脾肾气虚等病机变化。

脾胃气虚：脾胃同处中焦，脾气虚弱，最易引起胃气亏损，出现脾胃气虚的病机。这是临床最为多见的病机变化，可见脘痞腹胀，不思饮食，呕恶便溏等脾胃同虚的表现。治宜补中益气，调和脾胃。方选四君子汤，《小儿药证直诀》异功散，《妇人大全良方》六君子汤加减。

心脾两虚：心主血，脾气虚弱，不能化生心血，则会演变为心血虚、心脾两虚的病机。既可见纳呆食少、腹胀便溏，又见心悸失眠、多梦健忘等症状。治宜补脾益气，养心安神。方选《济生方》归脾汤加减。

脾肺气虚：脾与肺，母子相生，脾气虚弱，土不生金，可演变成肺气虚的病机。如《脾胃论·脾胃胜衰论》所云："肺金受邪，由脾胃虚弱不能生肺，乃所生受病也。故咳嗽、气短、气上、皮毛不能御寒、精神少而渴、情惨惨而不乐。"进一步发展，脾气虚与肺气虚并见，可形成脾肺气虚的病机。既见纳呆食少、腹胀便溏，又见咳喘无力，气短声低等症状。治宜健脾益气，补土生金。方选六君子汤合《永类钤方》补肺汤（人参、黄芪、桑白皮、紫菀、熟地黄、五味子）加减。

肝郁脾虚：脾主运化，肝主藏血、疏泄 。脾气虚弱，不能化生血液，滋养肝体，可引起肝血不足或肝体不舒，疏泄失常，形成肝郁脾虚的病机。既见纳呆腹胀便溏，又见头昏眼花、胸胁胀痛，情志不舒等症状。治宜疏肝开郁，健脾益气。方选《和剂局方》柴芍六君子汤（六君子加柴胡、白芍）加减。

脾肾气虚：肾藏先天之精气，必须得到脾胃化生的后天精气之资助，才能发挥其生理效应。脾气虚，不能化生精气，滋养先天，可引起肾的精气亏损，出现脾肾气虚的病机。既见纳呆腹胀，腹泻便溏，又见腰膝酸软、头昏耳鸣等肾功能减的等许多见症。治宜补益脾肾。方选六君子汤合金匮肾气丸加减。总之，脾胃执中央以运四旁，脾气虚弱，可致其它四脏失养，引起多种脏腑相兼的病机变化。

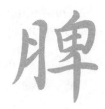

Chapter 2

Spleen Yáng Vacuity

脾阳虚

When spleen qì vacuity advances further, yáng qì is consumed and loses its ability to warm, stimulate, and propel. This can create the pathomechanism of spleen yáng vacuity. The chapter, "Five Evils" in the *Líng Shū* ("Magic Pivot"), explains: "When the evil is in the spleen and stomach, disease will make the flesh hurt… When yáng qì is insufficient and yīn qì superabundant, it causes cold strike, rumbling intestines, and abdominal pain." This is the earliest mention of the pathomechanism of spleen yáng vacuity.

Zhāng Zhòng-Jǐng elaborated in more detail on the various clinical manifestations of greater yīn disease that result from spleen yáng vacuity. In the chapter,"Identifying the Pulses, Patterns, and Treatments of Greater Yīn Disease" in the *Shāng Hán Lùn* ("On Cold Damage"), he stated: "When greater yīn is diseased, it causes abdominal fullness and vomiting, inability to get food down, exacerbated loose bowels, and periodic spontaneous abdominal pain." He also mentioned the corresponding treatment method and formula: "Spontaneous diarrhea without thirst is associated with greater yīn and is caused by cold in its viscus. One should warm it and use a variation of *sì nì tāng* (Counterflow Cold Decoction)." The *Qiān Jīn Yào Fāng* ("A Thousand Gold Pieces Prescriptions"), *Shèng Jì Zǒng Lù* ("Sages' Salvation Records"), and *Chóng Dìng Yán Shì Jì Shēng Fāng* ("Revised Life-Saving Formulas of Master Yán") all discussed the pathomechanism of spleen yáng vacuity in terms like "spleen visceral cold" or "spleen vacuity cold," but none of them directly mentioned the phrase spleen yáng vacuity.

During the Jīn-Yuán period, Lǐ Dōng-Yuán, the founder of the Earth-Supplementing School, greatly advanced the recognition of spleen yáng vacuity. In the "Treatise on the Exuberance and Debility of the Spleen and Stomach" in the *Pí Wèi Lùn* ("On the Spleen and Stomach"), he explains: "The source of spleen-stomach insufficiency is really found in an insufficiency of yáng qì." He further stated: "Insufficiency of the spleen and stomach is always a case of blood disease, which means an insufficiency of yáng qì and a superabundance of yīn qì."

Lǐ suggested that yáng vacuity is the main cause of spleen and stomach vacuity. From the perspective of the upbearing and downbearing of the qì dynamic, he also pointed out that insufficiency of spleen yáng, failure of clear yáng to bear upward, and vacuity fall of original qì are the main pathomechanisms of disease arising from internal damage to the spleen and stomach. He thereby laid a solid foundation for the later establishment of the Warming and Supplementing School.

Subsequently, no generation lacked scholars who continued in the tradition of Lǐ Dōng-Yuán's theories. His disciple Wáng Hào-Gǔ composed the *Yīn Zhèng Lüè Lì* ("Examples of Yin Patterns") based on an analysis of disease causes and symptoms and proposed that the main characteristics of spleen yáng vacuity are insufficiency of yáng qì and inability to transform grain. When setting forth the principles of internal damage heat effusion, in the section, "Miscellaneous Works by Míng Physicians: Internal Damage Heat Effusion" of his treatise, *Xuē Shì Yī Àn* ("Case Histories of Master Xuē"), Xuē Jǐ also pointed out:

> "Although the two patterns can be distinguished on the basis of yīn and yáng, in reality they are both caused by an insufficiency of yáng qì in the spleen and stomach"

What he referred to as "insufficiency of yáng qì in the spleen and stomach" mainly indicates an insufficiency of spleen yáng, which is identical with spleen yáng vacuity.

During the Míng period, Zhāng Jǐng-Yuè, the prominent founder of the Warming and Supplementing School, compiled *Jǐng Yuè Quán Shū* ("Jǐng-Yuè's Complete Compendium"). In the section, "Record of Transmitting Loyalty: Further Identification of Yáng Insufficiency"), he expounded:

> "Is there anything more important to engender than qì? And is there anything more important to engender in one's whole lifetime than yáng qì? That which is difficult to obtain and easy to lose refers only to yáng, just as that which when lost is difficult to recover refers only to yáng"

In his opinion, the most important aspect of the human body was yáng qì. Since spleen yáng was the foundation for later heaven yáng qì and was closely linked to the formation of yáng qì in the other organs, spleen yáng vacuity could thus easily damage yáng qì in the other organs. Therefore, he emphasized warming and supplementing spleen yáng in order to strengthen yáng qì in the whole body.

In the chapter, "Spleen and Stomach" in his work, *Lín Zhèng Zhǐ Nán Yī Àn* ("A Clinical Guide with Case Histories"), Yè Tiān-Shì explained:

> "If spleen yáng is insufficient, there will be cold-damp in the stomach. Thus, all the organs, one by one, should be treated by warming and drying, upbearing and moving, in careful observation of Lǐ Dōng-Yuán's method."

This is the earliest mention of the phrase "insufficiency of spleen yáng."

In the *Bǐ Huā Yī Jìng* ("Bihua's Medical Mirror"), Jiāng Bǐ-Huā described in more detail the clinical symptoms of spleen yáng vacuity. In modern times, the physician Táng Róng-Chuān also explained as follows in the chapter, "Pathomechanisms of the Viscera and Bowels" in the *Xuè Zhèng Lùn* ("On Blood Patterns"): "When spleen yáng is insufficient, the solids of grain and water are not transformed."

In his work, *Pú Fǔ-Zhōu Yī Liáo Jīng Yàn* ("Pú Fǔ-Zhōu's Medical Experience"), the famous contemporary physician Pú Fǔ-Zhōu points this out even more clearly, in the chapter, "Searching for the Root in Pattern Identification":

> "When spleen yáng is vacuous, it causes lack of warmth in the four limbs, periodic abdominal fullness, spontaneous diarrhea, puffy swelling in the face, bland taste in the mouth, aversion to water, shortage of qì, and laziness to speak"

This is an excellent summary of spleen yáng vacuity.

Spleen yáng vacuity can stem from an advanced development of spleen qì vacuity. Damage to spleen yáng can also result from excessive consumption of raw or cold foods or a direct strike of external cold. Other causes include feebleness in old age, constitutional insufficiency, enduring or severe illness, or overuse of bitter and cold medicinals. Lastly, debility of the life gate fire impairs the warming and steaming of spleen-earth, so it can also cause simultaneous vacuity of spleen yáng. Spleen yáng vacuity is most commonly involved in pathomechanisms such as grain and water failing to move, water-damp failing to transform, and impaired warming.

脾气虚进一步发展，阳气耗损，失于温煦、激发、推动，可形成脾阳虚衰的病机。《灵枢•五邪篇》说："邪在脾胃，则病肌肉痛。…阳气不足，阴气有余，则寒中肠鸣腹痛。"最早提出脾阳虚的病机。

张仲景更详细阐述了脾阳虚衰引起太阴病的各种临床表现。他在《伤寒论•辨太阴病脉证并治》中云:"太阴之为病,腹满而吐,食不下,自利益甚,时腹自痛。"并提出相应的治法和方药:"自利不渴者属太阴,以其脏有寒故也,当温之,宜四逆辈。"《千金要方》、《圣济总录》、《济生方》皆以"脾虚冷"、"脾脏冷"、"脾虚寒"等提法对脾阳虚的病机予以讨论,但均还未正式提出脾阳虚的名称。

金元时期,补土派大师李东垣对脾阳虚的认识有了很大发展,《脾胃论•脾胃胜衰论》说:"脾胃不足之源,乃阳气不足。"又说:"夫脾胃不足皆为血病,是阳气不足,阴气有余。"认为脾胃虚弱的主要原因是阳虚,并从气机升降的角度,指出脾阳不足,清阳不升,元气虚陷是脾胃内伤发病的主要病机,为后世温补派的创立奠定了坚实基础。其后禀承东垣之说者,代不乏人。其弟子王好古撰《阴证略例》从病因和症状分析,认为脾阳虚是以阳气不足、不能化谷为主要特征。薛己也在阐述内伤发热之理时指出:"二证虽有阴阳之分,实则皆因脾胃阳气不足所致"(《薛氏医案•明医杂著•内伤发热》)。这里所谓"脾胃阳气不足",主要是指脾阳不足,亦即脾阳虚。明代杰出的温补派大师张景岳说:"凡在生者无非生气为主,而一生之生气何莫非阳气为主...难得而易失者惟阳,既失难复者亦惟阳"(《景岳全书•传忠录•阳不足再辨》),认为人的一身以阳气为主,脾阳为后天阳气之本,与其它脏腑阳气的生成有密切的关系,脾阳虚则其它脏腑阳气易损,重视温补脾阳以增强全身阳气。叶天士在《临证指南医案•脾胃》中说:"若脾阳不足,胃有寒湿,一脏一腑,皆宜于温燥升运者,自当恪遵东垣之法。"最早提出了"脾阳不足"的名词。江笔花在《笔花医镜》中较为详细地描述了脾阳虚的临床症状。近代医家唐容川在《血证论•脏腑病机》亦有"脾阳不足,水谷固不化"之说。现代名医蒲辅周更明确地指出:"脾阳虚,四肢不温,腹时满,自下利,面浮肿,口淡无味,恶水,少气懒言"(《蒲辅周医疗经验•辨证求本》),是对脾阳虚病机的高度概括。

脾阳虚可由脾气虚损进一步发展而来;也可由过食生冷或外寒直中损伤脾阳所致;老年体弱、禀赋不足、久病重病、过用苦寒亦可引起;命门火衰,不能温蒸脾土,致使脾阳亦虚。脾阳虚衰,最易引起水谷失运、水湿不化、温煦失职等病机变化。

2.1 Grain and Water Failing to Move

During the Qīng period, Luó Hào stated in the chapter, "Further Discussion on the Spleen and Stomach" in the *Yī Jīng Yú Lùn* ("Additional Comments on Medical Classics"):

> "The spleen is earth. It is often damp in substance, so it uses yáng. Similarly, damp earth is unable to engender the myriad things when the yáng rays of the sun do not shine on it."

This quotation stresses that the spleen is rooted in yáng qì. Spleen yáng assists in the spleen's movement and transformation and ensures normal digestion, absorption, and transport of grain and water. If spleen yáng is vacuous and therefore unable to promote movement and transformation, spleen qì moves slowly and without force. Qì stagnates in the center burner, resulting in torpid intake and reduced eating, distention in the abdomen and stomach duct that likes pressure and is aggravated after meals, or distention even when hungry.

"Schema of Miscellaneous Patterns; Section on Food and Drink" in the *Jǐng Yuè Quán Shū* ("Jǐng-Yuè's Complete Compendium") states:

> "In all patterns of food and drink damaging the spleen… most easily recognize repletion patterns, but usually fail to recognize cold, enduring, or vacuity patterns. However, if the spleen is unable to transform, patterns of center vacuity are common. They result either in not eating and yet feeling satiated, or in distention after reduced eating, or in lack of satiety or hunger and no thought of food and drink, or in vomiting and abdominal fullness and expansion in spite of stomach vacuity."

This passage points out that enduring damage from food and drink, susceptibility of the spleen to vacuity cold, and impaired movement and transformation can cause symptoms such as no thought of food and drink or reduced eating with abdominal distention.

The chapter on "Glomus Fullness" of the same text also states: "Why is it that vacuity of the spleen and stomach frequently occurs simultaneously with cold patterns? The spleen and stomach belong to earth. When earth is vacuous, it is commonly caused by an absence of fire. When earth contracts cold, the transformation of qì will lack force, causing increased glomus and fullness, which is precisely what leads to the generation of cold in the center." Earth cold refers to spleen-stomach vacuity cold, spleen yáng vacuity, forceless qì transformation, and qì stagnation in the center, which cause glomus, binding, distention, and fullness below the heart.

When spleen yáng is vacuous, grain and water are dispersed only with difficulty. Thus, they collect and stagnate in the center burner and obstruct the qì dynamic. Qì and grain and water attack and contend with each other, and grain and water come and go in the intestinal area. This can lead to rumbling intestines. Congealing cold and stagnating qì can lead to dull pain in the stomach duct and abdomen.

The chapter, "Various Formulas for Treating Cool Qì in the Spleen and Vacuity Rumbling in the Abdomen" in the *Tài Píng Shèng Huì Fāng* ("Great Peace Sagacious Benevolence Formulary") comments as follows:

"When the viscera and bowels lack harmony and the spleen and stomach are vacuous and unable to disperse grain and water, this causes vacuity rumbling in the abdomen and intestines. This is always caused by the fact that an insufficiency of yáng qì and superabundance of yīn qì has allowed the qì of evil cold to hide out in the viscera and run to and fro without dissipating, causing vacuity rumbling in the abdomen and intestines."

As this passage points out, spleen yáng vacuity and a one-sided exuberance of yīn cold cause grain and water to move into the intestinal area, which can result in rumbling intestines.

The chapter, "Abdominal Pain" in the *Jiǎn Míng Yī Gòu* ("Concise Drawn Bow Book of Medicine"), proposes:

"Most patterns of abdominal pain are caused by excessive physical labor, dietary irregularities, insufficiency of center qì, and cold qì exploiting vacuity and intruding, which leads to great pain with a sudden onset."

This quotation explains that patients with insufficiency of spleen qì tend to contract cold invasion, spleen yáng vacuity, and congealing cold qì stagnation, which can lead to pain in the stomach duct and abdomen.

When spleen yáng is vacuous, movement and transformation are impaired. The spleen is unable to assist the stomach in the decomposition of grain and water and fails to benefit from the separation of the clear and turbid by the small intestine. Food and grain are transformed with difficulty, the clear and turbid are not separated, grain and water pour downward, and large intestinal conveyance breaks down. This can cause diarrhea, often manifesting in such symptoms as clear thin stool and nontransformation of whole grains.

The chapter, "Spleen Vacuity Cold Diarrhea" in the *Shèng Jì Zǒng Lù* ("Sages' Salvation Records") explains:

"When grain and water enter the stomach, the spleen is responsible for moving them. However, when spleen-stomach qì is vacuous, cold qì exploits. Then, grain and water fail to be transformed, the clear and turbid fail to be separated, and spreading cold enters the large intestine. When the large intestine contracts cold, it is unable to secure and constrain. This causes diarrhea."

As this passage points out, when spleen yáng is vacuous, warming and movement are impaired, grain and water are not transformed, and the clear and turbid are not separated. This can lead to diarrhea and thin sloppy stool.

When spleen yáng is vacuous and unable to move and transform grain and water, it is extremely likely to influence the harmonious down-bearing of stomach qì. This results in counterflow ascent of stomach qì. When this coincides with abdominal fullness, it can be accompanied by such symptoms as clear drooling from the mouth, nausea and vomiting, and belching and hiccupping.

The *Zhōng Zàng Jīng* ("Central Treasury Canon") chapter, "Discussing the Pulses and Patterns of Vacuity and Repletion, Cold and Heat, Life and Death, and Favorable and Unfavorable Shifts in the Spleen," explains: "Cold causes drooling and foaming from the mouth and inability to eat."

The *Qiān Jīn Yào Fāng* ("A Thousand Gold Pieces Prescriptions") has this comment in the chapter, "Spleen Vacuity Cold":

"When the right bar pulse is yīn and vacuous, it is the foot greater yīn channel. The patient suffers from outpour diarrhea, abdominal fullness and qì counterflow, cholera, vomiting, jaundice, vexation and inability to lie down, and rumbling intestines. This condition is called spleen vacuity cold."

Because spleen yáng vacuity spreads to stomach yáng and the pathome-chanism weighs more heavily on the spleen, it is more common to mention spleen yáng vacuity alone, while the phrase spleen-stomach yáng vacuity is less commonly used.

Grain and water failing to move is treated by warming the center and fortifying the spleen. The recommended formula for conditions that are mainly characterized by torpid intake and reduced eating is *lǐ zhōng wán* (Center-Rectifying Pill) from the *Shāng Hán Lùn* ("On Cold Damage") with additions.

Lǐ Zhōng Wán 理中丸
Center-Rectifying Pill [modified]

rén shēn (人参 ginseng, Ginseng Radix)
gān jiāng (干姜 dried ginger, Zingiberis Rhizoma)
bái zhú (白术 white atractylodes, Atractylodis Macrocephalae Rhizoma)
zhì gān cǎo (炙甘草 mix-fried licorice, Glycyrrhizae Radix cum
　　Liquido Fricta)
Plus:
mù xiāng (木香 costusroot, Aucklandiae Radix)
shā rén (砂仁 amomum, Amomi Fructus)

The recommended formula for conditions characterized by distention in the stomach duct and abdomen that likes pressure is *hòu pò wēn zhōng tāng* (Official Magnolia Bark Center-Warming Decoction) from the *Nèi*

Wài Shāng Biàn Huò Lùn ("Clarification of Perpexities about Internal and External Damage") with additions.

Hòu Pò Wēn Zhōng Tāng 厚朴温中汤 Officinal Magnolia Bark Center-Warming Decoction [modified]
hòu pò (厚朴 officinal magnolia bark, Magnoliae Officinalis Cortex) *gān jiāng* (干姜 dried ginger, Zingiberis Rhizoma) *cǎo dòu kòu* (草豆蔻 Katsumada's galangal seed, Alpiniae Katsumadai Semen) *chén pí* (陈皮 tangerine peel, Citri Reticulatae Pericarpium) *fú líng* (茯苓 poria, Poria) *mù xiāng* (木香 costusroot, Aucklandiae Radix) *zhì gān cǎo* (炙甘草 mix-fried licorice, Glycyrrhizae Radix cum Liquido Fricta) Plus: *rén shēn* (人参 ginseng, Ginseng Radix)

For conditions characterized by dull pain in the stomach duct and abdomen, recommended formulas are *xiǎo jiàn zhōng tāng* (Minor Center-Fortifying Decoction) from the *Shāng Hán Lùn* ("On Cold Damage"), or *huáng qí jiàn zhōng tāng* (Astragalus Center-Fortifying Decoction) from the *Jīn Guì Yào Lüè* ("Essential Prescriptions of the Golden Coffer") (This is *xiǎo jiàn zhōng tāng* (Minor Center-Fortifying Decoction) with the addition of *huáng qí* (Astragali Radix)).

Xiǎo Jiàn Zhōng Tāng 小建中汤 Minor Center-Fortifying Decoction
guì zhī (桂枝 cinnamon twig, Cinnamomi Ramulus) *bái sháo yào* (白芍药 white peony, Paeoniae Radix Alba) *shēng jiāng* (生姜 fresh ginger, Zingiberis Rhizoma Recens) *dà zǎo* (大枣 jujube, Jujubae Fructus) *zhì gān cǎo* (炙甘草 mix-fried licorice, Glycyrrhizae Radix cum Liquido Fricta) *yí táng* (饴糖 malt sugar, Maltosum)

For conditions characterized by severe pain in the stomach duct and abdomen, the recommended formula is *dà jiàn zhōng tāng* (Major Center-Fortifying Decoction) from the *Jīn Guì Yào Lüè* ("Essential Prescriptions of the Golden Coffer"), with additions.

Dà Jiàn Zhōng Tāng 大建中汤
Major Center-Fortifying Decoction [modified]

huā jiāo (花椒 zanthoxylum, Zanthoxyli Pericarpium)
gān jiāng (干姜 dried ginger, Zingiberis Rhizoma)
rén shēn (人参 ginseng, Ginseng Radix)
yí táng (饴糖 malt sugar, Maltosum)
Plus:
gāo liáng jiāng (高良姜 lesser galangal, Alpiniae Officinarum Rhizoma)
xiāng fù zǐ (香附子 cyperus, Cyperi Rhizoma)

For conditions that are mainly characterized by diarrhea, the recommended formula is *fù zǐ lǐ zhōng wán* (Aconite Center-Rectifying Pill) from the *Tài Píng Huì Mín Hé Jì Jú Fāng* ("Tài-Píng Imperial Grace Pharmacy Formulas").

Fù Zǐ Lǐ Zhōng Wán 附子理中丸
Aconite Center-Rectifying Pill

rén shēn (人参 ginseng, Ginseng Radix)
gān jiāng (干姜 dried ginger, Zingiberis Rhizoma)
bái zhú (白术 white atractylodes, Atractylodis Macrocephalae Rhizoma)
zhì gān cǎo (炙甘草 mix-fried licorice, Glycyrrhizae Radix cum Liquido Fricta)
fù zǐ (附子 aconite, Aconiti Radix Lateralis Praeparata)

For conditions that are mainly characterized by retching counterflow, the recommended formula is *dīng yú lǐ zhōng tāng* (Clove and Evodia Center-Rectifying Decoction) from the *Yī Zōng Jīn Jiàn* ("Golden Mirror of Medicine").

Dīng Yú Lǐ Zhōng Tāng 丁萸理中汤
Clove and Evodia Center-Rectifying Decoction

rén shēn (人参 ginseng, Ginseng Radix)
gān jiāng (干姜 dried ginger, Zingiberis Rhizoma)
bái zhú (白术 white atractylodes, Atractylodis Macrocephalae Rhizoma)
zhì gān cǎo (炙甘草 mix-fried licorice, Glycyrrhizae Radix cum Liquido Fricta)
dīng xiāng (丁香 clove, Caryophylli Flos)
wú zhū yú (吴茱萸 evodia, Evodiae Fructus)

水谷失运

清•罗浩《医经余论•续脾胃论》云："脾为己土，其体常湿，故其用阳，譬如湿土之地，非阳光之照，无以生万物也。"强调脾以阳气为本。脾阳可助脾运化，保证水谷正常消化、吸收、转输。若脾阳虚弱，不能推动脾气运化，可使脾气运迟，推动乏力，气滞中焦，引起纳呆食少、脘腹胀满、食后尤甚，或饥时反胀等症状。如《景岳全书•杂证谟•饮食门》曰："凡饮食伤脾之证…实者人皆易知，而寒者、久者、虚者人多不识。…惟其不能化者，则最有中虚之证。故或以不食亦知饥，少食即作胀；或以无饥无饱，全然不思饮食；或以胃虚兼呕而腹满膨膨。"指出饮食久伤，脾易虚寒，运化失职，可致不思饮食，食少腹胀等症状。该书《痞满篇》又曰："脾胃虚者，多兼寒证何也？盖脾胃属土，土虚者多因无火。土寒，则气化无权，故多痞满，此即寒生于中也。"土寒，是指脾胃虚寒，脾阳虚，气化无权，气滞于中，故为心下痞结胀满。

脾阳虚，水谷难消，停滞中焦，阻滞气机，气与水谷相互搏击，水谷往来于肠间，可致肠鸣；寒凝气滞，可致脘腹隐痛。如《太平圣惠方•治脾脏冷气腹内虚鸣诸方》云："脏腑不和，脾胃虚弱，不能消于水谷，则腹肠虚鸣也。此皆阳气不足，阴气有余，邪冷之气，伏留在脏，流走往来不散，故令腹内虚鸣也。"指出脾阳虚，阴寒偏盛，水谷行走于肠间，可引起肠鸣。《简明医彀•腹痛》提出："夫腹痛之证，多因劳役过甚，饮食失节，中气不足，寒气乘虚而客之，故卒然而作大痛。"说明脾气不足，易受寒侵，脾阳虚衰，寒凝气滞，可致脘腹疼痛。

脾阳虚，运化失职，不能助胃腐熟水谷，也不利于小肠分清泌浊，食谷难化，清浊不分，水谷下注，大肠传导失司，可为腹泄、下痢，易见大便清稀、完谷不化等症状。如《圣济总录•脾脏虚冷泄痢》所说："水谷入胃，脾为行之。今脾胃气虚，冷气乘之，则水谷不化，清浊不分，移寒入于大肠，大肠得冷，则不能固敛，故为泄痢。"指出脾阳虚，温运失职，使水谷不化，清浊不分，可致泄泻下痢，大便溏稀。

脾阳虚衰，不能运化水谷，极易影响胃气的和降，导致胃气上逆，可在腹满同时，兼见口吐清涎、恶心呕吐、嗳气呃逆等症状。如《中藏经•论脾脏虚实寒热生死逆顺脉证》说："寒则吐涎沫而不食。"《千金要方•脾虚冷》亦说："右手关上脉阴虚者，足太阴经也。病苦泄注，腹满气逆，霍乱，呕吐，黄疸，心烦不得卧，肠鸣，名曰脾虚冷也。"此因脾阳虚而波及胃阳，病机侧重于脾，习惯上多单提脾阳虚，较少把脾胃阳虚相提并论。

治宜温中健脾。以纳呆食少为主，用《伤寒论》理中丸（人参、干姜、白术、炙甘草）加木香、砂仁。

以脘腹胀满为主，用《内外伤辨惑论》厚朴温中汤（厚朴、干姜、草豆蔻、陈皮、茯苓、木香、炙甘草）加人参。

以脘腹隐痛为主，用《伤寒论》小建中汤（饴糖、桂枝、白芍、生姜、大枣），或《金匮要略》黄芪建中汤（小建中汤加黄芪）。

以脘腹剧痛为主，用《金匮要略》大建中汤（蜀椒、干姜、人参、饴糖）加良姜、香附。

以泄泻为主，用《和剂局方》附子理中丸（理中汤原方加附子）。

以呕逆为主，用《医宗金鉴》丁萸理中汤（理中汤原方加丁香、吴茱萸）治疗。

Literature Review of Grain and Water Failing to Move

📖 *Líng Shū* ("Magic Pivot"), "Five Evils"

> "When yáng qì is insufficient and yīn qì superabundant, it results in cold strike, rumbling intestines, and abdominal pain."

Cold strike means that yáng is vacuous and yīn exuberant. The spleen fails to warm and move, cold congeals and qì stagnates, and grain and water are not transformed. This results in the symptoms of rumbling intestines and abdominal pain.

📖 *Zhū Bìng Yuán Hòu Lùn* ("The Origin and Indicators of Disease"), "Symptoms of Enduring Abdominal Distention"

> "Enduring abdominal distention is caused by evil qì of wind or cold being present in the abdomen. It contends with the bowels and viscera, and the spleen becomes vacuous, causing distention.... When spleen vacuity and the accumulation of cold qì persist for a long time, spleen qì is weakened. Food therefore fails to be dispersed. Moreover, if the cold shifts into the large intestine, and the large intestine, as the path for the waste of grain and water, becomes vacuous and contracts cold, the condition will transform into dysentery."

This passage describes how enduring conditions of abdominal distention and dysentery are caused by spleen yáng vacuity and impaired warming and transportation.

📖 *Tài Píng Shèng Huì Fāng* ("Great Peace Sagacious Benevolence Formulary"), "Treatise on the Spleen"

> "The spleen is located in the center, is made effulgent by the four seasons, receives the essential qì of grain and water, transforms qì and

blood to make them luxuriant, nourishes the physical body, and irrigates the viscera and bowels. If it is vacuous, it engenders cold. Cold results in an exuberance of yīn qì. An exuberance of yīn qì results in distention and fullness in the heart and abdomen, non-dispersal of grain and water... abdominal pain and rumbling intestines, spontaneous diarrhea, and heaviness of the four limbs."

Cold engendered by spleen vacuity impairs movement and transformation and disables the transformation of grain and water. They collect and stagnate in the greater abdomen and percolate down into the intestinal tract, thereby causing abdominal fullness and pain, rumbling intestines, and diarrhea.

📖 *Jǐng Yuè Quán Shū* ("Jǐng-Yuè's Complete Compendium"), "Schema of Miscellaneous Patterns: Glomus and Fullness"

"Vacuity cold glomus can be caused by excessive anxiety and thought, by excessive taxation fatigue, by untimely satiety or hunger, by a failure to arouse spleen qì after an illness, or by the reckless use of cold and restraining preparations in patients with a constitutional spleen-stomach weakness. All of these can result in serious damage to spleen qì. This pattern does not result in distention or oppression, but merely a lack of hunger and no thought of food. When asked whether they suffer from distention or glomus in the chest and abdomen, such patients affirm that they feel it a little, but then again state that they do not have pronounced distention. This is because it is not really a case of distention, but the patients themselves mistake their lack of appetite for distention."

This passage describes how the overuse of bitter and cold treatments damages spleen yáng. Spleen qì fails to move and qì stagnates in the center burner, causing glomus and fullness below the heart.

📖 *Gǔ Jīn Yī Tǒng Dà Quán* ("Complete Compendium of Medical Works, Ancient and Modern"), "Section on Diarrhea"

"The pathocondition of duck-stool diarrhea is caused by cold arising in the lesser abdomen. The spleen is yīn within yīn. Spleen-stomach vacuity causes wind and cold to prevail, resulting in a great exuberance of yīn qì. Yīn exuberance then results in visceral cold, and visceral cold results in the nontransformation of waste, causing black stool that looks like duck slop."

This passage describes how spleen yáng vacuity causes an excessive exuberance of yīn cold. Grain and water fail to be transformed and move straight into the intestines, causing the stool to flow down clearly and thinly like duck slop.

📖 *Sì Shèng Xīn Yuán* ("Four Sages' Original Heart"), "The Origin of Diarrhea"

"Diarrhea means the collapse of the liver and spleen. When yáng is debilitated and earth is damp, spleen yáng is vanquished and unable to distill the qì of grain and water. Therefore, grain and water are mixed together and move down into the two intestines. This causes diarrhea."

This passage points out that diarrhea can be caused by spleen yáng vacuity and center qì fall, resulting in failure to move and transform grain and water so that they percolate down into the intestinal area.

📖 *Lèi Zhèng Zhì Cái* ("Systematized Patterns with Clear-Cut Treatments"), "Vomiting"

"Vomiting is a symptom caused by the failure of stomach qì to downbear... In cases of abdominal distention, pain, and vomiting that are caused by spleen yáng weakness and inability to move and transform, use acrid and warm medicinals to move the stagnation. [Select] *xiāng shā liù jūn zǐ tāng* (Costusroot and Amomum Six Gentlemen Decoction) with the addition of *yì zhì rén* (Alpiniae Oxyphyllae Fructus), *hòu pò* (Magnoliae Officinalis Cortex), and *shén qū* (Massa Medicata Fermentata)."

The pathomechanism of vomiting is caused by the failure of stomach qì to bear downward, but spleen yáng vacuity and impaired warming and movement can also cause the various symptoms of retching counterflow due to stomach qì failing to downbear.

文献评述

《灵枢•五邪》"阳气不足，阴气有余，则寒中肠鸣腹痛。"寒中，是阳虚阴盛，脾失温运，寒凝气滞，水谷不化，故可引起肠鸣腹痛等症状。

《诸病源候论•久腹胀候》："久腹胀者，此由风冷邪气在腹内不散，与脏腑相搏，脾虚故胀；…脾虚寒气积久，脾气衰弱，故食不消也；而冷移入大肠，大肠为水谷糟粕之道路，虚而受冷，故变为痢也。"论述久病腹胀下痢，是由脾阳虚衰，温运失职所致。

《太平圣惠方•脾脏论》："夫脾者，位居中央，王（旺）于四季，受水谷之精气，化气血以荣华，用养身形，灌溉脏腑者也。若虚则生寒，寒则阴气盛，阴气盛则心腹胀满，水谷不消…腹痛肠鸣，时自泻利，四肢沉重。"脾虚生寒，运化失职，水谷不化，停滞大腹，下渗肠道，故致腹满腹痛、肠鸣泄利诸症。

《景岳全书•杂证谟•痞满》："虚寒之痞，或过于忧思，或过于劳倦，饥饱失时，或病后脾气未醒，或脾胃素弱之人而妄用寒凉克伐之剂，以致重伤脾气者，皆能有之。其证则无胀无闷，但不知饥，亦不欲食。问其胸腹胀否，则曰亦觉有些，但又曰不甚胀，盖本非胀也，止(只)因不欲食而自疑为胀耳。"论述过用苦寒，损伤脾阳，脾气失运，气滞中焦，引起心下痞满的病机及临床表现。

《古今医统大全·泻泄门》："鹜泻者，少腹生寒而为此证。盖阴中之阴脾也，脾胃虚弱，为风寒所胜，则阴气大盛，阴盛则脏寒，脏寒则糟粕不化，大便黑，状似鹜溏者是也。"论述脾阳虚，阴寒太盛，水谷不化，直趋肠中，大便可泻下清稀如鹜溏。

《四圣心源·泄利根源》："泄利者，肝脾之陷也…。阳衰土湿，脾阳陷败，不能蒸水化气，则水谷混合，下趋二肠，而为泄利。"指出脾阳虚衰，中气下陷，不能运化水谷，下渗肠间，则为泄利。

《类证治裁·呕吐》："呕吐症，胃气失降使然也。…其脾阳衰，不能运化，腹胀腹痛呕吐者，用辛温行滞，香砂六君子汤加益智、厚朴、神曲。"呕吐的病机为胃气不降，但脾阳虚衰，温运失职，亦可引起胃气失降而致呕逆诸证。

Summary of Grain and Water Failing to Move
1. Spleen Failing to Warm and Move
Torpid intake and reduced eating, distention in the stomach duct and abdomen that likes pressure and is aggravated after meals, distention even when hungry.
2. Congealing Cold Qì Stagnation
Rumbling intestines, dull pain in the stomach duct and abdomen.
3. Inability to Transform Food
Diarrhea, clear thin stool, nontransformation of whole grains.
4. Counterflow Ascent of Stomach Qì
Clear drooling from the mouth, nausea and vomiting, belching and hiccup.

水谷失运
脾失温运——纳呆食少，脘腹胀满，食后尤甚，饥时反胀。
寒凝气滞——肠鸣，脘腹隐痛。
不能化食——腹泄下痢，大便清稀，完谷不化。
胃气上逆——口吐清涎，恶心呕吐，嗳气呃逆。

2.2 Water-Damp Failing to Transform

Through its warming action, spleen yáng assists in splenic movement and transformation by promoting the movement of water-humor. It causes the liquids to be distributed throughout the body and moistens the whole body. At the same time, it is also able to assist the spleen's movement by expelling water-damp. Spleen yáng causes turbid damp to be transported down to the bladder and form urine, and can also allow turbid damp to percolate down into the large intestine and follow the stool to be expelled outside the body. When spleen yáng is vacuous, qì transformation lacks force and yáng fails to transform the fluids. This can result in internal collection of water-damp.

When spleen yáng is vacuous and unable to move water, water collects below the heart, causing phlegm-rheum and symptoms of propping fullness in the chest and rib-side, palpitations and shortness of breath, the sound of quivering water below the heart, and aversion to cold in the back in an area the size of the palm of the hand.

As explained in the chapter, "Phlegm-rheum" in the *Qiān Jīn Fāng Yǎn Yì* ("Expanded Thousand Gold Formulas"):

> "When phlegm lodges below the heart, it causes aversion to cold in the back; when it lodges under the rib-side, it causes pain and tautness in the supraclavicular fossa. During periods of remission, it causes shortness of breath, thirst, and joint running pain in the four limbs; when it erupts, it causes panting and fullness, counterflow vomiting, aversion to cold and heat effusion, back and lumbar pain, and spontaneous tearing; when exacerbated, it causes shaking and twitching of the body. This is called deep-lying rheum. Deep-lying rheum refers to the deep-lying and static nature of lodged rheum."

Although the formation of deep-lying rheum is related to the lung, spleen, and kidney, spleen yáng vacuity causing failure to warm and transform and collecting water, cold, and liquid is the most direct pathomechanism. The fact that one can use *líng guì zhú gān tāng* (Poria, Cinnamon Twig, White Atractylodes, and Licorice Decoction) as an effective treatment also serves as secondary proof.

An insufficiency of spleen yáng and poor qì transformation mean that water qì cannot be transported normally. It soaks into the viscera and bowels, percolates out into the channels and network vessels, pours into ravines and valleys, and floods the skin and flesh, causing water swelling. As a result of spleen yáng vacuity, earth is unable to dam water, and water-damp rushes downward. Therefore, the water swelling is most pronounced below the lumbus, and pits when pressure is applied. When water qì floods the skin and flesh and fails to be transported down to the bladder so that the source of transformation is insufficient, it causes short voidings of scant urine.

The chapter, "Water swelling" in the *Chóng Dìng Yán Shì Jì Shēng Fāng* ("Revised Life-Saving Formulas of Master Yán"), states:

> "The disease of water swelling is always caused by a timidity and short-age of true yáng, spleen and stomach taxation damage, spleen and stom-ach cold, and cold accumulation transforming into water. The spleen is earth and the kidney is water. The kidney is able to contain water, and the spleen is able to house water. When kidney water fails to flow or when the spleen's housing is congested, the result is panting and cough above, swelling in the skin of the feet and knees below, puffy face and abdomi-nal distention, and inhibited urination."

Both spleen and kidney yáng vacuity can lead to water swelling, but this passage describes mainly the pathomechanism by which spleen yáng va-cuity causes cold to collect and transform into water, resulting in water swelling. It also explains the special significance of spleen yáng vacuity and nontransformation of water-damp in the process of forming water swelling.

When spleen yáng is vacuous, it is unable to warm and transform wa-ter-humor. Water-damp flows downward, and dampness and turbidity congeal and accumulate, transforming into white vaginal discharge. This can lead to an increase in white vaginal discharge. In an analysis of the pathomechanism of white vaginal discharge, the chapter, "Vaginal Dis-charge" in the *Nǚ Kē Cuō Yào* ("Synopsis of Gynecology"), points out: "Spleen and stomach depletion cause yáng qì to fall." The chapter, "White Vaginal Discharge and Red Strangury" in the *Xiān Xǐng Zhāi Yī Xué Guǎng Bǐ Jì* ("Broad-Ranging Medical Notes from the Studio of Early Awaking"), also explains:

> "An increase in white vaginal discharge means spleen vacuity. Liver qì depression causes damage to the spleen. When the spleen is damaged, the qì of damp earth falls. This means that spleen essence is not composed and unable to transport construction-blood, but instead discharges a white slippery substance below."

The pathocondition of vaginal discharge falls under the responsibility of spleen-earth. When spleen yáng is injured, the absorption of warmth is weakened and spleen essence loses its composure and is unable to trans-form essence into construction-blood. Instead, it causes damp qì to flow downward and change into a white slippery substance that is discharged straight down from the vagina in an unstoppable flow. This is an impor-tant pathomechanism for the generation of white vaginal discharge.

Spleen yáng vacuity causes an internal exuberance of yīn cold. Yáng qì is devitalized, the qì transformation is inhibited, and water-humor fails to move. Instead, it collects to form dampness and turn into water. Cold and water bind with each other, the clear and turbid are combined, the passage ways are stopped, the blood in the network vessels is stagnant and obstructed, and water and blood adhere to each other. When they are not transformed for a long time, they block the center burner, causing a slightly enlarged abdomen and drum distention. One can observe the symptoms of abdominal distention and fullness that feels like a bag of water when pressed and eases up slightly when heat is applied, a fatigued cumbersome essence-spirit, fear of cold and laziness to move, and scant urine and sloppy stool.

"Treatise on Center Fullness and Abdominal Distention" in the *Lán Shì Mì Cáng* ("Secret Treasure of the Orchid Chamber") points out:

> "[Abdominal fullness] is always due to spleen and stomach qì vacuity and inability to move and transform essence and to dam grain and water, causing them to accumulate instead of dissipating and to form distention and fullness... Cold distention is generally more common than heat distention."

This passage explains that abdominal distention is mainly caused by spleen yáng vacuity.

The chapter, "Origin of Swelling and Distention" in the *Zá Bìng Yuán Liú Xī Zhú* ("Incisive Light on the Source of Miscellaneous Disease"), further points out:

> "The condition of drum distention is rooted in the spleen.... It is potentially caused by anger damaging the liver and gradually eroding the person's spleen, to the point of extreme spleen vacuity. As a result, yīn and yáng fail to interact, the turbid and the clear are mixed together, and the sagging pathways are stopped.... Therefore, the person's abdomen is distended and enlarged, the center is empty of any substances, the external skin is stretched tight, and the person is unable to eat an evening meal when they have eaten in the morning."

In fact, the formation of drum distention is not only caused by the sole vacuity of spleen yáng, but is usually closely related to the cross counter-flow of liver qì. Therefore, Shěn Jīn-Áo summarized this pathomechanism as "vanquished earth and robbed wood."

Water-damp failing to transform is treated by warming the center and fortifying the spleen, and by eliminating dampness and disinhibiting water. When water collects below the heart, it is treated by warming the center and supplementing yáng, and by transforming phlegm and dispersing rheum. The recommended formula is *líng guì zhú gān tāng* (Poria, Cinnamon Twig, White Atractylodes, and Licorice Decoction) from the *Shāng Hán Lùn* ("On Cold Damage") with the addition of *fù zǐ* (Aconiti Radix Lateralis Praeparata).

Líng Guì Zhú Gān Tāng 苓桂术甘汤
Poria, Cinnamon Twig, White Atractylodes, and Licorice Decoction

fú líng (茯苓 poria, Poria)

guì zhī (桂枝 cinnamon twig, Cinnamomi Ramulus)

bái zhú (白术 white atractylodes, Atractylodis Macrocephalae Rhizoma)

zhì gān cǎo (炙甘草 mix-fried licorice, Glycyrrhizae Radix cum
   Liquido Fricta)

Plus:

fù zǐ (附子 aconite, Aconiti Radix Lateralis Praeparata)

Conditions that are mainly characterized by water swelling are treated with *shí pí sǎn* (Spleen-Firming Powder) from the *Chóng Dìng Yán Shì Jì Shēng Fāng* ("Revised Life-Saving Formulas of Master Yán").

Shí Pí Sǎn 实脾散
Spleen-Firming Powder

hòu pò (厚朴 official magnolia bark, Magnoliae Officinalis Cortex)

bái zhú (白术 white atractylodes, Atractylodis Macrocephalae Rhizoma)

mù guā (木瓜 chaenomeles, Chaenomelis Fructus)

mù xiāng (木香 costusroot, Aucklandiae Radix)

cǎo guǒ (草果 tsaoko, Tsaoko Fructus)

bīng láng (槟榔 areca, Arecae Semen)

fù zǐ (附子 aconite, Aconiti Radix Lateralis Praeparata)

fú líng (茯苓 poria, Poria)

gān jiāng (干姜 dried ginger, Zingiberis Rhizoma)

zhì gān cǎo (炙甘草 mix-fried licorice, Glycyrrhizae Radix cum
   Liquido Fricta)

Conditions that are mainly characterized by white vaginal discharge are treated by warming the center and transforming dampness, and by upbearing the clear and checking the discharge. The recommended formula is *wán dài tāng* (Discharge-Ceasing Decoction) from the *Fù Qīng Zhǔ Nǚ Kē* ("Fù Qīng-Zhǔ's Gynecology"), with additions.

Wán Dài Tāng 完带汤
Discharge-Ceasing Decoction

bái zhú (白术 white atractylodes, Atractylodis Macrocephalae Rhizoma)

shān yào (山药 dioscorea, Dioscoreae Rhizoma)

rén shēn (人参 ginseng, Ginseng Radix)

gān cǎo (甘草 licorice, Glycyrrhizae Radix)

bái sháo yào (白芍药 white peony, Paeoniae Radix Alba)

chē qián zǐ (车前子 plantago seed, Plantaginis Semen)

cāng zhú (苍术 atractylodes, Atractylodis Rhizoma)

chén pí (陈皮 tangerine peel, Citri Reticulatae Pericarpium)

jīng jiè tàn (荆芥炭 charred schizonepeta, Schizonepetae Herba et Flos Carbonisatae)

chái hú (柴胡 bupleurum, Bupleuri Radix)

Plus:

gān jiāng (干姜 dried ginger, Zingiberis Rhizoma)

lù jiǎo shuāng (鹿角霜 degelatinated deer antler, Cervi Cornu Degelatinatum)

qiàn shí (芡实 euryale, Euryales Semen)

Conditions characterized by drum distention are treated with modifications based on a combination of *fù zǐ lǐ zhōng wán* (Aconite Center-Rectifying Pill) with *wǔ líng sǎn* (Poria Five Powder). *Wǔ líng sǎn* comes from the *Shāng Hán Lùn* ("On Cold Damage").

Fù Zǐ Lǐ Zhōng Wán 附子理中丸
Aconite Center-Rectifying Pill

rén shēn (人参 ginseng, Ginseng Radix)

gān jiāng (干姜 dried ginger, Zingiberis Rhizoma)

bái zhú (白术 white atractylodes, Atractylodis Macrocephalae Rhizoma)

zhì gān cǎo (炙甘草 mix-fried licorice, Glycyrrhizae Radix cum Liquido Fricta)

fù zǐ (附子 aconite, Aconiti Radix Lateralis Praeparata)

Wǔ Líng Sǎn 五苓散
Poria Five Powder

bái zhú (白术 white atractylodes, Atractylodis Macrocephalae Rhizoma)

fú líng (茯苓 poria, Poria)

zhū líng (猪苓 polyporus, Polyporus)

zé xiè (泽泻 alisma, Alismatis Rhizoma)

guì zhī (桂枝 cinnamon twig, Cinnamomi Ramulus)

水湿不化

脾阳温煦，助脾运化，推动水液，使水津四布，滋润全身。同时又可协助脾运，排泄水湿，使浊湿下输膀胱，化生尿液，或使浊湿下渗大肠，随同大便，排出体外。脾阳虚衰，气化无权，阳不化津，可致水湿内停。脾阳虚不能行水，水停心下，则为痰饮，常见胸胁支满、心悸气短、心下有振水音、背恶寒如掌大等症状。如《千金方衍义•痰饮》说："留饮伏心下则背恶寒，留于胁下则痛引缺盆，平时则短气而渴，四肢历节痛，发则喘满吐逆，寒热，背痛腰疼，目泣自出，剧则振振身瞤，谓之伏饮，伏饮即留饮之伏而不动者。"伏饮的形成，虽与肺脾肾三脏均有关系，但脾阳虚衰，失于温化，水寒津停是最直接的病机。用苓桂术甘汤可取得治疗效果，亦是间接的证明。

脾阳不足，气化不行，水气不能正常输布，浸渍于脏腑，渗透于经络，流注于溪谷，泛溢于肌肤，发为水肿。由于脾阳虚，土不制水，水湿趋下，故水肿腰以下为甚，按之凹陷不起。水气泛溢肌肤，不能下输膀胱，化源不足，则小便短少。如《济生方•水肿》云："水肿为病，皆由真阳怯少，劳伤脾胃，脾胃既寒，积寒化水。盖脾者土也，肾者水也，肾能摄水，脾能舍水，肾水不流，脾舍埋塞，是以上为喘呼咳嗽，下为足膝胕肿，面浮腹胀，小便不利。"脾肾阳虚均可引起水肿，这里却重点阐述脾阳虚衰，积寒化水而形成水肿的病机，说明脾阳虚，水湿不化在形成水肿的过程中具有重要意义。

脾阳虚衰，不能温化水液，水湿下流，湿浊凝聚，化生白带，可引起白带增多。如《女科撮要•带下》在分析白带病机时指为："脾胃亏损，阳气下陷。"《先醒斋医学广笔记•白带赤淋》亦说："白带多是脾虚，盖肝气郁则脾受伤，脾伤则湿土之气下陷，是脾精不守，不能输为营血，而下白滑之物矣。"带下之症，责之脾土。其中脾阳损伤，温摄无力，脾精失守，不能化精微为营血，反为湿气下流，变成白滑之物由前阴直下，不能自止，是生成白带的重要病机。

脾阳虚衰，阴寒内盛，阳气不振，气化不利，水液不行，停聚为湿，积而成水，寒水互结，清浊相混，隧道不通，血络瘀阻，水血胶结，日久不化，阻塞中焦，其腹渐大，而成鼓胀。可见腹部胀满，按之如囊裹水，得热稍舒，精神困倦，畏寒懒动，小便少，大便溏等症状。《兰室秘藏•中满腹胀论》认为腹胀"皆由脾胃之气虚弱，不能运化精微而制水谷，聚而不散而成胀满。"而且"大抵寒胀多而热胀少"，说明腹胀主要由于脾阳虚所致。《杂病源流犀烛•肿胀源流》进一步指出："鼓胀病根在脾…或由怒气伤肝，渐蚀其脾，脾虚之极，故阴阳不交，清浊相混，坠道不通…故其腹胀大，中空无物，外皮绷急，且食不能暮食也。"其实鼓胀的形成，不独为脾阳自虚，常与肝气横逆有密切关系，故沈金鳌把这一病机过程概括为"土败木贼"。

治宜温中健脾，除湿利水。水停心下，治宜温中补阳，化痰消饮，用《伤寒论》苓桂术甘汤（茯苓、桂枝、白术、炙甘草）加附子。

以水肿为主，用《重订严氏济生方》实脾散（厚朴、白术、木瓜、木香、草果仁、大腹子、附子、茯苓、干姜、炙甘草）。

以白带为主，治宜温中化湿，升清止带，用《傅青主女科》完带汤（白术、山药、人参、甘草、白芍、车前子、苍术、陈皮、黑芥穗、柴胡）加干姜、鹿角霜、芡实。

以鼓胀为主，用附子理中丸合《伤寒论》五苓散（白术、茯苓、猪苓、泽泻、桂枝）加减进行治疗。

Literature Review of Water-Damp Failing to Transform

📖 *Sì Shèng Xīn Yuán* ("Four Sages' Original Heart"), "The Roots of Phlegm-Rheum"

"When phlegm-rheum is deeply lodged, it putrefies and congests, obstructs the pathways of qì and blood circulation, and blocks the communication of the essence-spirit. The various diseases all arise from this.. When original qì is depleted, they summarily result due to the vanquishing of spleen yáng. Going along the foot greater yīn spleen [channel], damp earth serves as leader, and the hand greater yīn lung [channel] transforms qì from damp earth. Dampness is effulgent and the spleen depleted, the dispersal of grain and water is delayed, lung and spleen qì is depressed and fails to diffuse, and phlegm-drool is engendered."

This passage describes in detail the pathomechanism by which spleen yáng vanquishes and water-damp fails to move, engendering phlegm-rheum.

📖 *Zhū Bìng Yuán Hòu Lùn* ("Origin and Indicators of Disease"), "The Various Symptoms of Women's Postpartum Conditions: The Symptom of Postpartum Diarrhea and Swelling"

"Childbirth-related taxation damages construction and defense and makes the spleen and stomach vacuous. Wind and cold exploit this, grain and water are not bound, and the large intestine is vacuous, causing diarrhea. Diarrhea is accompanied by swelling because the spleen governs earth and its indicator is the flesh. It is the nature of earth to overcome water. However, when spleen qì is debilitated, it is unable to overcome and disperse water. Water qì flows and spills over to dissipate into the skin, thereby causing swelling."

Debilitation of spleen qì means that spleen yáng is vacuous and unable to move and transform water-damp. Water qì spills and turns into water swelling.

📖 *Zhèng Yīn Mài Zhì* ("Pathoconditions: Causes, Pulses, and Treatments"), "Spleen Vacuity-Related Generalized Swelling"

"The pathocondition of spleen vacuity water swelling [is characterized by] clear and smooth flowing urination, sloppy stool and diarrhea, withered-yellow facial complexion, laziness and timidity in speaking, and swelling. These are the symptoms for spleen vacuity swelling... After major illness or enduring diarrhea, the true yīn of spleen-earth is damaged. It fails to perform its function of converting and transporting and is unable to move and transport grain and water, causing the various channels to congeal and congest, which results in the pathocondition of swelling."

Enduring illness or diarrhea can damage the spleen's true yīn and can also damage the spleen's true yáng. When spleen yáng is depleted, movement and transformation of the fluids breaks down. This can then cause the various channels to congeal and congest, and water swelling erupts.

📖 *Nǚ Kē Cuō Yào* ("Synopsis of Gynecology"), "Vaginal Discharge"

"Due to the six excesses and seven emotions, or by intoxication, over-eating, sexual taxation, [the consumption of] fatty meats, refined grains, and strong flavors, or the ingestion of dry formulas, spleen qì is depleted and yáng qì falls."

This passage points out that vaginal discharge originates from a number of causes that injure the spleen and stomach, deplete the spleen's yáng qì, and prevent water-damp from moving upward and instead cause it to fall downward, congeal, and accumulate, turning into white vaginal discharge.

📖 *Sì Shèng Xīn Yuán* ("Four Sages' Original Heart"), "The Roots of Drum Distention"

"Drum distention means the vanquishing of center qì... Once center qì is vanquished, qì fails to transform water and lies depressed in the lower body, which is what is called qì drum. When water spills upward instead of transforming into qì, it causes water swelling... The root cause of this situation lies in earth becoming damp and yáng becoming vanquished. When damp earth fails to move, metal and wood are depressed and the upbearing and downbearing is congested."

Vanquishing of center qì refers to spleen yáng being debilitated and failing to move and transform water-damp. As a result, liver qì is depressed, the qì dynamic is obstructed, qì and water become congested and bind, and the blood flow is inhibited. This causes drum distention.

文献评述

《四圣心源•痰饮根源》："盖痰饮伏留，腐败壅阻，碍气血环周之路，格精神交济之关，诸病皆起，变化无恒，随其本气所亏而发，而总由脾阳之败。缘足太阴脾以湿土为令，手太阴肺从湿土化气，湿旺脾亏，水谷消迟，肺脾之气，郁而不宣，淫生痰涎。"详细论述脾阳衰败，水湿不运，化生痰饮的病机。

《诸病源候论•妇人产后病诸候•产后利肿候》："因产劳伤营卫，脾胃虚弱，风冷乘之，水谷不结，大肠虚则泄成利也。利而肿者，脾主土，候肌肉，土性本克水，今脾气衰微，不能克消于水，水气流溢，散在皮肤，故令肿也。"脾气衰微，即是脾阳虚衰，不能运化水湿，水气泛溢，而成水肿。

《症因脉治•脾虚身肿》："脾虚水肿之症，小便清利，大便溏泄，面色萎黄，语音懒怯，常肿常退，此脾虚肿之症也。…大病后，久泻后，脾土之真阴受伤，转输之官失职，不能运化水谷，则诸经凝窒，而肿症作矣。"久病久泻，既可伤脾之真阴，又可伤脾之真阳。脾阳亏损，运化水液失司，才可能诸经凝窒，发为水肿。

《女科撮要•带下》："或因六淫七情，或因醉饱房劳，或因膏粱厚味，或服燥剂所致，脾胃亏损，阳气下陷。"指出带下是由各种原因，损伤脾胃，脾的阳气亏损，水湿不能上输，反而下陷，凝聚成为白带。

《四圣心源•鼓胀根源》："鼓胀者，中气之败也。…中气一败，则气不化水而抑郁于下，是谓气鼓；水不化气而泛溢于上，是为水胀。…而其根，总因土湿而阳败，湿土不运，则金木郁而升降窒故也。"中气败，即指脾阳衰败，不能运化水湿，肝气郁滞，气机阻碍，气水壅结，血行不畅，而成鼓胀。

Summary of Water-Damp Failing to Transform

1. Water Collecting Below the Heart

   Phlegm-rheum, propping fullness in the chest and rib-sides, palpitations and shortness of breath, a sound of quivering water below the heart, aversion to cold in the back in an area the size of the palm of the hand.

2. Spilling into the Skin and Flesh

   Water swelling that is most pronounced below the lumbus and pits when pressure is applied, short voidings of scant urine.

3. Water-Damp Flowing Downward

Increased white vaginal discharge.

4. Water and Blood Binding

Drum distention, abdominal distention and fullness that feels like a bag of water when pressed and eases up slightly when heat is applied, fatigued and cumbersome essence-spirit, fear of cold and laziness to move, scant urine and sloppy stool.

水湿不化

水停心下—痰饮，胸胁支满，心悸气短，心下振水音，背恶寒如掌大。

泛溢肌肤—水肿腰以下为甚，按之凹陷不起，小便短少。

水湿下流—白带增多。

水血胶结—鼓胀，腹部胀满，按之如囊裹水，得热稍舒，精神困倦，畏寒懒动，小便短少，大便溏稀。

2.4 Impaired Warming

The spleen governs upbearing of the clear. When spleen yáng is strong and effulgent, it is able to warm and transform the liquids and humors and distribute and dissipate them upward to enrich and moisten the mouth, nose, and throat. When spleen yáng is vacuous, its functions of warming, promoting movement, and distributing fluids are impaired. Thus, although there are fluids collecting inside the body, they are not distributed above to the mouth and throat. A patient with this condition will therefore suffer from dryness and discomfort in the throat, constant desire to drink water in the mouth, and slow swallowing to enrich and moisten the throat, possibly with dry mouth with desire to drink, but drinking only small amounts, or with thirst with a liking for hot drinks. When the tongue body loses its supply of warmth and nourishment, the tongue becomes stiff and difficult to turn. If the vocal tract is deprived of warmth, nourishment, and stimulation by yáng qì and moreover lacks the enrichment and moistening by the fluids, the quality of voice and enunciation are impaired. This manifests as low and deep speech and a hoarse voice.

"Treatise on Morbid Pulses of the Spleen" in the *Qiān Jīn Fāng* ("Thousand Gold Pieces Formulary") explains:

"Spleen damage results in cold. Cold results in vacuity. Vacuity results in generalized emaciation, a deep and hoarse voice, a sound as if hitting a drum, a stiff tongue that cannot be turned, a tendency to swallow and salivate, and a clenched jaw and black lips."

The condition of dry mouth and throat is not necessarily caused by heat exuberance damaging liquid, but can also result from spleen yáng vacuity, from qì failing to transform liquid, and from liquid failing to bear upward. Later generations often tended to wrongly identify heat exuberance or yīn depletion as main causes for this condition, resulting in faulty diagnoses. Thus, this condition must be identified very carefully.

When spleen yáng is insufficient, yáng vacuity causes yīn exuberance. Cold governs congealing and stagnation, contracture and tautness. Since the greater abdomen belongs to the spleen, the qì dynamic in the intestinal tract congeals and stagnates, the channels become hypertonic, and their flow is blocked and stopped, resulting in abdominal pain. This condition is characterized especially by cold pain in the abdominal area, possibly with severe pain that likes warmth and pressure. Upward counterflow of cold qì can result in heart pain; a downward attack can lead to lesser abdominal pain.

The chapter, "On the Pulses and Patterns of Vacuity and Repletion, Cold and Heat, Life and Death, and Favorable and Unfavorable Shifts in the Spleen" in the *Zhōng Zàng Jīng* ("Central Treasury Canon"), states:

> "When there is cold in the spleen and heat in the feet, they both cause pain in the patient's abdomen and inability to get food down. Moreover, the patient will suffer from a stiff tongue, halting speech, retracted testicles, and tautness and pain in the thighs."

The chapter, "Pain Caused by Attacks of Cold Qì from the Spleen on the Heart and Abdomen" in the *Shèng Jì Zǒng Lù* ("Sages' Salvation Records"), also explains:

> "It is said that foot greater yīn is the channel of the spleen. When wind and cold interfere with it, contend with the spleen viscus, and strike at right qì, upward surges to the heart cause heart pain, and attacks on the abdomen below cause abdominal pain. As a rule, one should use warming treatments to regulate it."

In clinic, the majority of cases manifest with abdominal pain, predominantly related to spleen yáng vacuity and congealing cold qì stagnation. When spleen yáng is vacuous, yáng fails to provide warmth, vacuity cold arises internally, and cold qì and right qì struggle, striking and attacking each other. This causes rumbling intestines.

The chapter, "Spleen Cold Qì-Related Vacuity Rumbling in the Abdomen" in the *Shèng Jì Zǒng Lù* ("Sages' Salvation Records") notes:

> "The spleen constitutes the central region.... If the spleen is vacuous, cold qì and right qì strike at each other, causing vacuity rumbling inside

the abdomen…. What is called "fulminant qì like thunder" in the *Nèi Jīng* ("Inner Canon") is caused by the heat and cold of yīn and yáng striking at each other."

Defensive yáng has the functions of regulating body temperature, opening and closing the sweat pores, and warming the viscera and bowels. It is generated in the lower burner, nourished in the center burner, and diffused by the upper burner. When spleen-stomach yáng qì is strong and effulgent, it provides a source for nourishment, and defensive yáng is therefore abundant. When spleen-stomach qì is vacuous, it fails to provide warmth and nourishment. It is unable to secure the external defenses, the skin and the viscera and bowels are not warmed, and the creation of heat is reduced. This can lead to such symptoms of vacuity cold as fear of cold, perspiration, and susceptibility to the common cold.

The spleen governs the four limbs, which are the root of all yáng. When spleen yáng is vacuous, yáng qì is unable to reach the limbs, which manifests as counterflow cold of the limbs.

When spleen yáng is vacuous, it fails to promote movement. As a result, qì and blood are unable to rise and provide luxuriance for the face, which manifests as a pale white facial complexion and pale lips and tongue. "Treatise on [the Effects of] Spleen-Stomach Vacuity on the Lung" in the *Pí Wèi Lùn* ("On the Spleen and Stomach") comments:

> "Spleen and stomach vacuity causes fatigue and somnolence and loss of use of the limbs… simultaneously manifesting in lung conditions, aversion to cold after a soaking, dullness and melancholy, and a hateful and disharmonious facial expression. These are the result of yáng qì failing to stretch."

This means that when spleen yáng is vacuous, it is unable to engender defensive yáng, so that yáng is vacuous and fails to provide warmth, resulting in the symptoms of fear of cold and a white face.

Impaired warming is treated by warming the center and dissipating cold. For conditions that are characterized by dryness of the mouth and throat, the recommended formula is *qī wèi bái zhú sǎn* (Seven-Ingredient White Atractylodes Powder) from the *Xiǎo Ér Yào Zhèng Zhí Jué* ("Key to Diagnosis and Treatment of Children's Diseases"), with the addition of *pào jiāng* (Zingiberis Rhizoma Praeparatum) and *shēng má* (Cimicifugae Rhizoma).

Qī Wèi Bái Zhú Sǎn 七味白朮散
Seven-Ingredient White Atractylodes Powder

bái zhú (白朮 white atractylodes, Atractylodis Macrocephalae Rhizoma)
rén shēn (人参 ginseng, Ginseng Radix)

gān cǎo (甘草 licorice, Glycyrrhizae Radix)

fú líng (茯苓 poria, Poria)

huò xiāng (藿香 agastache, Agastaches Herba)

mù xiāng (木香 costusroot, Aucklandiae Radix)

gé gēn (葛根 pueraria, Puerariae Radix)

Plus:

pào jiāng (炮姜 blast-fried ginger, Zingiberis Rhizoma Praeparatum)

shēng má (升麻 cimicifuga, Cimicifugae Rhizoma)

For conditions that are mainly characterized by a deep voice and a rigid tongue that cannot be turned, the recommended treatment is *má huáng sǎn* (Ephedra Powder) from the *Tài Píng Shèng Huì Fāng* ("Great Peace Sagacious Benevolence Formulary") with modifications.

Má Huáng Sǎn 麻黄散
Ephedra Powder

fù zǐ (附子 aconite, Aconiti Radix Lateralis Praeparata)

guì xīn (桂心 shaved cinnamon bark, Cinnamomi Cortex Rasus)

gān jiāng (干姜 dried ginger, Zingiberis Rhizoma)

bái zhú (白术 white atractylodes, Atractylodis Macrocephalae Rhizoma)

rén shēn (人参 ginseng, Ginseng Radix)

má huáng (麻黄 ephedra, Ephedrae Herba)

xì xīn (细辛 asarum, Asari Herba)

shí gāo (石膏 gypsum, Gypsum Fibrosum)

líng yáng jiǎo (羚羊角 antelope horn, Saigae Tataricae Cornu)

fáng fēng (防风 saposhnikovia, Saposhnikoviae Radix)

qín jiāo (秦艽 large gentian, Gentianae Macrophyllae Radix)

fáng jǐ (防己 fangji, Stephaniae Tetrandrae Radix)

chuān xiōng (川芎 chuanxiong, Chuanxiong Rhizoma)

xìng rén (杏仁 apricot kernel, Armeniacae Semen)

gān cǎo (甘草 licorice, Glycyrrhizae Radix)

For conditions characterized by abdominal cold and severe pain, the recommended formula is *fù zǐ gēng mǐ tāng* (Aconite and Rice Decoction) from the *Jīn Guì Yào Lüè* ("Essential Prescriptions of the Golden Coffer") with additions.

Fù Zǐ Gēng Mǐ Tāng (附子粳米汤
Aconite and Rice Decoction

fù zǐ (附子 aconite, Aconiti Radix Lateralis Praeparata)

bàn xià (半夏 pinellia, Pinelliae Rhizoma)

gān cǎo (甘草 licorice, Glycyrrhizae Radix)

dà zǎo (大枣 jujube, Jujubae Fructus)

gēng mǐ (粳米 non-glutinous rice, Oryzae Semen)

Plus:

chuān jiāo (川椒 zanthoxylum, Zanthoxyli Pericarpium)

gān jiāng (干姜 dried ginger, Zingiberis Rhizoma)

shā rén (砂仁 amomum, Amomi Fructus)

Conditions that are characterized by fear of cold and cold limbs and white face and pale limbs are best treated with *lǐ zhōng wán* (Center-Rectifying Pill) from the *Shāng Hán Lùn* ("On Cold Damage"), with the addition of *guì zhī* (Cinnamomi Ramulus) and *fù zǐ* (Aconiti Radix Lateralis Praeparata).

Lǐ Zhōng Wán 理中丸
Center-Rectifying Pill)

gān jiāng (干姜 dried ginger, Zingiberis Rhizoma)

rén shēn (人参 ginseng, Ginseng Radix)

bái zhú (白术 white atractylodes, Atractylodis Macrocephalae Rhizoma)

gān cǎo (甘草 licorice, Glycyrrhizae Radix)

Plus:

fù zǐ (附子 aconite, Aconiti Radix Lateralis Praeparata)

guì zhī (桂枝 cinnamon twig, Cinnamomi Ramulus)

温煦失职

脾主升清，脾阳健旺，能温化津液，向上布散，以滋润口、鼻、咽喉。脾阳虚弱，失于温煦、推动，津液输布障碍，虽然体内有津液停留，但因不能上布口咽，患者却感咽喉干燥不适，常常欲饮水于口中，慢慢下咽以滋润咽喉；或口干欲饮、饮水不多，或渴喜热饮；舌体失于温运和滋养，则舌强运转不便；或声道失于阳气的温养和激发，又缺少津液滋润，发音功能障碍，而见语声低沉、声音嘶哑。如《千金要方·脾脏病脉论》说：脾被"伤则寒，寒则虚，虚则举体消瘦，语音沉涩，如破鼓之声，舌强不转，而好咽唾，口噤唇黑。"所以口燥咽干不一定为热盛伤津而致，亦可因脾阳虚衰，气不化津，津不上承引起。后者最易误认为热盛或阴亏，导致诊断失误，必须仔细辨识。

脾阳不足，阳虚阴盛，寒主凝滞、收引，大腹属脾，肠道气机凝滞，经脉挛急，阻塞不通，引起腹痛。其特点是腹部冷痛，或剧痛，喜温喜按。寒气上逆，可引起心痛，下攻可牵引少腹疼痛。如

《中藏经•论脾脏虚实寒热生死逆顺之法》说："脾中寒，足热，则皆使人腹中痛，不下食，又病其舌强，语涩不转，卵缩牵阴，股中引痛。"《圣济总录•脾脏冷气攻心腹疼痛》亦说："论曰足太阴，脾之经也。风冷干之，搏于脾脏，与正气相击，上冲于心则心痛，下攻于腹则腹痛，法宜温以调之。"临床上大多数腹痛，多与脾阳虚，寒凝气滞有关。脾阳虚衰，阳失温煦，虚寒内生，冷气与正气相争，互相搏击，则为肠鸣。如《圣济总录•脾脏冷气腹内虚鸣》说："脾为中州...若脾虚，冷气与正气相击，则令腹内虚鸣...内经所谓暴气象雷者，以阴阳之冷热相击故也。"

卫阳有调节体温和开阖汗孔，温煦脏腑的作用。卫阳化生于下焦，滋养于中焦，宣发于上焦。脾胃阳气健旺，滋养有源，则卫阳充足。脾胃阳虚，失于温养，卫阳不足，不能卫外为固，皮肤脏腑失却温煦，产热减少，则会引起畏寒怕冷、汗出、易于感冒等虚寒症状。脾主四肢，四肢为诸阳之本，脾阳虚，阳气不能运达四肢，故见四肢逆冷。脾阳虚衰，失于推动，气血不能上荣于面，故见面色淡白，唇舌色淡等症状。如《脾胃论•肺之脾胃虚论》说："脾胃之虚，怠惰嗜卧，四肢不收... 兼见肺病，洒淅恶寒，惨惨不乐，面色恶而不和，乃阳气不伸故也。"此即脾阳虚，不能化生卫阳，阳虚失于温煦而引起的畏寒面白的症状。

治宜温中散寒。以口咽干燥为主，用《小儿药证直诀》七味白术散（四君子汤加藿香叶、木香、葛根）加炮干姜、升麻。

以声低语沉、舌强不转为主，用《太平圣惠方》麻黄散（附子、桂心、干姜、白术、人参、麻黄、细辛、石膏、羚羊角、防风、秦艽、防己、川芎、杏仁、甘草）加减。

以腹冷剧痛为主，用《金匮要略》附子粳米汤（附子、半夏、甘草、大枣、粳米）加川椒、干姜、砂仁。以畏寒肢冷、面白唇淡为主，用《伤寒论》理中丸加桂枝、附子进行治疗。

Literature Review of Impaired Warming

📖 *Jĭng Yuè Quán Shū* ("Jĭng-Yuè's Complete Compendium"), "Schema of Various Patterns: Ten Questions"

> "Whenever the mouth is thirsty and likes heat, but not cold, this is not a fire pattern, but evidently a cold strike."

Cold strike means cold damage to the interior, spleen yáng depletion, and poor qì transformation that is preventing it from providing warmth and steaming the fluids to bear upward. This causes a dry mouth that likes heat but does not like cold drinks.

📖 *Chóng Dìng Tōng Sú Shāng Hán Lùn* ("Revised Popular On Cold Damage"), "Inquiring about the Presence or Absence of Thirst"

> "All cases of thirst with a liking for hot drinks are associated with phlegm-rheum obstructing the center, or else with qì failing to transform liquid."

Phlegm-rheum is a yīn evil and is caused by damage to yáng qì. Phlegm-rheum obstructing the center means that spleen yáng is vacuous and therefore unable to warm and transform liquid to upbear it to the mouth. This causes a dry mouth and liking for hot drinks.

📖 *Zhōng Zàng Jīng* ("Central Treasury Canon"), "On the Methods for Treating Vacuity and Repletion, Cold and Heat, Life and Death, and Favorable and Unfavorable Shifts in the Spleen"

> "Again, spleen disease results in a stiff tongue and difficult speech... When it is a case of cold, it results in drool foaming at the mouth and inability to eat, pain in the four limbs, incessant efflux diarrhea, reversal of the extremities, and in severe cases, trembling and shivering as in malaria."

When the spleen is vacuous, it is unable to provide warmth, yīn cold is abnormally exuberant, and cold governs contracture and tautness. This results in stiffness of the tongue, cramping feet, and contraction of the scrotum. The spleen governs the four limbs; when yáng qì fails to reach the limbs, it causes counterflow cold of the limbs and pain. When spleen yáng is unable to contain the fluids, it causes drool foaming at the mouth.

📖 *Tài Píng Shèng Huì Fāng* ("Great Peace Sagacious Benevolence Formulary"), "Various Prescriptions for Treating Pain Caused by Cold Qì from the Spleen Attacking the Heart and Abdomen"

> "When visceral and bowel qì is vacuous, the spleen and stomach become vacuous, yáng qì insufficient, and yīn qì overabundant; the qì of evil cold strikes the foot greater yīn channel and lodges deeply without leaving; the spleen accumulates cold qì, which then overwhelms the heart; and right qì and evil qì fight with each other above and below. This causes heart and abdominal pain."

Spleen yáng vacuity causes qì accumulation inside the abdomen, contracture and tautness governed by cold, and congealing and stagnation, resulting in pain in the stomach duct and abdomen.

📖 *Yī Zōng Bì Dú* ("Indispensable Medical Reading"), "Reverse Flow of the Extremities"

> "Cold in the four limbs is referred to as 'fourfold counterflow' [i.e. counterflow cold of the limbs] and is also called 'reversal.' [For the treatment

of] reverse flow, a fine deep pulse, a curled-up lying position and aversion to cold, putting on additional clothes and covering up, and clear-food diarrhea, use *sì nì tāng* (Counterflow Cold Decoction). If the pulse fails to arrive, use *tōng mài sì nì tāng* (Vessel-Freeing Counterflow Cold Decoction). If the pulse is slow and weak, use *lǐ zhōng tāng* (Center-Rectifying Decoction). For slight cold in the extremities and fingers [referred to as "cool,"] use *lǐ zhōng tāng* (Center-Rectifying Decoction)."

In addition to being influenced by kidney yáng vacuity, counterflow cold of the limbs is also related to spleen yáng vacuity and the inability of yáng qì to reach the four limbs. The fact that *lǐ zhōng tāng* (Center-Rectifying Decoction) is used to treat this indeed serves as supporting evidence.

📖 *Gǔ Jīn Yī Tǒng Dà Quán* ("Great Compendium of Medical Orthodoxy, Ancient and Modern"), "Entry on Spontaneous Sweating: Spontaneous Sweating Yáng Vacuity"

"Spontaneous sweating that is irregular, slight and incessant, and exacerbated by activity is related to yáng vacuity and insecurity of the interstices. It is the responsibility of stomach qì."

Stomach qì refers to the qì of the spleen and stomach. When spleen yáng is vacuous and unable to transform and transport the essence of grain and water to nourish defense qì, the external defense is insecure and the interstices are loose. This causes spontaneous sweating.

📖 *Lǐ Xū Yuán Jiàn* ("Original Mirror of Rectifying Vacuity"), "The Three Despoliations of Yáng Vacuity Governed by the Spleen"

"I have seen the [following symptoms of] yáng vacuity: sweating without measure, wrapping oneself in cotton at the height of summer, aching lumbus and weak legs forming the pathocondition of wilting, kidney vacuity generating cold, wood repletion generating wind, spleen weakness and stagnating dampness, difficulty to bend the lumbus and back forward and backward, and inability to bend or stretch the calves and thighs, forming the pathocondition of impediment. These are possibly accompanied by a bright white facial complexion or a light and faint voice, in a great variety of manifestations, but the most critical symptom of all is a complete absence of food intake due to poor appetite, resulting in the non-transformation of spleen qì... For the treatment of this kind of yáng vacuity, one must carefully control the condition through the spleen."

This passage describes how spleen yáng vacuity and failure to provide warmth can lead to sweating without measure, fear of cold, a bright white facial complexion, and a light and faint voice.

文献评述

《景岳全书•杂证谟•十问篇》：”凡口虽渴而喜热不喜冷者，此非火证，中寒可知。”中寒，即指寒伤于里，脾阳亏损，气化不行，不能温煦、蒸腾津液上承，故口干喜热而不喜冷饮。

《重订通俗伤寒论•问口渴否》：”凡渴喜热饮者，皆属痰饮阻中，否则气不化津。”痰饮属阴邪，为阳气所伤，痰饮阻中，即是脾阳虚衰，脾阳不能温化水津上升于口，故口干而喜热饮。

《中藏经•论脾脏虚实寒热生死逆顺之法》：”又脾病则舌强语涩…寒则吐涎沫而不食，四肢痛，滑泄不已，手足厥，甚则颤栗如疟也。”脾阳虚，失于温煦，阴寒偏盛，寒主收引，则舌体强硬，足转筋，阴囊收缩。脾主四肢，阳气不达四肢，则四肢逆冷、疼痛。脾阳不能统摄津液，则口吐涎沫。

《太平圣惠方•治脾脏冷气攻心腹疼痛诸方》：”夫脏腑气虚，脾胃衰弱，阳气不足，阴气有余，邪冷之气，内搏于足太阴之经，伏留而不去，脾积冷气，乘之于心，正气与邪气交争，上下相击，故令心腹疼痛也。”脾阳虚，冷气积于腹中，寒主收引、凝滞，则脘腹疼痛。

《医宗必读•手足厥逆》：”四肢冷谓之四逆，即名为厥也。厥逆，脉沉细，踡卧恶寒，引衣自覆，不饮水，下利清谷，四逆汤。脉不至者，通脉四逆汤。脉迟弱，理中汤。手足指微冷，谓之清，理中汤。”四肢逆冷，除受肾阳虚的影响外，还与脾阳虚，阳气不能达于四肢有关，用理中汤治疗即是佐证。

《古今医统大全•自汗门•自汗阳虚》：”自汗者，无时而溅溅然出，动则为甚，属阳虚，腠理不固，胃气之所司也。”胃气是指脾胃之气，脾阳虚，不能化生、转输水谷精微充养卫气，卫外不固，腠理疏松，故而自汗。

《理虚元鉴•阳虚三夺统于脾》：”余尝见阳虚者，汗出无度；或盛夏裹绵，或腰酸足软而成痿症，或肾虚生寒，木实生风，脾弱滞湿，腰背难于俯仰，胻股不可屈伸，而成痹症。或面色白光[1]白，语音轻微，种种不一，然皆以胃口不进饮食，及脾气不化为最危。…此阳虚之治，所当悉统于脾也。”论述脾阳虚衰，温煦失职，可引起汗出无度、畏寒怕冷、面色(白光)语声轻微等症状。

---

[1] Author's note: This characters (白光) refer to a single character that cannot be rendered by computer; it is written as a combination of the words 白 and 光, and means white and bright.

Summary of Impaired Warming

1. Loss of Warmth in the Mouth and Throat

   In the throat: Dryness with desire to drink water or to swallow to moisten

   In the mouth: Dryness with desire to drink, but drinking only small amounts, thirst with a liking for hot drinks.

2. Loss of Warmth in the Tongue Body

   Stiff tongue that is difficult to move.

3. Loss of Warmth in the Vocal Tract

   Deep low voice, hoarse voice.

4. Congealing Cold Qì Stagnation

   Cold pain in the abdominal section, possibly severe pain that likes warmth and pressure; heart pain stretching down to induce lesser abdominal pain.

5. Loss of Warmth in the Whole Body

   Fear of cold, sweating, susceptibility to the common cold, counterflow cold of the limbs, pale white facial complexion, pale lips and tongue.

温煦失职

口咽失温——咽喉干燥，欲饮水或吞咽滋润； 口干欲饮、饮水不多，渴喜热饮。

舌体失温——舌强运转不便。

声道失温——语声低沉、声音嘶哑。

寒凝气滞——腹部冷痛，或剧痛，喜温喜按。

心痛，下引少腹疼痛。

全身失温——畏寒怕冷，汗出，易于感冒，四肢逆冷，面色淡白，唇舌色淡。

When spleen yáng vacuity advances further, it can form the pathomechanism of spleen and kidney yáng vacuity. This is due to the fact that spleen yáng constantly relies on warmth from kidney yáng to ripen and rot grain and water and to warm and transform water-humor without interruption. Therefore, when spleen yáng vacuity is enduring and without remission, it can wear on kidney yáng and develop into kidney yáng vacuity, leading to the pathomechanism of spleen-kidney yáng vacuity. In clinic, this manifests as enduring diarrhea, enduring dysentery, five watches diarrhea, or severe water swelling. It is treated by warming the spleen and supplementing the kidney. The recommended formula is a modified version of *fù zǐ lǐ zhōng tāng* (Aconite Center-Rectifying Decoction) in combination with *sì shén wán* (Four Spirits Pill) from the *Zhèng Zhì Zhǔn Shéng* ("Level-Line of Pattern Identification and Treatment").

Fù Zǐ Lǐ Zhōng Tāng 附子理中汤 + *Sì Shén Wán* 四神丸 Aconite Center-Rectifying Decoction with Four Spirits Pill
rén shēn (人参 ginseng, Ginseng Radix) *gān jiāng* (干姜 dried ginger, Zingiberis Rhizoma) *bái zhú* (白术 white atractylodes, Atractylodis Macrocephalae Rhizoma) *gān cǎo* (甘草 licorice, Glycyrrhizae Radix) *ròu dòu kòu* (肉豆蔻 nutmeg, Myristicae Semen) *bǔ gǔ zhī* (补骨脂 psoralea, Psoraleae Fructus) *wú zhū yú* (吴茱萸 evodia, Evodiae Fructus) *wǔ wèi zǐ* (五味子 schisandra, Schisandrae Fructus)

In addition, when spleen yáng is vacuous and unable to move and transform water-damp, causing an internal exuberance of cold-damp, it can develop into the pathomechanism of cold-damp encumbering the spleen; when spleen yáng is vacuous and unable to promote the movement of blood, it can lead to the pathomechanism of congealing cold blood stasis.

脾阳虚进一步发展，可形成脾肾阳虚的病机变化。这是因为脾阳常依赖肾阳的温煦方能不断地腐熟水谷，温化水液。故脾阳虚日久不愈，可消磨肾阳而发展为肾阳虚，进而引起脾肾阳虚的病机。临床常见久泻久痢，五更泻痢或严重水肿之病。治宜温脾补肾，方用附子理中汤合《证治准绳》四神丸（肉豆蔻、补骨脂、吴茱萸、五味子）加减。

此外，脾阳虚不能运化水湿，寒湿内盛，可发展为寒湿困脾的病机；脾阳虚，不能推动血行，可引起寒凝血瘀的病机。

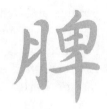

Chapter 3

Spleen Yīn Vacuity

脾阴虚

The pathomechanism of spleen yīn vacuity is first described in the *Nèi Jīng* ("Inner Canon"). The "Chapter on the Five Evils" in the *Líng Shū* ("Magic Pivot") states:

> "When the evil is located in the spleen and stomach, the patient suffers from flesh pain, a superabundance of yáng qì, and an insufficiency of yīn qì, causing heat strike and rapid hungering."

This describes the pathomechanism of dispersion-thirst disease, caused by a superabundance of stomach yáng and an insufficiency of spleen yīn.

In the *Shāng Hán Zá Bìng Lùn* ("On Cold Damage and Miscellaneous Diseases"), Zhāng Zhòng-Jǐng introduced the use of several yīn-enriching formulas, such as *shǔ yù wán* (Dioscorea Pill), *mài mén dōng tāng* (Ophiopogon Decoction), and *má zǐ rén wán* (Cannabis Seed Pill), aimed at treating the pathomechanism of spleen yīn vacuity. Thereby he expanded our knowledge about this pathomechanism from the clinical perspective of patterns and treatments.

During the Jīn-Yuán period, Zhū Dān-Xī, the famous leader of the Yīn-Supplementing School, explained in the chapter, "Drum Distention" in the *Dān Xī Xīn Fǎ* ("Dān Xī's Heart-Approach"):

> "When the yīn of spleen earth is damaged, the office of converting and transporting is impaired. As a result, the stomach receives grain, but is unable to move and transport it."

This quotation illustrates that an insufficiency of spleen yīn can lead to disturbances in the stomach's movement and transformation functions.

During the Míng period, Wáng Lún integrated the theories of Lǐ Dōng-Yuán and Zhū Dān-Xī and for the first time proposed a theory regarding spleen yīn vacuity. In "Treatise on *Zhǐ Zhú Qán* (Unripe Bitter

Orange and White Atractylodes Pill)" in the *Míng Yī Zá Zhù* ("Miscellaneous Works by Famous Physicians"), he explained: "The more effulgent stomach fire is, the more spleen yīn is damaged." In his work, (*Xiān Xǐng Zhāi Yī Xué Guǎng Bǐ Jì* ("Broad-Ranging Medical Notes from the Studio of Early Awaking"), "Further Treatise on Sand Papules"), Miào Zhòng-Chún also stated:

> "Ordinary people are only familiar with the technique of treating spleen vacuity with fragrant, dry, warming, and supplementing [drugs], but do not know that the spleen benefits from sweet, cooling, enriching, and moistening [drugs] to boost yīn."

He believed that such symptoms as inability to eat and drink, nontransformation of food, abdominal distention, and wilting limbs are invariably "symptoms of spleen yīn insufficiency." Thus, he emphasized the importance of recognizing the pathomechanism of spleen yīn vacuity.

During the Qīng period, Wú Chéng-Míng explicitly described the pathomechanism of spleen yīn vacuity. In "Comprehensive Treatise on Rectifying Spleen Yīn" in the *Bù Jū Jí* ("Non-limitation Collection"), he stated:

> "The ancient formulas for rectifying the spleen and fortifying the stomach mostly concentrated on supplementing yáng inside the stomach and failed to affect yīn inside the spleen."

These authors laid the foundations for the pathomechanism of spleen yīn vacuity.

In the "Chapter on Original Diseases; Lín's Commentary" in the *Zēng Bǔ Pìng Zhú Wēn Bìng Tiáo Bian* ("Supplemented Annotation to the Systematized Identification of Warm Diseases"), Wú Jū-Tōng, one of the four masters of the Warm Disease School, further noted: "Retching is a disease of spleen yīn." In "Chapter on the Center Burner; Cold-Damp" in the same text, he advocated:

[In diagnosing spleen-stomach disease, differentiate] "damage to spleen yáng, damage to spleen yīn, damage to stomach yáng, damage to stomach yīn, or damage to both the spleen and stomach."

Closer to our own time, the physician Táng Róng-Chuān explained as follows in the chapter, "Pathomechanisms of the Viscera and Bowels" in the *Xuè Zhèng Lùn* ("On Blood Patterns"): "When spleen yīn is insufficient, grain and water are not transformed," which pointed very explicitly to the pathomechanism of spleen yīn vacuity.

The contemporary famous physician Pú Fǔ-Zhōu directly mentions the term "spleen yīn vacuity" in the chapter, "Searching for the Root in Pattern Identification" in his *Pú Fǔ-Zhōu Yī Liáo Jīng Yàn* ("Pú Fǔ-Zhōu's Medical Experience"):

"Spleen yīn vacuity causes heat vexation in the extremities, dry mouth with no desire to drink, vexation and fullness, and no thought of food."

In the 1970s and 1980s, a lengthy academic dialog was undertaken regarding the pathomechanism of spleen yīn vacuity. Since then, a gradual consensus has been reached that accepts the objective existence of spleen yīn vacuity.

The causes of spleen yīn vacuity are complex. Externally contracted summer-heat heat, damp-heat, dryness evil, or the evils of the six excesses can transform into fire, and the damage can affect spleen yīn; dietary irregularities and the excessive consumption of hot-spicy, acrid, and fried foods, fatty meats, refined grain, or strong flavors can form heat, and the damage can affect spleen yīn; taxation fatigue and excessive thought and preoccupation can also transform into heat and damage yīn. As the chapter on "Vacuity Taxation; *guī pí tāng* (Spleen-Returning Decoction) in the *Gū Sòng Yuán Yī Jìng* ("Gū Sòng-Yuán's Mirror of Medicine") notes: "When taxation fatigue damages the spleen, damage to the yīn aspect of the spleen is frequent." Enduring illness, severe illness, diseases that have shifted from other organs, as well as overuse of warm drying, inappropriate sweating, and inappropriate precipitation, can all damage spleen yīn, resulting in the pathomechanism of spleen yīn vacuity.

Because governing movement and transformation and forming qì, blood, and fluids are important physiological functions of the spleen, the pathomechanism of spleen yīn vacuity constantly includes the aspects of breakdown of movement and transformation, loss of nourishment, and internal generation of vacuity heat.

脾阴虚的病机，《内经》已有初步描述。《灵枢•五邪篇》"邪在脾胃，则病肌肉痛，阳气有余，阴气不足，则热中善饥。"即是对胃阳有余，脾阴不足之消渴病的病机阐述。张仲景在《伤寒杂病论》中针对脾阴虚的病机，创立了薯蓣丸、麦门冬汤、麻子仁丸等不少有滋脾阴作用的方剂，从临床证治的角度发展了对脾阴虚病机的认识。金元时期著名补阴派大师朱丹溪在《丹溪心法•鼓胀》中说："脾土之阴受伤，转输之官失职，胃虽受谷，不能运化。"指明脾阴不足，可引起脾的运化功能失调。明•王伦结合东垣、丹溪之说，最早提出有关"脾阴"的理论。他在《明医杂著•枳术丸论》中说："胃火益旺，脾阴愈伤"。缪仲淳亦说："世人徒知香燥温补为治脾虚之法，而不知甘凉滋润益阴之有益于脾也"（《先醒斋医学广笔记•痧疹续论》）。认为饮食不进，食不消化，腹胀，肢痿等往往是"脾阴不足之候"，强调对脾阴虚病机认识的重要。清代吴澄明确地阐述了脾阴虚的病机，他在《不居集•理脾阴总论》中说："古方理脾健

胃，多偏补胃中之阳，而不及脾中之阴。"至此脾阴虚的病机已基本
建立。温病四大家之一的吴鞠通在《增补评注温病条辨•原病篇•霖
按》中亦说："哕，脾阴病也。"主张诊断脾胃病要注意"有伤脾阳，
有伤脾阴，有伤胃阳，有伤胃阴，有两伤脾胃。"(《增补评注温病
条辨•中焦篇•寒湿》)。近代医家唐容川在《血证论•脏腑病机》中
说："脾阴不足，水谷仍不化也"，比较明确地提出了脾阴虚的病
机。现代名医蒲辅周在《蒲辅周医疗经验•辨证求本》中说："脾阴
虚，手足烦热，口干不欲饮，烦满，不思食"，才算正式点出"脾阴
虚"的名字。七十、八十年代以来，中医学术界对脾阴虚的病机开展
广泛争论。现在已逐渐取得共识，承认脾阴虚的客观存在。

引起脾阴虚的病因颇为复杂，外感暑热、湿热、燥邪，或六淫之邪
化火，伤及脾阴；饮食不节，过食辛辣煎炒、膏粱厚味可化热伤及
脾阴；劳倦、思虑过度，亦可化热伤阴。如《顾松园医镜•虚劳•归
脾汤》说："劳倦伤脾，乃脾之阴分受伤者多"；久病、重病，其它
脏腑疾病的传变，以及过用温燥、误汗、误下均可伤及脾阴，引起
脾阴虚的病机。由于脾的主要生理功能是主运化，化生气血津液。
故脾阴虚的病机常有运化失职、失于滋润和虚热内生的区分。

3.1 Breakdown of Movement and Transformation

The spleen's function of governing movement and transformation depends on the movement-promoting action of spleen qì for its force, as
well as on the nourishing action of spleen yīn for its material basis. In
spleen yīn vacuity, the spleen's movement and transformation function
lacks its necessary material basis, which can lead to disturbances in the
digestive function. If grain and water cannot be digested and absorbed
promptly after meals, this can manifest as torpid intake and reduced eating or eating without tasting food. If the qì dynamic fails to spread out
after meals and collects and stagnates inside the abdomen, it manifests in
such symptoms as abdominal distention and fullness that is exacerbated
after meals and likes soft pressure.

The chapter, "Determining Treatment for the Spleen and Stomach" in
the *Lèi Zhèng Zhì Cái* ("Systematized Patterns with Clear-Cut Treatments"), explains:

> "When spleen-stomach yīn is vacuous, there is absence of hunger, inabil-
> ity to eat, and a bland taste in the mouth. Nourish it by clearing and mois-
> tening."

"Treatise on the Differences and Similarities between Men and Women"
in the *Xuè Zhèng Lùn* ("On Blood Patterns") explains:

> "When spleen yáng is insufficient, grain and water certainly cannot be transformed; when spleen yīn is insufficient, grain and water still fail to be transformed. One can compare this to cooking rice in a cauldron. If there is no fire underneath the cauldron, it will certainly not get cooked. If there is no water inside the cauldron, it will also not get cooked."

This analogy explains how spleen yīn vacuity can lead to the pathomechanism of indigestion.

In addition, when spleen yīn, as the material basis, is depleted and unable to form spleen qì, the spleen's movement and transformation function is impaired. Grain and water are not transformed, but spill down into the large intestine, which can lead to diarrhea and sloppy stool. Lín Yè recognized that sloppy stool can result from a pathomechanism caused by spleen yīn vacuity. Thus in his notes for "Chapter on Original Diseases" in the *Zēng Bǔ Pìng Zhú Wēn Bìng Tiáo Biàn* ("Supplemented Annotation to the Systematized Identification of Warm Diseases"), he clearly states:

> "When diarrhea and abdominal fullness are severe, this means that spleen yīn suffers from a serious disease and that it is also related to a dual disease of yīn and yáng."

While this passage fails to clarify in detail the exact pathomechanism by which spleen yīn vacuity leads to abdominal fullness and diarrhea, it makes it possible to differentiate the nature of this condition and therefore carries great significance in clinical practice.

Breakdown of movement and transformation is treated by supplementing and nourishing spleen yīn, and by assisting movement and opening the stomach. Conditions that are mainly characterized by torpid intake and reduced eating are best treated with *liù shén tāng* (Six Spirits Decoction) from the *Sān Yīn Jí Yī Bìng Zhèng Fāng Lùn* ("Unified Treatise on Diseases, Patterns, and Remedies According to the Three Causes"), with the addition of *gǔ yá* (Setariae Fructus Germinatus), *jī nèi jīn* (Galli Gigeriae Endothelium Corneum), and *shān zhā* (Crataegi Fructus).

Liù Shén Tāng 六神汤 Six Spirits Decoction
rén shēn (人参 ginseng, Ginseng Radix)
bái zhú (白术 white atractylodes, Atractylodis Macrocephalae Rhizoma)
fú líng (茯苓 poria, Poria)
gān cǎo (甘草 licorice, Glycyrrhizae Radix)
shān yào (山药 dioscorea, Dioscoreae Rhizoma)
biǎn dòu (扁豆 lablab, Lablab Semen Album)

Plus:

gǔ yá (谷芽 millet sprout, Setariae Fructus Germinatus)

jī nèi jīn (鸡内金 gizzard lining, Galli Gigeriae Endothelium Corneum)

jiāo shān zhā (焦山楂 scorch-fried crataegus, Crataegi Fructus Ustus)

Conditions mainly characterized by abdominal fullness that likes pressure are treated with *liù shén tāng* (Six Spirits Decoction) with the addition of *zhǐ qiào (ké)* (Aurantii Fructus), *jú hóng* (Citri Reticulatae Pericarpium Rubrum), *tán xiāng* (Santali Albi Lignum), and *chén xiāng* (Aquilariae Lignum Resinatum).

Conditions mainly characterized by diarrhea and sloppy stool are treated with *shēn líng bái zhú sǎn* (Ginseng, Poria, and White Atractylodes Powder) from the *Tài Píng Huì Mín Hé Jì Jú Fāng* ("Tài-Píng Imperial Grace Pharmacy Formulas"), without *chén pí* (Citri Reticulatae Pericarpium), *shā rén* (Amomi Fructus), and *dǎng shēn* (Codonopsis Radix), and with the addition of *tài zǐ shēn* (Pseudostellariae Radix), *shí hú* (Dendrobii Herba), *qiàn shí* (Euryales Semen), and *gǔ yá* (Setariae Fructus Germinatus).

Shēn Líng Bái Zhú Sǎn 参苓白术散
Ginseng, Poria, and White Atractylodes Powder [modified]

fú líng (茯苓 poria, Poria)

bái zhú (白术 white atractylodes, Atractylodis Macrocephalae Rhizoma)

shān yào (山药 dioscorea, Dioscoreae Rhizoma)

biǎn dòu (扁豆 lablab, Lablab Semen Album)

lián zǐ ròu (莲子肉 lotus fruit, Nelumbinis Semen)

yì yǐ rén (薏苡仁 coix, Coicis Semen)

jié gěng (桔梗 platycodon, Platycodonis Radix)

gān cǎo (甘草 licorice, Glycyrrhizae Radix)

Plus:

tài zǐ shēn (太子参 pseudostellaria, Pseudostellariae Radix)

shí hú (石斛 dendrobium, Dendrobii Herba)

qiàn shí (芡实 euryale, Euryales Semen)

gǔ yá (谷芽 millet sprout, Setariae Fructus Germinatus)

运化失职

脾主运化的功能，依赖作为动力的脾气的推动作用，亦同样依赖作为物质基础的脾阴的濡养作用。脾阴虚，脾的运化功能缺乏必要的物质基础，则会引起消化功能减退。食后水谷不能及时消化吸收，可表现为纳呆食少、食而无味之症状。食后气机失布，停滞腹中，则见腹部胀满、食后尤甚、喜柔按等症状。如《类证治裁•脾胃论治》说：”脾胃阴虚，不饥不食，口淡无味，宜清润以养之。”《血证论•男女异同论》说：”脾阳不足，水谷固不化；脾阴不足，水谷仍不化也。譬如釜中煮饭，釜底无火固不熟，釜中无水亦不熟也。”形像地运用比喻，说明脾阴虚可导致消化不良的病机。

此外，作为物质基础的脾阴亏虚，不能化生脾气，脾的运化功能减退，水谷不化，下渗大肠，可致腹泻便溏。如叶霖对便溏可因脾阴虚而引起的病机有所认识，他在《增补评注温病条辨•原病篇》的补注中明确提出：”泄而腹满甚，脾阴病重也，亦系阴阳皆病。”虽未详细阐明脾阴虚引起腹满腹泻的详细病机，但能辨别这种性质，已具有非常重要的临床意义。

治宜补养脾阴，助运开胃。以纳呆食少为主，用《三因极一病证方论》六神汤（四君子加山药、扁豆）加谷芽、鸡内金、焦山楂。以腹满喜按为主，用六神汤加枳壳、橘红、檀香、沉香。以腹泻便溏为主。用《和剂局方》参苓白术散去陈皮、砂仁、党参，加太子参、石斛、芡实、谷芽。

Literature Review of Breakdown of Movement and Transformation

📖 *Lèi Zhèng Zhì Cái* ("Systematized Patterns with Clear-Cut Treatments"), "Food and Drink"

"Spleen-stomach yīn vacuity causes absence of hunger, inability to eat, and bland taste in the mouth. Nourish [spleen-stomach yīn] by clearing and moistening. [Use medicinals] like *shā shēn* (Adenophorae seu Glehniae Radix), *biǎn dòu zǐ* (Cassiae Mimosoidis Semen), *shí hú* (Dendrobii Herba), *yù zhú* (Polygonati Odorati Rhizoma), *dāng guī* (Angelicae Sinensis Radix), *bái sháo* (Paeoniae Radix Alba), *huǒ má rén* (Cannabis Semen), *jīng mǐ* (Oryzae Semen), and *xiǎo mài* (Tritici Fructus)."

When spleen yīn is vacuous, spleen qì is deprived of nourishment from spleen yīn, movement and transformation break down, and digestion slows, causing absence of hunger, torpid intake and stagnation in the stomach, a bland taste in the mouth, and reduced food intake.

📖 *Bù Jū Jí* ("Non-limitation Collection"), "Treatise on No Pleasure in Food and Drink"

"Failure to take pleasure in food and drink is mostly caused by depletion in the spleen and stomach... In patients with vacuity detriment, spleen yīn is insufficient and stomach yáng is depleted. They eat greater amounts of rich, oily, sticky, and stagnating food, believing them to be supplementing and boosting. Whether they stagnate or pour down, they are difficult to digest, eating is reduced, and food damage and aversion to food result."

When spleen yīn is depleted, spleen qì is nourished improperly and movement and transformation are disturbed. Careless eating causes digestive difficulties. This can lead to inability to taste food, reduced food intake, food damage, or aversion to food.

📖 *Bù Jū Jí* ("Non-limitation Collection"), "Comprehensive Treatise on Rectifying Spleen Yīn"

"*Shēng bǔ zhōng hé tāng* (Lifting and Supplementing Harmonious Center Decoction) treats vacuity taxation cold and heat, reduced food intake and diarrhea, failure to control upbearing, and brushwood[2] [emaciation]. The formula consists of *rén shēn* (Ginseng Radix), *hé yè* (Nelumbinis Folium), *gōu téng* (Uncariae Ramulus cum Uncis), *shān yào* (Dioscoreae Rhizoma), *gǔ yá* (Setariae Fructus Germinatus), *fú shén* (Poria cum Pini Radice), *lǎo mǐ* (Oryzae Semen), *hóng zǎo* (Jujubae Fructus), and *gān cǎo* (Glycyrrhizae Radix)."

The ingredients *rén shēn*, *hé yè*, and *gōu téng* upbear stomach yáng; *shān yào*, *gǔ yá*, *fú shén*, and *lǎo mǐ* upbear spleen yīn. Therefore, the formula is able to treat spleen-stomach yīn vacuity, clear yáng fall, and such resulting symptoms of vacuity taxation as reduced food intake and diarrhea.

📖 *Xiān Xǐng Zhāi Yī Xué Guǎng Bǐ Jì* ("Broad-Ranging Medical Notes from the Studio of Early Awaking"), "Further Treatise on Sand Papules"

"Young Master Gù Míng-Liù had a weak constitution. When only a few years old, he suffered from spleen vacuity signs and would not allow food or drink to touch his lips. When his parents forced him, he would still only eat half a bowl of rice gruel in an entire day. His body was completely whittled away... I used *rén shēn* (Ginseng Radix) as the sovereign and *fú líng* (Poria), *shān yào* (Dioscoreae Rhizoma), *jú hóng* (Citri Reticulatae Pericarpium Rubrum), *bái sháo* (Paeoniae Radix Alba), *lián zǐ* (Nelumbinis Semen), and *bái biǎn dòu* (Lablab Semen Album) as assistants. ...After a hundred days, his eating and drinking abruptly increased and after half a year his flesh was bountiful and full. Ordinary people are only familiar with the technique of treating spleen vacuity with fragrant, dry, warming and supplementing [drugs], but do not know that the spleen benefits from sweet, cold, enriching and moistening [drugs] to boost yīn."

---

[2] The word used here is *chái* 柴—literally, firewood or brushwood. Its use in this context is taken to mean emaciation, in reference to thinness and dessication one would associate with wood used for burning.

After the disease of sand papules,[3] heat toxin had damaged spleen yīn, the appetite was visibly reduced, and the whole body was emaciated. The fact that a formula that supplements and nourishes spleen yīn achieved obvious results is proof that one must pay attention to the pathomechanism of spleen yīn vacuity. Otherwise one only knows how to fortify the spleen and boost qì with sweetness and warmth, but does not know the treatment method of enriching yīn and nourishing the spleen with sweetness and cold. In that case, it will be very difficult to obtain satisfactory results.

📖 *Shèn Róu Wǔ Shū* ("Shèn Róu Five Books"), "Vacuity Detriment"

> "When the pulse is intermittent and moderate, it means that stomach qì is not yet expired and can still be rectified. Use *sì jūn zǐ tāng* (Four Gentlemen Decoction) with the addition of *shān yào* (Dioscoreae Rhizoma) to conduct it into the spleen channel. Supplement only spleen yīn and apply it according to the accompanying symptoms."

This describes the use of *sì jūn zǐ tāng* (Four Gentlemen Decoction) for supplementing and boosting spleen-stomach qì. With the addition of *shān yào* (Dioscoreae Rhizoma), it becomes an important medicine for supplementing and boosting spleen yīn and therefore proves effective for treating such spleen yīn vacuity-related symptoms as torpid intake and reduced eating, and abdominal distention and sloppy stool.

文献评述

《类证治裁•饮食》："脾胃阴虚，则不饥不食，口淡无味者，宜清润以养之。如沙参、扁豆子、石斛、玉竹、当归、白芍、麻仁、粳米、大麦仁。"脾阴虚，脾气失于脾阴的滋养，运化失职，消化迟钝，故心中无饥饿感，胃纳呆滞而口淡无味，进食减少。

《不居集•饮食不甘论》："饮食不甘，多因脾胃有亏损。…虚损之人脾阴不足，胃阳又亏，多食肥浓凝滞之物，以为补益，孰知停注难消，饮食渐减而伤食恶食也。"脾阴亏损，脾气失养，运化失调，饮食不慎，难于消化，故可引起饮食无味、纳食减少，伤食恶食等症状。

《不居集•理脾阴总论》："升补中和汤，治虚劳寒热，食少泄泻，不任升、柴者，此方主之。人参、荷叶、钩藤、山药、谷芽、茯神、老米、红枣、甘草。"方中人参、荷叶、钩藤升胃中之阳，山

---

[3] Sand papules, 沙疹 *shā zhěn*: Any rash occurring in febrile disease characterized by small papules the size of millet seeds.

药、谷芽、茯神、老米升脾中之阴，故能治脾胃阴虚，清阳下陷，而所引起的食少腹泻等虚劳病证。

《先醒斋医学广笔记•痧疹续论》："顾鸣六乃郎，禀赋素弱，年数岁，患脾虚证，饮食绝不沾唇，父母强之，终日不满稀粥半盂，形体倍削。...以人参为君，茯苓、山药、橘红、白芍药、莲肉、扁豆为佐。...百日后，饮食顿加，半年肌体丰满。世人徒知香燥温补为治脾虚之治，而不知甘寒滋润益阴之有益于脾也。"麻疹后，热毒伤脾阴，食欲明显减退，全身消瘦，用补养脾阴的方药治疗收到显著效果，证明必须重视脾阴虚的病机。否则只知甘温健脾益气，不知甘寒滋阴养脾的治法就很难取得较好的疗效。

《慎柔五书•虚损》："脉代缓，是胃气未绝，尤可调理，用四君子加山药，引入脾经，单补脾阴，再随所兼之症而用之。"论述四君子汤有补益脾胃之气的作用，若加入山药，则为补益脾阴之要药，对脾阴虚所致纳呆食少、腹胀便溏等症状有较好的疗效。

Summary of Breakdown of Movement and Transformation
1. Nontransformation of Grain and Water   Torpid intake and reduced eating, eating without tasting food.
2. Qì Stagnation in the Abdomen: Abdominal distention and fullness that is exacerbated after eating and likes soft pressure.
3. Reduced Movement and Transformation: Diarrhea and sloppy stool.
运化失职
水谷不运——纳呆食少，食而无味。
气滞腹中——腹部胀满，食后尤甚，喜柔按压。
运化减弱——腹泻便溏。

3.2 Loss of Nourishment

Spleen yín includes construction blood and the fluids. When spleen yīn is vacuous, it is unable to absorb and move and transport, formation of qì and blood is insufficient, the fluids are depleted, and the body is deprived of nourishment. This can result in malfunctions in the entire body, including the bowels and viscera. It manifests as loss of nourishment and moisture in the face and a withered yellow lusterless facial complexion.

When the body's external structure is deprived of nourishment, this manifests as emaciation and lack of strength in the limbs. When the heart spirit is deprived of the nourishment provided by yīn blood, this manifests as fatigue and lassitude of the spirit, encumbrance, and somnolence. When the offices and orifices are deprived of nourishment, this manifests as dry skin, dry nose and lips, and hair loss or withered hair.

"Treatise on Showing Breadth of Vision" in the *Sù Wèn* ("Plain Questions") notes: "Fatigue of the four limbs means that essence is not moving." The chapter, "Methods for Rectifying Spleen Yīn" in the *Bù Jū Jí* ("Non-limitation Collection") explains:

> "The ancient formulas for rectifying the spleen and fortifying the stomach mostly concentrated on supplementing yáng in the stomach and failed to affect yīn in the spleen. However, in patients with vacuity detriment, the fluids become insufficient because of the scorching of yīn fire. The sinews, channels, skin, and bones all are deprived of nourishment, and the essence-spirit is also gradually emaciated and weakened, causing the hundred pathoconditions to arise from this."

Both quotations describe how spleen yīn vacuity can manifest in loss of nourishment to the external structure of the body, to the four limbs, or to the skin, channels, sinews, and bones.

When spleen yīn is depleted, the fluids are insufficient and therefore cannot enrich the large intestine below. This can manifest as dry and rough stagnant stool, and in serious cases as constipation.

"Chapter on Yáng Míng Diseases" in the *Shāng Hán Lùn* ("On Cold Damage") states:

> "When the instep yáng pulse is floating and rough, the floating means a strong stomach qì and the roughness means frequent urination. Floating and roughness contend with each other, causing hardening of the stool and a straitened spleen. Use *má rén wán* (Cannabis Seed Pill) to treat."

Later physicians largely believed that the symptom of straitened spleen is caused by spleen yīn vacuity and failure to enrich the large intestine. As the chapter, "Differentiating the Pulse, Symptoms, and Treatments of Yáng Brightness Disease" in the *Shāng Hán Lùn Tōng Sú Jiǎng Huà* ("Popular Guide to 'On Cold Damage'"), points out:

> "When a patient presents with a floating and rough instep yáng pulse, the floating means an abnormal exuberance of yáng qì, and the roughness means a yīn humor deficit. This disease is characterized by strong yáng brightness stomach qì and weak greater yīn spleen yīn. The strength of stomach yáng is aggravated by the weakness of spleen yīn, causing the stomach to be straitened and fettered. Consequently, it is unable to move the fluids for the stomach, the fluids are unable to enter the stomach, and the stomach and intestines are not moistened; they become dry and produce hard stool."

This is a penetrating elucidation of the pathomechanism by which spleen yīn vacuity leads to dry and rough stool or constipation.

In the "Chapter on the Center Burner; Cold-Damp" in the *Zēng Bǔ Pìng Zhú Wēn Bìng Tiáo Bian* ("Supplemented Annotation to the Systematized Identification of Warm Diseases"), Wú Jū-Tóng noted in detail:

> "When spleen yīn is damaged, the tongue will be ashen and glossy in the front, but yellow and dry in the back, and the stool will be hard and bound."

The chapter, "*Zhǐ Zhú Wán* (Unripe Bitter Orange and White Atractylodes Pill)" in the *Míng Yī Zá Zhù* ("Miscellaneous Works by Famous Physicians"), notes:

> "Contemporary discussions of spleen and stomach treatments fail to distinguish between yīn and yáng and qì and blood…. The medicines they use are all preparations for assisting fire and dispersing yīn with acridity, warmth, dryness, and heat. Subsequently, the more effulgent they make stomach fire, the more they damage spleen yīn. The clear, pure, central, and harmonious qì becomes dry and hot, the stomach and stomach duct become desiccated, and the large intestine becomes dry and bound."

This passage stresses the importance of differentiating the pathomechanism of spleen yīn vacuity from a clinical perspective.

Loss of nourishment is treated by supplementing and boosting spleen yīn, and by enriching yīn and moistening dryness. Conditions that are characterized by improper nourishment of the head, face, structure of the body, or offices and orifices are best treated with sweet, bland, and moistening medicinals like *rén shēn* (Ginseng Radix), *bái biǎn dòu* (Lablab Semen Album), *huáng jīng* (Polygonati Rhizoma), *bái sháo* (Paeoniae Radix Alba), *qiàn shí* (Euryales Semen), *shí lián zǐ* (Nelumbinis Fructus), *gé gēn* (Puerariae Radix), and *gān cǎo* (Glycyrrhizae Radix). Conditions that are characterized mainly by constipation are best treated with *má zǐ rén wán* (Cannabis Seed Pill) from the *Shāng Hán Lùn* ("On Cold Damage").

Má Zǐ Rén Wán 麻子仁丸
Cannabis Seed Pill

huǒ má rén (火麻仁 cannabis seed, Cannabis Semen)
xìng rén (杏仁 apricot kernel, Armeniacae Semen)
bái sháo yào (白芍药 white peony, Paeoniae Radix Alba)
zhǐ shí (枳实 unripe bitter orange, Aurantii Fructus Immaturus)
hòu pò (厚朴 officinal magnolia bark, Magnoliae Officinalis Cortex)
dà huáng (大黄 rhubarb, Rhei Radix et Rhizoma)

失于滋养

脾阴包括营血、津液。脾阴虚，不能吸收、运化，气血生成不足，津液亏损，失于滋养，可引起全身脏腑功能低下。表现为面部失于滋养而见面色萎黄无华；形体失于滋养而见形体消瘦、四肢乏力；心神失于阴血滋养而见神疲倦怠、困倦嗜卧。官窍失于滋养而见皮肤干燥、鼻干唇燥、毛发脱落或憔悴。如《素问•示从容论》说："四肢懈惰，此脾精之不行也。"《不居集•理脾阴之法》中说："古方理脾健胃，多偏补胃中之阳，而不及脾中之阴。然虚损之人，为阴火所灼，津液不足，筋脉皮骨皆无所养，而精神亦渐羸弱，百症丛生焉。"两者均阐述了脾阴虚，可引起形体、四肢、皮脉筋骨失于滋养的表现。

脾阴亏损，津液不足，不能下滋大肠，又可出现大便干涩，甚至秘结。《伤寒论•阳明病篇》"趺阳脉浮而涩，浮则胃气强，涩则小便数，浮涩相搏，大便则硬，其脾为约，麻仁丸主之。"后世许多医家均认为是脾阴虚，大肠失滋而引起的脾约证。如《伤寒论通俗讲话•辨阳明病脉证并治》指出："病人趺阳脉浮而涩，浮为阳气偏盛，涩是阴液偏衰，说明其病为阳明胃气强，太阴脾阴弱。以胃阳之强，加于脾阴之弱，使脾为之约束，而不能为胃行其津液，津液不能入胃中，胃肠失润而干燥，则大便硬。"较为精辟地阐明脾阴虚引起大便干涩，或秘结的病机。吴鞠通在《增补评注温病条辨•中焦篇•寒湿》中则明确提出："伤脾阴则舌先灰滑，后反黄燥，大便坚结。"《明医杂著•枳术丸》说："近世论治脾胃者，不分阴阳气血…所用之药又皆辛温燥热助火消阴之剂，遂使胃火益旺，脾阴愈伤，清纯中和之气变为燥热，胃脘干枯，大肠燥结。"更从临床的角度强调辨识脾阴虚病机的重要意义。

治宜补益脾阴，滋阴润燥。以头面形体官窍失养为主，选人参、扁豆、黄精、白芍、芡实、石莲子、葛根、甘草等甘淡濡润之品治疗。以便秘为主，用《伤寒论》麻子仁丸（麻仁、杏仁、芍药、枳实、厚朴、大黄）治疗。

Literature Review of Loss of Nourishment

📖 *Xiān Xǐng Zhāi Yī Xué Guǎng Bǐ Jì* ("Broad-Ranging Medical Notes from the Studio of Early Awaking"), "Women"

"Lady Wáng Shàn-Zhǎng suffered from postpartum leg pain and inability to walk or stand. When this endured, she was unable to get down food or drink and reached an extreme point of exhaustion. Zhōng Chún performed a diagnosis and said, 'This is a symptom of spleen yīn insufficiency. The spleen governs the four limbs and when yīn is insufficient, the disease affects the lower body. In spite of the fact that she has been drinking many medicines all along, they have all been bitter and drying preparations and have been unable to boost yīn. Use *shí hú* (Dendrobii Herba), *mù guā* (Chaenomelis Fructus), *niú xī* (Achyranthis Bidentatae Radix), *bái sháo* (Paeoniae Radix Alba), and *suān zǎo rén* (Ziziphi Spinosi Semen) as sovereigns, *shēng dì huáng* (Rehmanniae Radix Exsiccata seu Recens), *gǒu qǐ zǐ* (Lycii Fructus), *fú líng* (Poria), and *huáng bǎi* (Phellodendri Cortex) as ministers, and *gān cǎo* (Glycyrrhizae Radix) and *chē qián zǐ* (Plantaginis Semen) as couriers.'"

This passage points out that limpness and fatigue of the body, lack of strength in the limbs, inability to walk, and reduced intake of food and drink can be caused by an insufficiency of spleen yīn and a breakdown of movement and transformation, which results in loss of nourishment in the limbs. Therefore, a spleen-yīn supplementing formula can be used to treat this condition with success.

📖 *Yī Biǎn* ("Lancing Stones of Medicine"), "Constipation"

"When a person suffers from constipation, dry mouth and cracked lips, inability to digest food, unbearable abdominal pain that is exacerbated by pressure, and short inhibited voidings of urine, people assume that it means that the stool is blocked by fire, but who is aware that it is the disturbing influence of spleen fire? They do not know that when earth is too soft, there are landslides; when earth is too hard, there is parching. Landslides cause wasted land and parching causes scorched earth. Nevertheless, if scorched earth is not a case of yáng brightness flaming downward, it must be life gate fire flaming upward. The two fires attack together, and the spleen's fluids dry up completely. When grain and water enter, they are barely enough to provide for the functions of the spleen. How could they also separately moisten the large intestine?"

This passage discusses how constipation can be caused by spleen fire damaging the liquids, spleen yīn failing to be moistened, and the large intestine failing to be moistened.

文献评述

《先醒斋医学广笔记•妇人》："王善长夫人产后腿疼，不能行立，久之，饮食不进，困惫之极，仲淳诊之曰：此脾阴不足之候。脾主四肢，阴不足故病下体，向所饮药虽多，皆苦燥之剂，不能益阴。用石斛、木瓜、牛膝、白芍药、酸枣仁为主，生地黄、甘枸杞、白茯苓、黄柏为臣，甘草、车前为使。"指出身软倦怠，肢体乏力，不能行走，饮食减少，可由脾阴不足，运化失职，肢体失养所致，故用补脾阴的方药治疗而获效。

《医碥·大便闭结》："人有大便闭结，口干唇裂，食不能消，腹痛难忍，按之益痛，小便短涩，人以为大便之火闭也，谁知是脾火之作祟哉？…不知土太柔则崩，土太刚则燥；土崩则成废土，土燥则成焦土也。然而土焦非阳明之焰下逼，必命门之火上炎，二火合攻，脾之津液涸矣。水谷之入，仅足供脾之用，何能分润于大肠乎？"论述便秘可由脾火伤津，脾阴失濡，大肠失润引起。

Summary of Loss of Nourishment
1. Loss of Nourishment in the Face 　　Withered-yellow and lusterless facial complexion
2. Loss of Nourishment in the Structure of the Body 　　Emaciation, lack of strength in the four limbs.
3. Loss of Nourishment in the Heart Spirit 　　Fatigue and lassitude of the spirit, encumbrance, and somnolence.
4. Loss of Nourishment in the Offices and Orifices 　　Dry skin, dry nose and lips, hair loss or withered hair.
5. Loss of Nourishment in the Large Intestine 　　Dry and inhibited stool, in serious cases constipation.

失于滋养
面部失养——面色萎黄无华。
形体失养——形体消瘦，四肢乏力。
心神失养——神疲倦怠，困倦嗜卧。
官窍失养——皮肤干燥，鼻干唇燥，毛发脱落或憔悴。
大肠失养——大便干涩，甚至秘结。

3.3 Internal Generation of Vacuity Heat

When spleen yīn is vacuous, it is unable to form yīn blood. When yīn blood is insufficient, yáng qì becomes exuberant, leading to an internal generation of vacuity heat. This results in symptoms like heat effusion and night sweating. When vacuity heat harasses the heart internally, one can observe vexation and fullness in the heart and chest. The spleen governs the four limbs, and when vacuity heat harasses and stirs the extremities, the result is vexation heat in the extremities.

"Treatise on the Pathomechanisms of the Viscera and Bowels" in the *Xuè Zhèng Lùn* ("On Blood Patterns") explains:

> "The spleen is called damp earth. When earth is damp, it enriches and engenders the myriad things; when the spleen is moistened, it is able to nourish the viscera and bowels. Stomach earth uses dryness to absorb things, and spleen earth uses dampness to transform qì. When spleen qì is not distributed, the stomach is dry and unable to intake food. When food intake is reduced and food cannot be transformed, it is like cooking things in a cauldron without adding water. Therefore, it causes morbid food blockage, difficult defecation, dry mouth and scorched lips, inability to generate blood, blood vacuity fire effulgence, and heat effusion and night sweating."

Táng Róng-Chuān suggested that tidal heat and night sweating arise due to blood vacuity fire effulgence, that blood vacuity is caused by spleen yīn failing to be enriched, and that therefore spleen yīn vacuity can manifest as vacuity heat harassing the inside. Since the spleen is associated with earth and the lung is associated with metal, when spleen yīn is vacuous, earth fails to engender metal and vacuity fire harasses lung-metal above. One can then observe the symptoms of cough and counterflow qì ascent, scant sticky phlegm that is not easy to expectorate, inhibition in the throat, and dryness and pain in the throat. When vacuity fire surges up into the lips and tongue, it causes lip and tongue erosion; when vacuity fire harasses internally, it causes frenetic movement of blood, possibly resulting in symptoms like nosebleed, spontaneous bleeding of the flesh, and profuse menstruation.

The chapter, "On Lung Wilting, Lung Pain, Cough, and Ascending Qì" in the *Jīn Guì Yào Lüè* ("Essential Prescriptions of the Golden Coffer") states:

> "Fire counterflow qì ascent causes inhibition in the throat. Stop the counterflow and precipitate qì. *Mài mén dōng tāng* (Ophiopogon Decoction) treats it."

For treatment of this type of vacuity-heat-related lung wilting, Zhòng-Jǐng advises to enrich the spleen and boost yīn, based on the principle that the lung can only be nourished when the spleen's yīn humor is transported up to the lung. And it is only by this method that the symptoms of vacuity fire flaming upward, like inhibition in the throat or cough and counterflow qì ascent can be eliminated. This in turn proves that spleen yīn vacuity can cause the pathomechanism of vacuity heat harassing upward.

In the chapter, "Blood Ejection" in the *Xuè Zhèng Lùn* ("On Blood Patterns"), Táng Róng-Chuān also explained:

> "If spleen yīn is vacuous, it causes a rapid pulse, generalized heat, a sore pharynx, and a hoarse voice. The *Shèn Róu Wǔ Shū* ("Shèn Róu Five Books") uses *yǎng zhēn tāng* (Nourish the True Decoction). Using the action of blandness to supplement the spleen is a secret method for nourishing spleen yīn."

This explains further how spleen yīn vacuity can lead to the pathomechanism of internal generation of vacuity heat.

This pathomechanism is treated by boosting the spleen and engendering liquids, and by enriching yīn and clearing heat. Conditions characterized by vacuity heat symptoms like vexing heat in the five hearts and night sweating are treated with *sì jūn zǐ tāng* (Four Gentlemen Decoction) with the addition of *shān yào* (Dioscoreae Rhizoma), *guī bǎn* (Testudinis Plastrum), *bái wēi* (Cynanchi Atrati Radix), *dì gǔ pí* (Lycii Cortex), and *yín chái hú* (Stellariae Radix).

Conditions characterized by dry cough and qì counterflow are treated with *mài mén dōng tāng* (Ophiopogon Decoction) from the *Jīn Guì Yào Lüè* ("Essential Prescriptions of the Golden Coffer"), taken internally.

Mài Mén Dōng Tāng 麦门冬汤 Ophiopogon Decoction
rén shēn (人参 ginseng, Ginseng Radix)
mài mén dōng (麦门冬 ophiopogon, Ophiopogonis Radix)
bàn xià (半夏 pinellia, Pinelliae Rhizoma)
gēng mǐ (粳米 non-glutinous rice, Oryzae Semen)
dà zǎo (大枣 jujube, Jujubae Fructus)
gān cǎo (甘草 licorice, Glycyrrhizae Radix)

Conditions characterized by bleeding symptoms like nosebleed and spontaneous bleeding of the flesh are treated with a modified version of *lǐ pí yīn zhèng fāng* (Rectify the Spleen and Correct Yin Formula) from the *Bù Jū Jí* ("Non-limitation Collection").

Lǐ Pí Yīn Zhèng Fāng 理脾阴正方 Rectify the Spleen and Correct Yin Formula
rén shēn (人参 ginseng, Ginseng Radix)
zǐ hé chē (紫河车 placenta, Hominis Placenta)
bái sháo yào (白芍药 white peony, Paeoniae Radix Alba)
shān yào (山药 dioscorea, Dioscoreae Rhizoma)
biǎn dòu (扁豆 lablab, Lablab Semen Album)

lián ròu (莲肉 lotus seed, Nelumbinis Semen)

hé yè (荷叶 lotus leaf, Nelumbinis Folium)

fú líng (茯苓 poria, Poria)

jú hóng (橘红 red tangerine peel, Citri Reticulatae Exocarpium Rubrum)

gān cǎo (甘草 licorice, Glycyrrhizae Radix)

lǎo mǐ (老米 old rice, (Oryzae Semen Vetum)

Plus:

xuè yú tàn (血余炭 charred hair, Crinis Carbonisatus)

bái máo gēn (白茅根 imperata, Imperatae Rhizoma)

ǒu jié (藕节 lotus root node, Nelumbinis Rhizomatis Nodus)

虚热内生

脾阴虚，不能化生阴血，阴血不足，阳气亢盛，可致虚热内生，引起发热盗汗等症状。虚热内扰心中，可见心胸烦满；脾主四肢，虚热扰动手足，则为手足烦热。如《血证论•脏腑病机论》说：”脾称湿土，土湿则滋生万物，脾润则长养脏腑。胃土以燥纳物，脾土以湿化气，脾气不布，则胃燥而不能食，食少而不能化，譬如釜中无水而不能熟物也。故病隔食，大便难，口燥唇焦，不能生血，血虚火旺，发热盗汗”。唐容川认为潮热盗汗是因”血虚火旺”而起，血虚是由脾阴失滋所致，故脾阴虚可导致虚热内扰的表现。脾属土，肺属金，脾阴虚，土不生金，虚火上扰肺金，可见咳逆上气、痰少而黏、不易咯出、咽喉不利、或咽干疼痛等症状；虚火上冲唇舌，则唇舌糜烂；虚火内扰，迫血妄行，或引起鼻衄、肌衄、月经过多等症状。如《金匮要略•肺痿肺痛咳嗽上气篇》说：”火逆上气，咽喉不利，止逆下气，麦门冬汤主之。”对这种虚热性肺痿的治疗，仲景参以滋脾益阴，则是根据脾之阴液上输于肺，才能使肺得以滋养，而消除虚火上炎引起的咽干不利，咳逆上气诸症，从而反证脾阴虚，可引起虚热上扰的病机。唐容川《血证论•吐血》亦说”若脾阴虚，脉数身热，咽痛声哑，<慎柔五书>用养真汤，煎去头煎，止服二三煎，取无味之功以补脾，为得滋养脾阴之秘法。”进一步说明脾阴虚，可引起虚热内生的病机。

治宜益脾生津，滋阴清热。以五心烦热、盗汗等虚热症状为主，用四君子汤加山药、龟板、白薇、地骨皮、银柴胡。以干咳气逆为主，用《金匮要略》麦门冬汤（人参、麦冬、半夏、粳米、大枣、甘草）内服。以鼻衄、肌衄等出血症状为主，用《不居集》理脾阴正方（人参、河车、白芍、山药、扁豆、莲肉、荷叶、老米、茯苓、橘红、甘草）加血余炭、白茅根、藕节进行治疗。

Literature Review of Internal Generation of Vacuity Heat

📖 *Bù Jū Jí* ("Non-limitation Collection"), "Comprehensive Treatise on Rectifying Spleen Yīn"

"*Lǐ pí yì yíng tāng* (Spleen-Rectifying Construction-Boosting Decoction) treats spleen vacuity blood scantness and yīn vacuity heat effusion… [It consists of] *hǎi shēn* (Stichopus Japonicus), *lián zǐ* (Nelumbinis Semen), *shān yào* (Dioscoreae Rhizoma), *bái biǎn dòu* (Lablab Semen Album), and *hēi dòu* (Sojae Semen Atrum)."

This quotation describes how spleen yīn vacuity, yīn blood insufficiency, and failure of yīn to restrain yáng can result in manifestations of internally generated vacuity heat, like vexing heat in the five hearts, tidal heat, and night sweating. The formula uses *lián zǐ* (Nelumbinis Semen), *shān yào* (Dioscoreae Rhizoma), and *bái biǎn dòu* (Lablab Semen Album) to nourish spleen yīn, enabling the spleen to move the fluids for the stomach. Consequently, yīn blood receives nourishment and the vacuity heat can be eliminated.

文献评述

《不居集•理脾阴总论》："理脾益营汤，治脾虚血少，阴虚发热。…海参、莲肉、山药、扁豆、黑料豆。"论述脾阴虚，阴血不足，阴不制阳，可致五心烦热、潮热盗汗等虚热内生的表现。治疗用莲肉、山药、扁豆以养脾阴，脾能为胃行其津液，则阴血得养，虚热可除。

Summary of Internal Generation of Vacuity Heat

1. Liquid Forced Outward

   Heat effusion and night sweating.

2. Internally Harassing the Heart

   Vexation and fullness in the heart and chest.

3. Harassing and Stirring the Extremities

   Vexing heat in the extremities.

4. Upwardly Harassing Lung-Metal

   Cough and counterflow qì ascent, scant sticky phlegm that is difficult to expectorate, inhibition in the throat, dry and sore throat.

5. Surging Upward to the Lips and Tongue

Erosion of the lips and tongue.

6. Causing Frenetic Movement of the Blood

Nosebleed, spontaneous bleeding of the flesh, profuse menstruation.

虚热内生
迫津外出——发热盗汗。
内扰心中——心胸烦满。
扰动手足——手足烦热。
上扰肺金——咳逆上气，痰少而粘，不易咯出，咽喉不利，咽干疼痛。
上冲唇舌——唇舌糜烂。
迫血妄行——鼻衄，肌衄，月经过多。

Spleen yīn vacuity is a condition that progresses slowly and develops gradually. When spleen yīn is vacuous and unable to form spleen qì, this can cause spleen qì vacuity; at the same time, when spleen qì is vacuous and qì is unable to transform the liquids, this can cause spleen yīn vacuity. Therefore, the pathomechanisms of spleen yīn vacuity and spleen qì vacuity often coincide, which is called dual vacuity of spleen qì and spleen yīn. When spleen yīn vacuity and stomach yīn vacuity arise at the same time in mutual dependence, it is called spleen-stomach yīn vacuity. Spleen yīn vacuity and lung yīn vacuity or heart yīn vacuity can interact, as cause and effect and influence each other. However, from the perspective of clinical experience, spleen yīn vacuity is not too closely related to liver or kidney yīn vacuity and understanding the mechanism of their interaction will benefit from further research.

脾阴虚是一慢性过程，发展缓慢。脾阴虚不能化生脾气，可使脾气虚弱；同时脾气虚，气不化津，可引起脾阴虚，故脾阴虚常与脾气虚的病机并存，称为脾的气阴两虚；脾阴虚与胃阴虚常同时发生，相互依存，称为脾胃阴虚；脾阴虚与肺阴虚、心阴虚之间可以互为因果，相互影响。不过，从临床实践观察，脾阴虚与肝、肾阴虚的关系不很密切，机理何在，有待进一步探讨。

Index

abdominal distention, 7, 8, 14, 17, 19, 20, 22-24, 29, 31-32, 34-36, 40, 43- 44, 46, 49-50, 52, 54, 56-57, 63, 66-70, 74, 82-83, 86, 90, 102-103, 115, 142-145, 153, 159, 161, 164-165, 172, 184, 186, 191
abdominal distention and fullness, 14, 20, 22, 36, 40, 44, 46, 52, 54, 57, 115, 165, 172, 186
abdominal distention and pain, 29, 50, 70
abdominal fullness, 7, 19, 36, 38, 40, 46, 74, 79, 82, 149, 151, 153, 155, 160, 187, 188
abdominal hardness, 14
abdominal pain, 2, 8, 9, 19-20, 22-24, 28, 30, 32, 36, 38-39, 46, 48, 54, 74, 83, 149, 154, 159, 160, 173, 178, 181, 196
abdominal pain and diarrhea, 20
abdominal pain that refuses pressure, 36, 39, 48, 54
absence of hunger, 2, 9, 18, 22, 81, 82, 186, 189
absence of thirst, 178
accumulated rheum, 93
accumulations and gatherings, 19, 20, 39, 40
aching lumbus, 145, 179
aching lumbus and weak legs, 179
aching of the lower legs, 13
aching pain, 26, 86, 95
achyranthes, *niú xī*, 牛膝, Achyranthis Bidentatae Radix, 196
Achyranthis Bidentatae Radix, *niú xī*, 牛膝, achyranthes, 196
acid swallowing, 8, 64, 74
Aconite and Rice Decoction, *fù zǐ gēng mǐ tāng*, 附子粳米汤, 175
Aconite Center-Rectifying Decoction, *fù zǐ lǐ zhōng tāng*, 附子理中汤, 182
Aconite Center-Rectifying Pill, *fù zǐ lǐ zhōng wán*, 附子理中丸, 157, 167
aconite main tuber, *chuān wū tóu*, 川乌头, Aconiti Radix, 25, 26, 27, 146, 157, 165, 166, 167, 175, 176
aconite, *fù zǐ*, 附子, Aconiti Radix Lateralis Praeparata, 19, 25, 26, 27, 37, 41, 146, 157, 165, 166, 167, 175, 176, 182
Aconiti Radix Lateralis Praeparata, *fù zǐ*, 附子, aconite, 19, 25, 26, 27, 37, 41, 146, 157, 165, 166, 167, 175, 176, 182
Aconiti Radix Lateralis Praeparata, *zhì fù zǐ*, 制附子, processed aconite, 25, 27, 146, 157, 165, 166, 167, 175, 176
Aconiti Radix Lateralis Tosta, *pào fù zǐ*, 炮附子, blast-fried aconite, 26
Aconiti Radix, *chuān wū tóu*, 川乌头, aconite main tuber, 25-27, 146, 157, 165-167, 175-176
Acori Tatarinowii Rhizoma, *shí chāng pú*, 石菖蒲, acorus, 62, 70

acorus, *shí chāng pú*, 石菖蒲, Acori Tatarinowii Rhizoma, 62, 70
acquired constitution, 5, 73, 121
adenophora/glehnia, *shā shēn*, 沙参, Adenophorae seu Glehniae Radix, 67, 189
Adenophorae seu Glehniae Radix, *shā shēn*, 沙参, adenophora/glehnia, 67, 189
affect-mind, 20
agastache leaf, *huò xiāng yè*, 藿香叶, Agastaches Folium, 49, 84, 87
agastache, *huò xiāng*, 藿香, Agastaches Herba, 49-51, 62, 84, 87, 175
Agastaches Herba, *huò xiāng*, 藿香, agastache, 51, 62, 175
Agrimoniae Herba, *xiān hè cǎo*, 仙鹤草, agrimony, 118
agrimony, *xiān hè cǎo*, 仙鹤草, Agrimoniae Herba, 118
ài yè, 艾叶, mugwort, Artemisiae Argyi Folium, 118
Akebiae Trifoliatae Caulis, *mù tōng*, 木通, trifoliate akebia, 63, 69
alcohol, *jiǔ jīng*, 酒精, Alcohol, 45, 73
alisma, *zé xiè*, 泽泻, Alismatis Rhizoma, 25, 27, 69, 84, 91, 101-102, 131, 146, 167
Alismatis Rhizoma, *zé xiè*, 泽泻, alisma, 25, 27, 69, 84, 91, 101-102, 131, 146, 167
Allii Fistulosi Herba, *cōng*, 葱, scallion, 127, 130
alpinia, *yì zhì rén*, 益智仁, Alpiniae Oxyphyllae Fructus, 107-108, 161
Alpiniae Galangae Rhizoma, *dà liáng jiāng*, 大良姜, galangal, 25, 156-157
Alpiniae Katsumadai Semen, *cǎo dòu kòu*, 草豆蔻, Katsumada's galangal seed, 24-25, 156
Alpiniae Officinarum Rhizoma, *gāo liáng jiāng*, 高良姜, lesser galangal, 157
Alpiniae Oxyphyllae Fructus, *yì zhì rén*, 益智仁, alpinia, 107-108, 161
Amomi Fructus Rotundus, *bái dòu kòu*, 白豆蔻, cardamom, 62, 84
Amomi Fructus, *shā rén*, 砂仁, amomum, 36-37, 62, 83-84, 88-89, 103, 108-109, 130, 155, 161, 176, 188
amomum, *shā rén*, 砂仁, Amomi Fructus, 36-37, 62, 83-84, 88-89, 103, 108-109, 130, 155, 161, 176, 188
ancestral qì, 4, 128
Angelicae Pubescentis Radix, *dú huó*, 独活, pubescent angelica, 27
Angelicae Sinensis Radix, *dāng guī*, 当归, Chinese angelica, 41, 68, 69, 100, 102, 107-109, 118, 124, 129, 144, 189

anger, 6, 20, 165

anger damaging the liver, 165

antelope horn, *líng yáng jiǎo*, 羚羊角, Saigae Tataricae Cornu, 175

anxiety and thought, 18, 120, 160

appetite, 33, 48, 52, 54, 64, 86, 95, 160, 179, 191

Apricot Kernel and Talcum Decoction, *xìng rén huá shí tāng*, 杏仁滑石汤, 58

apricot kernel, *xìng rén*, 杏仁, Armeniacae Semen, 50, 58, 175, 194

apricot, *xìng zǐ*, 杏子, Armeniacae Fructus, 50, 58, 175, 194

aquilaria, *chén xiāng*, 沉香, Aquilariae Lignum Resinatum, 188

Aquilariae Lignum Resinatum, *chén xiāng*, 沉香, aquilaria, 188

arborvitae leaf, *cè bǎi yè*, 侧柏叶, Platycladi Cacumen, 118

areca husk, *dà fù pí*, 大腹皮, Arecae Pericarpium, 19, 62, 91

areca, *bīng láng*, 槟榔, Arecae Semen, 19, 26, 58, 62, 91, 166

Arecae Pericarpium, *dà fù pí*, 大腹皮, areca husk, 19, 62, 91

Arecae Semen, *bīng láng*, 槟榔, areca, 19, 26, 58, 62, 91, 166

Armadillidium, *shǔ fù*, 鼠妇, wood louse, 41

Armeniacae Fructus, *xìng zǐ*, 杏子, apricot, 50, 58, 175, 194

Armeniacae Semen, *xìng rén*, 杏仁, apricot kernel, 50, 58, 175, 194

Artemisiae Argyi Folium, *ài yè*, 艾叶, mugwort, 118

Artemisiae Scopariae Herba, *yīn chén hāo*, 茵陈蒿, virgate wormwood, 27, 60, 63

Asari Herba, *xì xīn*, 细辛, asarum, 175

asarum, *xì xīn*, 细辛, Asari Herba, 175

Asini Corii Colla, *ē jiāo*, 阿胶, ass hide glue, 42, 118

Asparagi Radix, *tiān mén dōng*, 天门冬, asparagus, 124

asparagus, *tiān mén dōng*, 天门冬, Asparagi Radix, 124

ass hide glue, *ē jiāo*, 阿胶, Asini Corii Colla, 42, 118

aster, *zǐ wǎn*, 紫菀, Asteris Radix, 145

Asteris Radix, *zǐ wǎn*, 紫菀, aster, 145

Astragali Radix, *huáng qí*, 黄芪, astragalus, 41, 49-50, 58, 62-63, 69, 84, 100, 102, 107-109, 118, 124, 129-131, 136, 140, 144, 156

Astragalus Center-Fortifying Decoction, *huáng qí jiàn zhōng tāng*, 黄耆*建中汤, 131, 156

Astragalus Decoction, *huáng qí tāng*, 黄耆*汤, 84

astragalus, *huáng qí*, 黄耆, Astragali Radix, 41, 49-50, 58, 62-63, 69, 84, 100, 102, 107-109, 118, 124, 129-131, 136, 140, 144, 156

atractylodes, *cāng zhú*, 苍术, Atractylodis Rhizoma, 7, 19, 20, 24-27, 32, 37, 42, 68, 83-84, 86-87, 89, 91, 100, 102-103, 107-109, 118,

124, 129-130, 143-145, 155, 157, 166-167, 174-176, 182, 187-188

Atractylodis Macrocephalae Rhizoma, *bái zhú*, 白术, white atractylodes, 7, 20, 25-27, 32, 34, 42, 68, 83-84, 86-87, 89, 91, 100, 102-103, 107-109, 112, 118, 120, 124, 129-130, 143-145, 155, 157, 163, 165-167, 174-176, 182, 184, 187-188, 194

Atractylodis Rhizoma, *cāng zhú*, 苍术, atractylodes, 7, 19-20, 24-27, 32, 37, 42, 68, 83-84, 86-87, 89, 91, 100, 102-103, 107-109, 118, 124, 129-130, 143-145, 155, 157, 166-167, 174-176, 182, 187-188

Atramentum, *mò*, 墨, ink, 57, 118

Aucklandiae Radix, *mù xiāng*, 木香, costusroot, 19-20, 25-26, 36-37, 57-58, 83, 87-89, 103, 118, 124, 130, 144, 155-156, 161, 166, 175

Aurantii Fructus Immaturus, *zhǐ shí*, 枳实, unripe bitter orange, 19, 20, 24-27, 32, 34, 37, 41-42, 50, 57-58, 84, 87, 89, 91, 102, 104, 143, 145, 166, 184, 194

Aurantii Fructus, *zhǐ qiào ké*, 枳壳, bitter orange, 19-20, 24-27, 32, 34, 37, 41-42, 50, 57-58, 60-61, 84, 87, 89, 91, 102-104, 108-109, 143, 145, 166, 188, 194

Aurum, *huáng jīn*, 黄金, gold, 14, 46, 67, 74, 79, 122-123, 134, 149, 155, 163, 173, 194

aversion to cold, 57, 139, 163, 171, 174, 179

aversion to food, 36, 56, 68-69, 190

aversion to water, 151

aversion to wind, 5, 10, 63

back and lumbar pain, 163

back pain, 40

bad breath, 48

bái dòu kòu, 白豆蔻, cardamom, Amomi Fructus Rotundus, 62, 84

bái fú líng, 白茯苓, white poria, Poria Alba, 26

bái jí, 白及, bletilla, Bletillae Rhizoma, 118

bái máo gēn, 白茅根, imperata, Imperatae Rhizoma, 200

bái sháo yào, 白芍药, white peony, Paeoniae Radix Alba, 20, 26, 37, 67-68, 100, 130-131, 145, 156, 166, 189, 190, 194, 196, 199

bái sháo, 白芍, white peony, Paeoniae Radix Alba, 19-20, 24-27, 32, 37, 41, 49-50, 57-58, 67-68, 70, 84, 87, 89, 91, 100, 130-131, 145, 156, 166, 176, 182, 189-190, 194, 196, 199

bái wēi, 白薇, black swallowwort, Cynanchi Atrati Radix, 199

bái zhú, 白术, white atractylodes, Atractylodis Macrocephalae Rhizoma, 7, 20, 25-27, 32, 34, 42, 68, 83-84, 86-87, 89, 91, 100, 102-103, 107-109, 112, 118, 120, 124, 129-130, 143-145, 155, 157, 163, 165-167, 174-176, 182, 184, 187-188, 194

bamboo shavings, *zhú rú*, 竹茹, Bumbusae Caulis in Taenia, 50

bàn xià, 半夏, pinellia, Pinelliae Rhizoma, 32, 42, 50, 57-58, 60-61, 70, 87, 89-90, 102-103, 108-109, 112, 143, 145, 176, 199

bar pulse, 14, 20, 46, 155

barley sprout, *mài yá*, 麦芽, Hordei Fructus Germinatus, 37, 84

bèi mǔ, 贝母, fritillaria, Fritillariae Bulbus, 62

běi shú mǐ, 北秫米, sorghum, Sorghi Semen, 55

běi tíng lì, 北葶苈, lepidium, Lepidii Semen, 42

belamcanda, *shè gān*, 射干, Belamcandae Rhizoma, 41, 62

Belamcandae Rhizoma, *shè gān*, 射干, belamcanda, 41, 62

belching, 14, 21, 69, 155, 162

biǎn dòu, 扁豆, lablab, Lablab Semen Album, 83-84, 187-190, 194, 199, 201

Biǎn Què, 90

biē jiǎ jiān wán, 鳖甲煎丸, Turtle Shell Decocted Pill, 41

biē jiǎ, 鳖甲, turtle shell, Trionycis Carapax, 41

bile, 23-24, 29, 59-60, 64, 66

binding depression of liver qì, 44

binding depression of spleen qì, 43

bīng láng, 槟榔, areca, Arecae Semen, 19, 26, 58, 62, 91, 166

bitter orange, *zhǐ qiào (ké)*, 枳壳, Aurantii Fructus, 34, 37, 41, 50, 57-58, 60-61, 84, 103, 108-109, 188, 194

bitter taste in the mouth, 68

black soybean, *hēi dà dòu*, 黑大豆, Sojae Semen Atrum, 201

black stool, 160

black swallowwort, *bái wēi*, 白薇, Cynanchi Atrati Radix, 199

bladder, 56-57, 65-66, 89-90, 93, 104, 106-107, 112-113, 163-164

bland taste in the mouth, 31, 35-36, 39, 128, 130, 151, 186, 189

blast-fried aconite, *pào fù zǐ*, 炮附子, Aconiti Radix Lateralis Tosta, 26

blast-fried ginger, *pào jiāng*, 炮姜, Zingiberis Rhizoma Praeparatum, 26, 174-175

bleeding, 10, 116-117, 120-121, 199

bletilla, *bái jí*, 白及, Bletillae Rhizoma, 118

Bletillae Rhizoma, *bái jí*, 白及, bletilla, 118

bloating, 38, 92

blood depletion, 135

blood desertion, 4, 117, 120

blood disease, 150

blood ejection, 4, 10, 117-118, 120, 199

blood loss, 120

blood stasis, 13, 17, 43, 70, 182

blood vacuity, 76, 143, 198

bloody stool, 4, 10, 38-39, 117-118, 120

bloody urine, 4, 117-118, 121

blurred vision, 126, 129

bò hé, 薄荷, mint, Menthae Herba, 62, 68

boost qì, 191

boost yīn, 184, 190, 196, 198

bound stool, 56, 66

bowel and visceral pattern identification, 7

Braseniae Caulis et Folium, *chún*, 莼, water shield, 29, 59, 184, 196

breast milk, 116

bright white facial complexion, 179, 180

brighten the eyes, 126

bǔ fèi tāng, 补肺汤, Lung-Supplementing Decoction, 144

bǔ gǔ zhī, 补骨脂, psoralea, Psoraleae Fructus, 182

bǔ zhōng yì qì tāng, 补中益气汤, Center-Supplementing Qì-Boosting Decoction, 97, 100-102, 107-109, 112-113, 124, 129, 131, 135-136, 139

Bubali Cornu, *shuǐ niú jiǎo*, 水牛角, water buffalo horn, 49

Bumbusae Caulis in Taenia, *zhú rú*, 竹茹, bamboo shavings, 50

Bupleuri Radix, *chái hú*, 柴胡, bupleurum, 26, 42, 49, 68-69, 87, 100-104, 107-109, 124, 129-130, 145, 167, 199

Bupleurum and Peony Six Gentlemen Decoction, *chái sháo liù jūn zǐ tāng*, 柴芍六君子汤, 145

bupleurum, *chái hú*, 柴胡, Bupleuri Radix, 26, 42, 49, 68-69, 87, 100-104, 107-109, 124, 129-130, 145, 167, 199

Campsis Flos, *líng xiāo huā*, 凌霄花, campsis flower, 42

campsis flower, *líng xiāo huā*, 凌霄花, Campsis Flos, 42

campsis, *zǐ wēi gēn*, 紫葳根, Campsitis Radix, 42

Campsitis Radix, *zǐ wēi gēn*, 紫葳根, campsis, 42

camptotheca, *hàn lián*, 旱莲, Camptothecae Fructus seu Radix, 118

Camptothecae Fructus seu Radix, *hàn lián*, 旱莲, camptotheca, 118

cāng ěr zǐ, 苍耳子, xanthium, Xanthii Fructus, 130

cāng ěr, 苍耳, xanthium stem and leaf, Xanthii Herba, 130

cāng zhú, 苍术, atractylodes, Atractylodis Rhizoma, 7, 19-20, 24-27, 32, 37, 42, 68, 83-84, 86-87, 89, 91, 100, 102-103, 107-109, 118, 124, 129-130, 143-145, 155, 157, 166-167, 174-176, 182, 187-188

Cannabis Fructus, *huǒ má rén*, 火麻仁, cannabis fruit, 50, 84, 189, 194

Cannabis Fruit Pill, *má zǐ rén wán*, 麻子仁丸, 50, 183, 193-194

cannabis fruit, *huǒ má rén*, 火麻仁, Cannabis Fructus, 50, 84, 189, 194

cǎo dòu kòu, 草豆蔻, Katsumada's galangal seed, Alpiniae Katsumadai Semen, 24-25, 156

cǎo guǒ, 草果, tsaoko, Tsaoko Fructus, 26, 166

cardamom, *bái dòu kòu*, 白豆蔻, Amomi Fructus Rotundus, 62, 84

Carthami Flos, *hóng huā*, 红花, carthamus, 19-20, 27, 37, 41, 50, 58, 61, 70, 83-84, 124, 143, 145, 156-157, 167, 176, 182, 188

carthamus, *hóng huā*, 红花, Carthami Flos, 19-20, 27, 37, 41, 50, 58, 61, 70, 83-84, 124, 143, 145, 156-157, 167, 176, 182, 188

Caryophylli Flos, *dīng xiāng*, 丁香, clove, 157

Catharsius, *qiāng láng*, 蜣螂, dung beetle, 42

cè bǎi yè, 侧柏叶, arborvitae leaf, Platycladi
Cacumen, 118

center burner, 3, 9, 18, 21, 23, 34, 36, 56, 59, 61,
86, 89, 92, 98, 101, 112, 129, 142, 153, 160,
165, 174

center burner qì stagnation, 98, 101, 114

center fullness, 48, 92, 165

Center Harmony Decoction, *zhōng hé tāng*, 中和
汤, 190

center qì, 55, 57, 101, 105-106, 117, 120, 129,
170

center qì fall, 97, 107, 139, 140, 161

Center-Rectifying Decoction, *lǐ zhōng tāng*, 理中
汤, 117, 179, 182

Center-Rectifying Pill, *lǐ zhōng wán*, 理中丸,
155, 157, 167, 176

Center-Regulating Qì-Boosting Decoction, *tiáo
zhōng yì qì tāng*, 调中益气汤, 123

Center-Supplementing Qì-Boosting Decoction, *bǔ
zhōng yì qì tāng*, 补中益气汤, 97, 100-101,
107-109, 112-113, 124, 129-131, 135-136, 139

Central Treasury Canon, *Zhōng Zàng Jīng*, 7, 33,
74, 79, 91, 133, 155, 173, 178

Cervi Cornu Degelatinatum, *lù jiǎo shuāng*, 鹿角
霜, degelatinated deer antler, 167

Cervi Cornu, *lù jiǎo*, 鹿角, deerhorn, 167

chá yè, 茶叶, tea, Theae Folium, 22, 54

chaenomeles, *mù guā*, 木瓜, Chaenomelis
Fructus, 26, 166, 196

Chaenomelis Fructus, *mù guā*, 木瓜,
chaenomeles, 26, 166, 196

Chaenomelis Fructus, *shēng mù guā*, 生木瓜, raw
chaenomeles, 26, 166, 196

chái hú, 柴胡, bupleurum, Bupleuri Radix, 26,
42, 49, 68-69, 87, 100-104, 107-109, 124, 129-
130, 145, 167, 199

chái sháo liù jūn zǐ tāng, 柴芍六君子汤,
Bupleurum and Peony Six Gentlemen
Decoction, 145

channel qì, 86

channels and network vessels, 33, 89, 93-94, 163

chǎo mài yá, 炒麦芽, stir-fried barley sprout,
Hordei Fructus Germinatus Frictus, 84

charred hair, *xuè yú tàn*, 血余炭, Crinis
Carbonisatus, 200

charred imperata, *máo gēn tàn*, 茅根炭, Imperatae
Rhizoma, 200

charred schizonepeta, *jīng jiè tàn*, 荆芥炭,
Schizonepetae Herba et Flos Carbonisatae, 167

charred trachycarpus, *zōng lǘ tàn*, 棕榈炭,
Trachycarpi Stipulae Fibra Carbonisata, 118

charred trachycarpus, *zōng tàn*, 棕炭, Trachycarpi
Petiolus Carbonisatus, 118

chē qián zǐ, 车前子, plantago seed, Plantaginis
Semen, 26, 69, 167, 196

chē qián, 车前, plantago, Plantaginis Herba, 26,
69, 167, 196

Chebulae Fructus, *hē zǐ*, 诃子, chebule, 108

chebule, *hē zǐ*, 诃子, Chebulae Fructus, 108

chén cāng mǐ, 陈仓米, old rice, Oryzae Semen
Vetum, 200

chén pí, 陈皮, tangerine peel, Citri Reticulatae
Pericarpium, 19-20, 22, 26, 32, 37, 42, 50, 57-
58, 60-61, 83-84, 87, 89-91, 100, 102-103, 107-
109, 113, 124, 129, 143, 145, 156, 167, 188,
190, 200

chén xiāng, 沉香, aquilaria, Aquilariae Lignum
Resinatum, 188

chì fú líng, 赤茯苓, red poria, Poria Rubra, 50

chì sháo, 赤芍, red peony, Paeoniae Radix Rubra,
41

chì xiāo, 赤硝, red niter, Nitrum Rubrum, 42

children's diseases, 7, 14, 47, 49, 74, 83, 86, 142,
174

Chinese angelica, *dāng guī*, 当归, Angelicae
Sinensis Radix, 41, 68- 69, 100, 102, 107-109,
118, 124, 129, 144, 189

Chinese lovage, *gǎo běn*, 本, Ligustici Rhizoma,
27

cholera, 7, 23, 57, 69, 155

chuān bèi mǔ, 川贝母, Sichuan fritillaria,
Fritillariae Cirrhosae Bulbus, 62

chuān wū tóu, 川乌头, aconite main tuber,
Aconiti Radix, 25-27, 146, 157, 165-167, 175-
176

chuān xiōng, 川芎, chuanxiong, Chuanxiong
Rhizoma, 27, 41, 100, 175

Chuanxiong Rhizoma, *chuān xiōng*, 川芎,
chuanxiong, 27, 41, 100, 175

chuanxiong, *chuān xiōng*, 川芎, Chuanxiong
Rhizoma, 27, 41, 100, 175

chún, 莼, water shield, Braseniae Caulis et
Folium, 29, 59, 184, 196

cimicifuga, *shēng má*, 升麻, Cimicifugae
Rhizoma, 49, 84, 87, 100-104, 107-108, 109,
124, 129-130, 174-175

Cimicifugae Rhizoma, *shēng má*, 升麻,
cimicifuga, 49, 84, 87, 100-104, 107-109, 124,
129-130, 174-175

Cinnamomi Cortex Rasus, *guì xīn*, 桂心, shaved
cinnamon bark, 175

Cinnamomi Cortex, *ròu guì*, 肉桂, cinnamon
bark, 146, 175

Cinnamomi Ramulus, *guì zhī*, 桂枝, cinnamon
twig, 25, 41, 91, 131, 156, 163, 165-167, 176

cinnamon bark, *ròu guì*, 肉桂, Cinnamomi
Cortex, 146, 175

cinnamon twig, *guì zhī*, 桂枝, Cinnamomi
Ramulus, 25, 41, 91, 131, 156, 163, 165-167,
176

Citri Fructus, *jú*, 橘, tangerine, 19-20, 24-26, 32,
37, 42, 50, 58, 61, 83-84, 87, 89-91, 100, 102-
103, 107-109, 124, 129, 143, 145, 156-157,
167, 188, 190, 200

Citri Fructus, *xiāng yuán*, 香橼, citron, 20

Citri Reticulatae Exocarpium Rubrum, *jú hóng*,
橘红, red tangerine peel, 84, 188, 190, 200

Citri Reticulatae Pericarpium Viride, *qīng pí*, 青皮
, unripe tangerine peel, 19-20, 25, 27, 32, 37,
58, 61, 113, 167

Citri Reticulatae Pericarpium, *chén pí*, 陈皮, tangerine peel, 19-20, 24-27, 32, 37, 42, 50, 57-58, 60-61, 83-84, 87, 89-91, 100, 102-103, 107-109, 113, 124, 129, 143, 145, 156, 167, 188, 190, 200

citron, *xiāng yuán*, 香橼, Citri Fructus, 20

Classified Case Histories of Famous Physicians, *míng yī lèi àn*, 93, 111, 134

clear thin stool, 154, 162

clear yáng, 98-100, 106-107, 122, 126, 135-136, 138, 141, 150, 190

clear-food diarrhea, 179

clenched jaw, 173

clinical, 13, 14, 15, 20, 24, 55, 73, 76, 86, 96, 97, 141, 149, 151, 183, 187, 194, 202

Clinical Guide with Case Histories, *lín zhèng zhǐ nán yī àn* (1766 (Qīng), Yè Guì 叶桂 [Tiān-Shì 天士]), 20, 24, 55, 96, 97, 151

Clove and Evodia Center-Rectifying Decoction, *dīng yú lǐ zhōng tāng*, 丁萸理中汤, 157

clove, *dīng xiāng*, 丁香, Caryophylli Flos, 157

clover fern, *píng*, 苹, Marsileae Herba, 8, 19, 24, 26, 36, 37, 49-50, 52, 83, 134, 145, 154, 157, 159, 175, 178, 188

Cnidii Fructus, *shé chuáng zǐ*, 蛇床子, cnidium seed, 113

cnidium seed, *shé chuáng zǐ*, 蛇床子, Cnidii Fructus, 113

Codonopsis Radix, *dǎng shēn*, 党参, codonopsis, 188

codonopsis, *dǎng shēn*, 党参, Codonopsis Radix, 188

Coicis Semen, *yì yǐ rén*, 薏苡仁, coix, 83-84, 86-87, 188

coix, *yì yǐ rén*, 薏苡仁, Coicis Semen, 83-84, 86-87, 188

cold accumulation, 164

cold damage, 7, 29, 50, 58, 60, 79, 90, 149, 155, 156, 165, 167, 176, 178, 183, 193, 194

cold diarrhea, 154

cold evil, 29

cold in the back, 163, 171

cold in the uterus, 105

cold limbs, 23, 30, 176

cold pain, 173

cold patterns, 153

cold strike, 111, 149, 159, 178

cold-damp, 14, 18, 22-24, 29, 44, 151, 182

cold-damp encumbering the spleen, 18, 22, 24, 28, 30, 44, 182

common cold, 5, 174, 181

Compendium of Good Remedies for Women, *fù rén dà quán liáng fāng* (*Fù Rén Liáng Fāng* 妇人良方), 24, 102, 116, 142

complete absence of food intake, 179

concretions and conglomerations, 39

cōng, 葱, scallion, Allii Fistulosi Herba, 127, 130

congealing cold, 154, 162, 173, 181-182

congealing cold qì stagnation, 154, 173

constipation, 2, 9, 48, 50, 54, 67, 82, 84, 95, 193-194, 196-197

constitutional insufficiency, 6, 80, 151

construction and defense, 139, 169

construction-blood, 4, 164

consummate yīn, 134-135

consumption, 22, 45, 47, 151, 170, 185

contract cold, 154

contract dampness evil, 55

contracture and tautness, 173, 178

conveyance and transformation, 82

cooked rehmannia, *shú dì huáng*, 熟地黄, Rehmanniae Radix Praeparata, 145-146

copious phlegm, 31, 35

copious sweat, 99

Coptidis Rhizoma, *huáng lián*, 黄连, coptis, 49-50, 57, 58, 69-70, 84

Coptis and Officinal Magnolia Bark Beverage, *lián pò yǐn*, 连朴饮, 69

coptis, *huáng lián*, 黄连, Coptidis Rhizoma, 49-50, 57-58, 69-70, 84

Corni Fructus, *shān zhū yú*, 山茱萸, cornus, 146

cornus, *shān zhū yú*, 山茱萸, Corni Fructus, 146

Correction of Errors in Medical Classics, *yī lín gǎi cuò*, 41

Corydalis Rhizoma, *yán hú suǒ*, 延胡索, corydalis, 41

corydalis, *yán hú suǒ*, 延胡索, Corydalis Rhizoma, 41

Costusroot and Amomum Six Gentlemen Decoction, *xiāng shā liù jūn zǐ tāng*, 香砂六君子汤, 88, 103, 130, 161

Costusroot and Amomum Stomach-Calming Powder, *xiāng shā píng wèi sǎn*, 香砂平胃散, 36

costusroot, *mù xiāng*, 木香, Aucklandiae Radix, 19-20, 25-26, 36-37, 57-58, 83, 87-89, 103, 118, 124, 130, 144, 155-156, 161, 166, 175

cough, 2, 9, 20, 31, 35, 88, 95, 164, 198-199, 201

cough and counterflow qì ascent, 198

cough and oppression in the chest, 31

cough and panting, 2, 9

Counterflow Cold Decoction, *sì nì tāng*, 四逆汤, 149, 179

counterflow cold of the limbs, 174, 178-179, 181

counterflow qì ascent, 198, 201

crab, *xiè*, 蟹, Eriocheiris Caro et Viscera, 7-8, 20, 25, 27, 47, 49-50, 68-69, 84, 91, 101-102, 131, 146, 167

cracked lips, 196

cramp, 49, 52, 178

Crataegi Fructus Ustus, *jiāo shān zhā*, 焦山楂, scorch-fried crataegus, 84, 188

Crataegi Fructus, *shān zhā*, 山楂, crataegus, 37, 60-61, 84, 187-188

crataegus, *shān zhā*, 山楂, Crataegi Fructus, 37, 60-61, 84, 187-188

Crinis, *xuè yú*, 血余, hair, 111, 123, 138, 144, 193, 197, 200

Crinis Carbonisatus, *xuè yú tàn*, 血余炭, charred hair, 200

crustacean lindernia, *mǔ cǎo*, 母草, Linderniae Crustaceae Herba, 118 curcuma, *yù jīn*, 郁金, Curcumae Radix, 19, 20, 25, 27, 32, 58, 167

Curcumae Radix, *yù jīn*, 郁金, curcuma, 19, 20, 25, 27, 32, 58, 167

cuttlefish bone, *hǎi piāo xiāo*, 海螵蛸, Sepiae Endoconcha, 118

Cynanchi Atrati Radix, *bái wēi*, 白薇, black swallowwort, 199

Cyperi Rhizoma, *xiāng fù zǐ*, 香附子, cyperus, 19-20, 25-27, 32, 37, 41, 58, 61, 83-84, 91, 124, 145, 157, 167, 188

cyperus, *xiāng fù zǐ*, 香附子, Cyperi Rhizoma, 19-20, 25-27, 32, 37, 41, 58, 61, 83-84, 91, 124, 145, 157, 167, 188

dà fù pí, 大腹皮, areca husk, Arecae Pericarpium, 19, 62, 91

dà huáng, 大黄, rhubarb, Rhei Radix et Rhizoma, 41, 49-50, 60, 194

dà jiàn zhōng tāng, 大建中汤, Major Center-Fortifying Decoction, 156-157

dà liáng jiāng, 大良姜, galangal, Alpiniae Galangae Rhizoma, 25, 156-157

dà qīng yè, 大青叶, isatis leaf, Isatidis Folium, 49

dà zǎo, 大枣, jujube, Jujubae Fructus, 32, 51, 118, 131, 144, 156, 176, 190, 199

damage the spleen and stomach, 38, 39, 111

damage to stomach yīn, 184

damage to yáng, 24, 178

damp obstruction, 142

damp phlegm, 32, 34

damp qì, 82, 86, 93, 164

damp swelling, 93

damp turbidity, 2, 86, 95

damp-heat, 14, 45, 46, 54, 55, 56, 57, 59, 60, 62, 63, 64, 65, 67, 68, 69, 70, 185

damp-heat brewing in the spleen, 46, 54, 57, 60, 67

dampness damage, 86

dampness disease, 31, 86

dampness evil, 45, 54, 55

Dampness-Overcoming Decoction, *shèng shī tāng*, 胜湿汤, 26

dàn dòu chǐ, 淡豆豉, fermented soybean, Sojae Semen Praeparatum, 57, 70

dān zhī xiāo yáo sǎn, 丹栀逍遥散, Moutan and Gardenia Free Wanderer Powder, 68

dāng guī, 当归, Chinese angelica, Angelicae Sinensis Radix, 41, 68-69, 100, 102, 107-109, 118, 124, 129, 144, 189

dǎng shēn, 党参, codonopsis, Codonopsis Radix, 188

deafness, 127, 130, 135, 138

debilitation of the spleen and stomach, 31, 75, 80, 123, 133, 140

debility in old age, 80

deep pulse, 179

deep-lying rheum, 163

deerhorn, *lù jiǎo*, 鹿角, Cervi Cornu, 167

defense qì, 4, 64, 179

defensive yáng, 174

degelatinated deer antler, *lù jiǎo shuāng*, 鹿角霜, Cervi Cornu Degelatinatum, 167

Dendrobii Herba, *gān shí hú*, 干石斛, dried dendrobium, 67, 188-189, 196

Dendrobii Herba, *shí hú*, 石斛, dendrobium, 67, 188-189, 196

dendrobium, *shí hú*, 石斛, Dendrobii Herba, 67, 188-189, 196

depression in the chest, 120

desiccated, 79, 123, 138, 194

desire to defecate, 82, 95

desire to vomit, 23, 30, 36, 46

deviated mouth, 93

devitalized essence-spirit, 23, 30

dì gǔ pí, 地骨皮, lycium root bark, Lycii Cortex, 199

dì huáng, 地黄, rehmannia, Rehmanniae Radix, 67, 69, 124, 145-146, 196

dì yú, 地榆, sanguisorba, Sanguisorbae Radix, 118

Dianthi Herba, *qū mài*, 瞿麦, dianthus, 42

dianthus, *qū mài*, 瞿麦, Dianthi Herba, 42

diarrhea, 2-3, 7-9, 14, 20, 22-24, 29, 30-36, 38-40, 44, 46, 56-58, 64, 66, 69, 73-74, 79-80, 82, 88, 90, 92, 95, 97, 105-106, 108, 115, 120, 145, 149, 151, 154-155, 157, 160-162, 169-170, 178-179, 182, 187-188, 190, 192

diarrhea and dysentery, 2, 105

dietary irregularities, 6, 45, 92, 107, 111, 126, 154, 185

difficult defecation, 14, 198

difficult speech, 93, 178

difficult to cure, 41

difficult to expectorate, 201

difficult urination, 90

dīng xiāng, 丁香, clove, Caryophylli Flos, 157

dīng yú lǐ zhōng tāng, 丁萸理中汤, Clove and Evodia Center-Rectifying Decoction, 157

Dioscorea Pill, *shǔ yù wán*, 薯蓣丸, 183

dioscorea, *shān yào*, 山药, Dioscoreae Rhizoma, 26, 67, 83-84, 107-109, 113, 146, 166, 183, 187-188, 190-191, 199, 201

Dioscoreae Rhizoma, *shān yào*, 山药, dioscorea, 26, 67, 83-84, 107-109, 113, 146, 166, 183, 187-188, 190-191, 199, 201

Dipsaci Radix, *xù duàn*, 续断, dipsacus, 118

dipsacus, *xù duàn*, 续断, Dipsaci Radix, 118

Discharge-Ceasing Decoction, *wán dài tāng*, 完带汤, 25, 166

disinhibit water, 90

dispel phlegm, 129

dispersion-thirst, 48, 53, 183

disquieted, 17, 74, 79, 120

distention and pain, 29, 50, 70, 145

distention and pain in the chest, 145

dizziness, 46, 57, 99, 111, 114, 126, 129, 138-139, 145

dizziness and headache, 99

dizziness of the head, 3, 57, 68

dizzy head and vision, 3

double yīn, 29

downbear turbidity, 3, 34

dream emission, 112

dribbling (in infants), 4, 47, 54

dried dendrobium, *gān shí hú*, 干石斛, Dendrobii Herba, 67, 188-189, 196

dried ginger, *gān jiāng*, 干姜, Zingiberis Rhizoma, 25-27, 32, 37, 41, 51, 87, 91, 131, 155-157, 166-167, 174-176, 182

dried rehmannia, *gān dì huáng*, 干地黄, Rehmanniae Radix, 67, 69, 124, 145-146, 196

dried/fresh rehmannia, *shēng dì huáng*, 生地黄, Rehmanniae Radix Exsiccata seu Recens, 67, 69, 124, 196

drool, 128-129, 178

drool foaming at the mouth, 178

drooling, 46, 93, 138

drooling from the corners of the mouth, 128-129, 131

drooling from the mouth, 155, 162

drooping eyelid, 126, 129, 138

drum distention, 9, 40-41, 63-64, 165, 167, 170-171, 183

dry cough, 199

dry mouth, 8, 48-49, 56, 172-173, 178, 185, 196, 198

dry mouth and thirst, 56

dry mouth and throat, 173

dry nose, 193, 197

dry skin, 123, 193

dry stool, 49, 82

dry tongue, 47, 54

dú huó, 独活, pubescent angelica, Angelicae Pubescentis Radix, 27

dual vacuity of qì and yīn, 142

dual vacuity of the heart and spleen, 142, 143

duck-stool diarrhea, 160

dull pain, 56, 66, 82, 153, 156, 162

dung beetle, *qiāng láng*, 蜣螂, Catharsius, 42

dysentery, 2, 46, 97, 105, 116, 159, 182

ē jiāo, 阿胶, ass hide glue, Asini Corii Colla, 42, 118

easy to expectorate, 31, 32, 34, 35, 198

eclipta, *mò hàn lián*, 墨旱莲, Ecliptae Herba, 118

Ecliptae Herba, *mò hàn lián*, 墨旱莲, eclipta, 118

Effective Use of Set Formulas, *chéng fāng qiè yòng*, 106

efflux diarrhea, 105, 178

eliminate great heat with warmth and sweetness, 139

encrusted skin, 123, 124, 138

enduring depression, 47

enduring diarrhea, 3, 9, 80, 105, 106, 108, 170, 182

enduring dysentery, 182

engender blood, 116

engender qì, 5

enlarged abdomen, 165

enlarged tongue, 23

enuresis, 113

ephedra, *má huáng*, 麻黄, Ephedrae Herba, 175

Ephedrae Herba, *má huáng*, 麻黄, ephedra, 175

epidemic toxin, 112

èr chén tāng, 二陈汤, Two Matured Ingredients Decoction, 32, 34

Eriocheiris Caro et Viscera, *xiè*, 蟹, crab, 7-8, 20, 25, 27, 47, 49-50, 68-69, 84, 91, 101-102, 131, 146, 167

eroding mouth sore, 129

essence of grain and water, 2-3, 13, 81-82, 96, 98, 107, 112, 121-123, 126, 127, 133-135, 179

Essential Prescriptions of the Golden Coffer, *jīn guì yào lüè* (*Jīn Guì Yào Lüè Fāng Lùn* 金匮要略方論), 4, 41, 46, 74, 156, 175, 198-199

Eupatorii Herba, *pèi lán*, 佩兰, eupatorium, 50-51

eupatorium, *pèi lán*, 佩兰, Eupatorii Herba, 50-51

Eupolyphaga seu Steleophaga, *zhè chóng*, 蟅虫, ground beetle, 42

euryale, *qiàn shí*, 芡实, Euryales Semen, 67, 84, 109, 167, 188, 194

Euryales Semen, *qiàn shí*, 芡实, euryale, 67, 84, 109, 167, 188, 194

evodia, *wú zhū yú*, 吴茱萸, Evodiae Fructus, 157, 182

Evodiae Fructus, *wú zhū yú*, 吴茱萸, evodia, 157, 182

excessive consumption of raw or cold foods, 151

excessive taxation, 6, 38-39, 73, 99, 106, 160

excessive thought and preoccupation, 18, 19, 45, 185

expectoration of blood, 4, 10, 117, 120, 121

expel water, 85

external cold, 29, 151

external contraction, 6

external dampness, 55, 88

external evil, 5, 13, 134

extreme of the flesh, 134

exuberance and debilitation, 31, 75, 79-80, 133

eye disease, 126

faint (loose consciousness), 64, 82, 95, 103, 179, 180

fáng fēng, 防风, saposhnikovia, Saposhnikoviae Radix, 20, 27, 49, 175

fáng jǐ, 防己, fangji, Stephaniae Tetrandrae Radix, 175

fangji, *fáng jǐ*, 防己, Stephaniae Tetrandrae Radix, 175

fatigue and lack of strength, 31, 35, 64

fatigue and somnolence, 5, 10, 14, 60, 140, 174

fatigued limbs, 32, 40, 48

fatigued spirit, 5, 10, 82, 95, 117, 139

fatigued spirit and lack of strength, 5, 10, 95, 139

fatness, 23, 30, 31, 48, 123

fear of cold, 23, 165, 172, 174, 176, 180

febrile disease, 191

fecal qì, 19, 22

fěn fáng jǐ, 粉防己, mealy fangji, Stephaniae Tetrandrae Radix, 175

fēng mì, 蜂蜜, honey, Mel, 67, 84

fermented soybean, *dàn dòu chǐ*, 淡豆豉, Sojae Semen Praeparatum, 57, 70

fibrous gypsum, *lǐ shí*, 理石, Gypsum Fibrosum, 49, 175

fire formation due to excess among the five
    minds, 45, 47
five flavors, 36, 48, 53
five minds (joy anger anxiety thought fear), 45
five notes, 126
five phases, 146
five viscera (heart lung spleen liver and kidney),
    1, 14, 74, 75, 79, 116, 125, 126, 135, 142
five-phase theory, 60
flatus, 19, 102, 115
flesh impediment, 133, 134
flesh wilting, 46
flooding, 4, 10, 90, 117, 118, 121
flooding and spotting, 4, 10, 117, 118, 121
flowery knotweed, *hé shǒu wū*, 何首乌, Polygoni
    Multiflori Radix, 124
flowery vision, 99, 111, 126, 129, 138, 139, 145
foaming at the mouth, 178
food accumulation, 47
food damage, 36, 190
food diarrhea, 179
food intake, 18, 22, 103, 123, 126, 198
food stagnation, 32, 34
foot pain, 52
forgetfulness, 116, 143
forsythia, *lián qiáo*, 连翘, Forsythiae Fructus, 62
Forsythiae Fructus, *lián qiáo*, 连翘, forsythia, 62
fortify the spleen, 191
fortify the spleen and boost qì, 191
foul smell, 39, 56, 66
Four Gentlemen Decoction, *sì jūn zǐ tāng*, 四君子
    汤, 101, 130, 142, 191, 199
four seas, 4, 159
four seasons, 4, 159
Four Spirits Pill, *sì shén wán*, 四神丸, 182
free the stool, 50
free the waterways, 90
frenetic movement, 4, 117, 120, 198, 202
frequent belching, 21
frequent desire to defecate, 3, 9, 105, 107, 115
frequent retching, 21
frequent sighing, 22
frequent urination, 2, 9, 58, 113, 193
fresh ginger, *shēng jiāng*, 生姜, Zingiberis
    Rhizoma Recens, 32, 37, 51, 87, 131, 156
fresh rehmannia, *xiān dì huáng*, 鲜地黄,
    Rehmanniae Radix Recens, 69, 124
fritillaria, *bèi mǔ*, 贝母, Fritillariae Bulbus, 62
Fritillariae Bulbus, *bèi mǔ*, 贝母, fritillaria, 62
Fritillariae Cirrhosae Bulbus, *chuān bèi mǔ*, 川贝
    母, Sichuan fritillaria, 62
fú líng guì zhī bái zhú gān cǎo tāng, 茯苓桂枝白
    术甘草汤, Poria, Cinnamon Twig, White
    Atractylodes, and Licorice Decoction, 163, 165,
    166
fú líng pí, 茯苓皮, poria skin, Poriae Cutis, 62, 91
fú líng, 茯苓, poria, Poria, 24-27, 32, 42, 49-50,
    60-62, 68, 83-84, 87, 89-91, 101-103, 109, 112,
    118, 130-131, 143-146, 156, 163, 165-167, 175,
    187-188, 190, 196, 200
fú shén, 茯神, root poria, Poria cum Pini Radice,
    49, 190

fù zǐ gēng mǐ tāng, 附子粳米汤, Aconite and Rice
    Decoction, 175-176
fù zǐ lǐ zhōng tāng, 附子理中汤, Aconite Center-
    Rectifying Decoction, 182
fù zǐ lǐ zhōng wán, 附子理中丸, Aconite Center-
    Rectifying Pill, 157, 167
fù zǐ, 附子, aconite, Aconiti Radix Lateralis
    Praeparata, 19, 25-27, 37, 41, 146, 157, 165-
    167, 175-176, 182
fullness below the heart, 92, 101, 112, 115, 153,
    160
fullness in the chest and rib-side, 163, 171

galangal, *dà liáng jiāng*, 大良姜, Alpiniae
    Galangae Rhizoma, 25, 156-157
galenite, *qiān*, 铅, Galenitum, 14, 46, 74, 79, 122-
    123, 134, 149, 155, 163, 173
Galenitum, *qiān*, 铅, galenite, 14, 46, 74, 79, 122-
    123, 134, 149, 155, 163, 173
gallbladder qì, 40, 59, 60, 66
Gallbladder-Warming Decoction, *wēn dǎn tāng*,
    温胆汤, 50
Galli Gigeriae Endothelium Corneum, *jī nèi jīn*,
    鸡内金, gizzard lining, 187-188
gān cǎo, 甘草, licorice, Glycyrrhizae Radix, 19,
    24-27, 37, 41-42, 49-51, 58, 67-69, 83-84, 87,
    89, 91, 100, 102-103, 107-109, 118, 124, 129,-
    131, 143-145, 155-157, 163, 165-167, 175-176,
    182, 187-188, 190, 194, 196, 199-200
gān dì huáng, 干地黄, dried rehmannia,
    Rehmanniae Radix, 67, 69, 124, 145-146, 196
gān jiāng, 干姜, dried ginger, Zingiberis
    Rhizoma, 25-27, 32, 37, 41, 51, 87, 91, 131,
    155-157, 166-167, 174-176, 182
gān lù xiāo dú dān, 甘露消毒丹, Sweet Dew
    Toxin-Dispersing Elixir, 62
gān shí hú, 干石斛, dried dendrobium, Dendrobii
    Herba, 67, 188-189, 196
gān sore, 107
ganoderma, *líng zhī*, 灵芝, Ganoderma, 41
Ganoderma, *líng zhī*, 灵芝, ganoderma, 41
gǎo běn, 本, Chinese lovage, Ligustici Rhizoma,
    27
gāo liáng jiāng, 高良姜, lesser galangal, Alpiniae
    Officinarum Rhizoma, 157
gardenia, *shān zhī zǐ*, 山栀子, Gardeniae Fructus,
    49, 57, 60, 68-70, 113
Gardeniae Fructus, *shān zhī zǐ*, 山栀子, gardenia,
    49, 57, 60, 68-70, 113
gathering place of the ancestral vessels, 127
gathering place of the ancestral vessels, 127
gé gēn qín lián tāng, 葛根芩连汤, Pueraria,
    Scutellaria, and Coptis Decoction, 58
gé gēn, 葛根, pueraria, Puerariae Radix, 58, 87,
    130, 175, 194
gé xià zhú yū tāng, 膈下逐瘀汤,
    Infradiaphragmatic Stasis-Expelling Decoction,
    41
generalized heaviness, 17, 23, 52
generalized pain, 62
generalized pain and heaviness, 6, 13, 29

gēng mǐ gān, 粳米泔, rice water, Oryzae Aqua, 106, 115

gēng mǐ, 粳米, non-glutinous rice, Oryzae Semen, 175-176, 189-190, 199-200

genital sores, 109

Gentian Liver-Draining Decoction, *lóng dǎn xiè gān tāng*, 龙胆泻肝汤, 68

gentian, *lóng dǎn*, 龙胆, Gentianae Radix, 68, 69, 175

Gentianae Macrophyllae Radix, *qín jiāo*, 秦艽, large gentian, 175

Gentianae Radix, *lóng dǎn*, 龙胆, gentian, 68, 69, 175

getting soaked in the rain or wading through water, 22

ginger skin, *jiāng pí*, 姜皮, Zingiberis Rhizomatis Cortex, 91

ginger, *jiāng*, 姜, Zingiberis Rhizoma, 25-27, 32, 37, 41, 51, 87, 91, 131, 151, 155-157, 166-167, 174-176, 182

Ginseng Radix, *rén shēn*, 人参, ginseng, 26, 42, 83-84, 87, 89, 91, 100, 102-103, 107-109, 118, 124, 129-130, 136, 140, 143-145, 155-157, 166-167, 175-176, 182, 187-188, 190, 194, 199

Ginseng, Poria, and White Atractylodes Powder, *shēn líng bái zhú sǎn*, 参苓白术散, 83, 130, 188

ginseng, *rén shēn*, 人参, Ginseng Radix, 26, 42, 83-84, 87, 89, 91, 100, 102-103, 107-109, 118, 124, 129-130, 136, 140, 143-145, 155-157, 166-167, 175-176, 182, 187-188, 190, 194, 199

gizzard lining, *jī nèi jīn*, 鸡内金, Galli Gigeriae Endothelium Corneum, 187-188

Glaucidii Caro, *xiāo*, 鸮, 42, 62, 68, 118

glomus and fullness, 23, 36, 38, 153, 160

glomus and oppression in the stomach duct, 86

glomus blockage, 40, 44, 56, 101, 112

glomus in the chest, 160

glomus qì, 40, 43

glutinous rice, *nuò mǐ*, 糯米, Oryzae Glutinosae Semen, 176, 199

Glycyrrhizae Radix cum Liquido Fricta, *zhì gān cǎo*, 炙甘草, mix-fried licorice, 26-27, 42, 89, 91, 100, 102-103, 107-109, 124, 129-131, 143, 145, 155-157, 166-167

Glycyrrhizae Radix, *gān cǎo*, 甘草, licorice, 19, 20, 24-26, 32, 37, 41-42, 57-58, 83-84, 87, 89, 91, 100, 102-103, 107-109, 118, 124, 129-130, 136, 140, 143-145, 155-157, 166-167, 175-176, 182, 187-188, 190, 194, 199, 200

gold, *huáng jīn*, 黄金, Aurum, 14, 46, 67, 74, 79, 122-123, 134, 149, 155, 163, 173, 194

Golden Coffer Kidney Qì Pill, *jīn guì shèn qì wán*, 金匮肾气丸, 146

Gōng Tíng-Xián, 116

gǒu qǐ zǐ, 枸杞子, lycium, Lycii Fructus, 196

gōu téng, 钩藤, uncaria, Uncariae Ramulus cum Uncis, 190

grain and water are not transformed, 82, 151, 154, 159, 184

grain and water qì, 122

grain qì, 65, 97, 139, 140

Great Peace Sagacious Benevolence Formulary, *tài píng shèng huì fāng* (992 (Sòng), Wáng Huái-Yǐn 王懷隱 et al. ed.), 49

Greater Dictionary of Chinese Medicine, *zhōng guó yī xué dà cí diǎn*, 88

ground beetle, *zhè chóng*, 蟅虫, Eupolyphaga seu Steleophaga, 42

gǔ yá, 谷芽, millet sprout, Setariae Fructus Germinatus, 187-188, 190

guǎng huò xiāng, 广藿香, patchouli, Pogostemonis Herba, 49, 84, 87

guest qì, 112

guī bǎn, 龟版, tortoise shell, Testudinis Carapax et Plastrum, 199

guī pí tāng, 归脾汤, Spleen-Returning Decoction, 118, 143-144, 185

guì xīn, 桂心, shaved cinnamon bark, Cinnamomi Cortex Rasus, 175

guì zhī, 桂枝, cinnamon twig, Cinnamomi Ramulus, 25, 41, 91, 131, 156, 163, 165-167, 176

Gypsum Fibrosum, *lǐ shí*, 理石, fibrous gypsum, 49, 175

Gypsum Fibrosum, *shí gāo*, 石膏, gypsum, 49, 175

gypsum, *shí gāo*, 石膏, Gypsum Fibrosum, 49, 175

hǎi piāo xiāo, 海螵蛸, cuttlefish bone, Sepiae Endoconcha, 118

hǎi shēn, 海参, sea cucumber, Stichopus Japonicus, 201

hair loss, 193, 197

hair, *xuè yú*, 血余, Crinis, 111, 123, 138, 144, 193, 197, 200

hairy mistletoe, *shì jì shēng*, 柿寄生, Loranthi Yadoriki Ramus, 118, 143, 149, 164, 166

halting speech, 173

hàn lián, 旱莲, camptotheca, Camptothecae Fructus seu Radix, 118

hard stool, 193

hé shǒu wū, 何首乌, flowery knotweed, Polygoni Multiflori Radix, 124

hé yè, 荷叶, lotus leaf, Nelumbinis Folium, 190, 200

hē zǐ, 诃子, chebule, Chebulae Fructus, 108

headache, 20, 99, 114, 126, 139

heart and chest, 52, 198, 201

heart blood, 143

heart blood vacuity, 143

heart pain, 173, 181

heart palpitations, 5, 10, 105, 143

heart qì, 19, 88

heart vexation, 7

heart yīn vacuity, 202

heat depression, 62

heat disease, 46, 57, 62

heat distention, 165

heat effusion, iv, 8, 57, 61, 62, 97, 138, 139, 140, 141, 150, 163, 197, 198, 201

heat in the bladder, 65

heat in the stomach, 60

heat strike (stroke), 111, 183
heat toxin, 191
heat vexation, 185
heat vomiting, 46
hēi dà dòu, 黑大豆, black soybean, Sojae Semen Atrum, 201
hemorrhoids, 36
hiccup, 102, 115, 162
hoarse voice, 172, 173, 181, 199
Hominis Placenta, *zǐ hé chē*, 紫河车, placenta, 199
honey, *fēng mì*, 蜂蜜, Mel, 67, 84
hóng huā, 红花, carthamus, Carthami Flos, 19-20, 27, 37, 41, 50, 58, 61, 70, 83-84, 124, 143, 145, 156-157, 167, 176, 182, 188
Hordei Fructus Germinatus Frictus, *chǎo mài yá*, 炒麦芽, stir-fried barley sprout, 84
Hordei Fructus Germinatus, *mài yá*, 麦芽, barley sprout, 37, 84
hornet's nest, *lù fēng fáng*, 露蜂房, Vespae Nidus, 42
host qì, 99
hòu pò wēn zhōng tāng, 厚朴温中汤, Officinal Magnolia Bark Center-Warming Decoction, 24-25, 155-156
hòu pò, 厚朴, officinal magnolia bark, Magnoliae Officinalis Cortex, 19-20, 24-26, 37, 42, 50, 57-58, 60-61, 69-70, 103-104, 155-156, 161, 166, 194
huā jiāo, 花椒, zanthoxylum, Zanthoxyli Pericarpium, 157, 176
huá shí, 滑石, talcum, Talcum, 58, 62, 63
Huá Tuó, 7
huáng bǎi, 黄柏, phellodendron, Phellodendri Cortex, 60-61, 130, 196
huáng jīn, 黄金, gold, Aurum, 14, 46, 67, 74, 79, 122-123, 134, 149, 155, 163, 173, 194
huáng jīng, 黄精, polygonatum, Polygonati Rhizoma, 67, 194
huáng lián wēn dǎn tāng, 黄连温胆汤, Coptis Gallbladder-Warming Decoction, 50
huáng lián, 黄连, coptis, Coptidis Rhizoma, 49-50, 57-58, 69-70, 84
huáng qí jiàn zhōng tāng, 黄耆*建中汤, Astragalus Center-Fortifying Decoction, 131, 156
huáng qí tāng, 黄耆*汤, Astragalus Decoction, 84
huáng qí, 黄芪, astragalus, Astragali Radix, 41, 49-50, 58, 62-63, 69, 84, 100, 102, 107-109, 118, 124, 129-130, 131, 136, 140, 144, 156
huáng qín huá shí tāng, 黄芩滑石汤, Scutellaria and Talcum Decoction, 62
huáng qín, 黄芩, scutellaria, Scutellariae Radix, 41, 49-50, 58, 62-63, 69
hunger with no desire to eat, 67
huǒ má rén, 火麻仁, cannabis fruit, Cannabis Fructus, 50, 84, 189, 194
huò xiāng yè, 藿香叶, patchouli leaf, Pogostemonis Folium, 49, 84, 87

huò xiāng, 藿香, agastache, Agastaches Herba, 51, 62, 175
huò xiāng, 藿香, patchouli, Pogostemonis Herba, 49-51, 62, 84, 87, 175

impairment of splenic movement and transformation, iii, 55, 56, 66
impediment of the flesh, 134
imperata, *bái máo gēn*, 白茅根, Imperatae Rhizoma, 200
Imperatae Rhizoma, *bái máo gēn*, 白茅根, imperata, 200
Imperatae Rhizoma, *máo gēn tàn*, 茅根炭, charred imperata, 200
inability to defecate, 82
inability to detect fragrance or fetor, 128
inability to get food down, 8, 149, 173
inability to lie down, 7, 21, 46, 155
inability to lift the limbs, 31, 80
inability to rest, 52
inability to taste food, 120, 190
inability to turn sides, 52
inability to walk, 52, 133, 195, 196
inappropriate precipitation, 185
inappropriate sweating, 185
incessant diarrhea, 74, 106, 115
Incisive Light on the Source of Miscellaneous Disease, *zá bìng yuán liú xī zhú* (1773 (Qīng), Shěn Jīn-Áo 沈金鳌), 23, 31-32, 39, 112, 129, 165
incontinence, 113
indigestion, 79, 187
Indispensable Medical Reading, *yī zōng bì dú* (1637 (Míng), Lǐ Zhōng-Zǐ 李中梓 [Shì-Cái 士材]), 93, 133, 179
Infradiaphragmatic Stasis-Expelling Decoction, *gé xià zhú yū tāng*, 膈下逐瘀汤, 41
inhibited speech, 33
inhibited throat, 52
inhibited urination, 7, 17, 52, 59, 65, 164
ink, *mò*, 墨, Atramentum, 57, 118
insecurity of kidney qì, 113
insecurity of the interstices, 179
insomnia, 5, 10, 143
instep yáng pulse, 7, 74, 193
insufficiency of center qì, 99, 105, 154
insufficiency of liver blood, 145
insufficiency of original qì, 140
insufficiency of qì, 140
insufficiency of qì and blood, 135
insufficiency of yáng qì, 28, 150, 154
insufficient, 52, 75, 79-80, 82, 97, 99, 128-129, 149, 151, 159, 164, 173, 178, 184, 187, 189, 192-193, 196-197
internal dampness, 22, 23, 29, 88
internal heat, 48, 53, 140
internal obstruction (of the eye), 127
internal wind, 20
intestinal afflux, 36, 38
intestinal tract, 56, 160, 173
irregular eating, 36
Isatidis Folium, *dà qīng yè*, 大青叶, isatis leaf, 49
isatis leaf, *dà qīng yè*, 大青叶, Isatidis Folium, 49

itchy skin, 134

jaundice, 7, 23-24, 27, 29-30, 40, 43-44, 46, 59-60, 64- 66, 68, 155
jī nèi jīn, 鸡内金, gizzard lining, Galli Gigeriae Endothelium Corneum, 187, 188
jī xuè téng, 鸡血藤, spatholobus, Spatholobi Caulis, 124
jiāng pí, 姜皮, ginger skin, Zingiberis Rhizomatis Cortex, 91
jiāng, 姜, ginger, Zingiberis Rhizoma, 25-27, 32, 37, 41, 51, 87, 91, 131, 151, 155-157, 166-167, 174-176, 182
jiāo shān zhā, 焦山楂, scorch-fried crataegus, Crataegi Fructus Ustus, 84, 188
jié gěng, 桔梗, platycodon, Platycodonis Radix, 83-84, 108-109, 188
jīn guì shèn qì wán, 金匮肾气丸, Golden Coffer Kidney Qì Pill, 146
jīng jiè tàn, 荆芥炭, charred schizonepeta, Schizonepetae Herba et Flos Carbonisatae, 167
jīng jiè, 荆芥, schizonepeta, Schizonepetae Herba, 26, 167
jiǔ jīng, 酒精, alcohol, Alcohol, 45, 73
jiǔ, 酒, liquor, Vinum seu Spiritus, 22, 33, 37, 46, 54, 73
joint pain, 14
joint running, 163
jú hóng, 橘红, red tangerine peel, Citri Reticulatae Exocarpium Rubrum, 84, 188, 190, 200
jú, 橘, tangerine, Citri Fructus, 19-20, 24-26, 32, 37, 42, 50, 58, 61, 83-84, 87, 89-91, 100, 102-103, 107-109, 124, 129, 143, 145, 156-157, 167, 188, 190, 200
Jujubae Fructus, *dà zǎo*, 大枣, jujube, 32, 51, 118, 131, 144, 156, 176, 190, 199
jujube, *dà zǎo*, 大枣, Jujubae Fructus, 32, 51, 118, 131, 144, 156, 176, 190, 199

Katsumada's galangal seed, *cǎo dòu kòu*, 草豆蔻, Alpiniae Katsumadai Semen, 24-25, 156
kidney qì, 105, 113, 146
kidney qì vacuity, 90
kidney vacuity, 6, 179
kidney water, 164
kidney yáng vacuity, 164, 179, 181
kidney yīn vacuity, 202

Lablab Semen Album, *biǎn dòu*, 扁豆, lablab, 83-84, 187-190, 194, 199, 201
lablab, *biǎn dòu*, 扁豆, Lablab Semen Album, 83-84, 187-190, 194, 199, 201
lack of warmth, 151
large appetite with rapid hungering, 48
large gentian, *qín jiāo*, 秦艽, Gentianae Macrophyllae Radix, 175
large pulse, 139
lassitude of the spirit, 193, 197
laziness to speak, 5, 10, 14, 99, 114, 139, 151
leg pain, 195
Leonuri Herba, *yì mǔ cǎo*, 益母草, leonurus, 118

leonurus, *yì mǔ cǎo*, 益母草, Leonuri Herba, 118
Lepidii Semen, *běi tíng lì*, 北葶苈, lepidium, 42
Lepidii/Descurainiae Semen, *tíng lì zǐ*, 葶苈子, lepidium/descurainiae, 42
lepidium, *běi tíng lì*, 北葶苈, Lepidii Semen, 42
lepidium/descurainiae, *tíng lì zǐ*, 葶苈子, Lepidii/Descurainiae Semen, 42
lesser abdominal pain, 173, 181
lesser galangal, *gāo liáng jiāng*, 高良姜, Alpiniae Officinarum Rhizoma, 157
lǐ shí, 理石, fibrous gypsum, Gypsum Fibrosum, 49, 175
lǐ zhōng tāng, 理中汤, Center-Rectifying Decoction, 117, 179
lǐ zhōng wán, 理中丸, Center-Rectifying Pill, 155, 176
lián pò yǐn, 连朴饮, Coptis and Officinal Magnolia Bark Beverage, 69-70
lián qiáo, 连翘, forsythia, Forsythiae Fructus, 62
lián ròu, 莲肉, lotus seed, Nelumbinis Semen, 83-84, 188, 190, 200-201
lián zǐ ròu, 莲子肉, lotus fruit, Nelumbinis Semen, 83-84, 188, 190, 200-201
lián zǐ, 莲子, lotus fruit/seed, Nelumbinis Semen, 83, 84, 188, 190, 194, 200, 201
licorice, *gān cǎo*, 甘草, Glycyrrhizae Radix, 19-20, 24-27, 32, 37, 41-42, 49-51, 57-58, 67-69, 83-84, 87, 89, 91, 100, 102-103, 107-109, 118, 124, 129-131, 143, 144-145, 156-157, 163, 165-167, 175-176, 182, 187-188, 190, 194, 196, 199-200
life gate fire, 151, 196
Ligustici Rhizoma, *gǎo běn*, 本, Chinese lovage, 27
liking for pressure, 56, 66
liking for warmth, 135
limp aching lumbus and knees, 145
limp legs, 52
limp tongue, 128, 131, 138
lindera, *wū yào*, 乌药, Linderae Radix, 19, 41, 103-104
Linderae Radix, *wū yào*, 乌药, lindera, 19, 41, 103-104
Linderniae Crustaceae Herba, *mǔ cǎo*, 母草, crustacean lindernia, 118
líng guì zhú gān tāng, 苓桂术甘汤, Poria, Cinnamon Twig, White Atractylodes, and Licorice Decoction, 163, 165-166
líng xiāo huā, 凌霄花, campsis flower, Campsis Flos, 42
líng yáng jiǎo, 羚羊角, antelope horn, Saigae Tataricae Cornu, 175
líng zhī, 灵芝, ganoderma, Ganoderma, 41
líng, 菱, water caltrop, Trapae Fructus et Radix, 4, 17, 21, 24-28, 32, 41-42, 50, 52, 60-62, 68, 74, 79, 83-84, 87, 89-91, 96, 101-103, 109, 112, 118, 123, 127-128, 130-131, 143-146, 149, 156, 159, 163, 165-167, 175, 183, 187-188, 190, 196, 200
liquid failing to bear upward, 173
liquor jaundice, 46

liquor, *jiǔ*, 酒, Vinum seu Spiritus, 22, 33, 37, 46, 54, 73

liù jūn zǐ tāng, 六君子汤, Six Gentlemen Decoction, 41-42, 87, 90-91, 101-102, 142-144, 146

liù shén tāng, 六神汤, Six Spirits Decoction, 187-188

liù wèi huí yáng yǐn, 六味回阳饮, Six-Ingredient Yáng-Returning Beverage, 120

liver depression and spleen vacuity, 142, 145

liver qì exploiting the spleen, 20

liver-gallbladder damp-heat, 68

liver-spleen disharmony, 20

living in damp places, 22

lodged rheum, 163

lóng dǎn xiè gān tāng, 龙胆泻肝汤, Gentian Liver-Draining Decoction, 68-69

lóng dǎn, 龙胆, gentian, Gentianae Radix, 68-69, 175

lóng yǎn ròu, 龙眼肉, longan flesh, Longan Arillus, 118, 144

Longan Arillus, *lóng yǎn ròu*, 龙眼肉, longan flesh, 118, 144

longan flesh, *lóng yǎn ròu*, 龙眼肉, Longan Arillus, 118, 144

Loranthi Yadoriki Ramus, *shì jì shēng*, 柿寄生, hairy mistletoe, 118, 143, 149, 164, 166

loss of use of the limbs, 14, 17, 40, 43, 174

lotus leaf, *hé yè*, 荷叶, Nelumbinis Folium, 190, 200

lotus root node, *ǒu jié*, 藕节, Nelumbinis Rhizomatis Nodus, 200

lotus root, *ǒu*, 藕, Nelumbinis Rhizoma, 200

lotus seed, *lián ròu*, 莲肉, Nelumbinis Semen, 83-84, 188, 190, 200-201

low food intake, 18, 22, 103, 123

low voice, 52, 99, 114, 144, 181

lower body gān sore, 107

lù fēng fáng, 露蜂房, hornet's nest, Vespae Nidus, 42

lú gēn, 芦根, phragmites, Phragmitis Rhizoma, 57, 67, 70

lù jiǎo shuāng, 鹿角霜, degelatinated deer antler, Cervi Cornu Degelatinatum, 167

lù jiǎo, 鹿角, deerhorn, Cervi Cornu, 167

lumbar pain, 46, 163

lung qì, 99, 127

lung qì vacuity, 144

lung wilting, 198

lung yīn vacuity, 202

Lung-Supplementing Decoction, *bǔ fèi tāng*, 补肺汤, 144

lusterless facial complexion, 5, 10, 23, 192, 197

Lycii Cortex, *dì gǔ pí*, 地骨皮, lycium root bark, 199

Lycii Fructus, *gǒu qǐ zǐ*, 枸杞子, lycium, 196

lycium root bark, *dì gǔ pí*, 地骨皮, Lycii Cortex, 199

lycium, *gǒu qǐ zǐ*, 枸杞子, Lycii Fructus, 196

má huáng, 麻黄, ephedra, Ephedrae Herba, 175

madder, *qiàn cǎo gēn*, 茜草根, Rubiae Radix, 118

Magic Pivot, *líng shū* (1st century C), 4, 52

magnolia flower, *xīn yí*, 辛夷, Magnoliae Flos, 130, 136

Magnoliae Flos, *xīn yí*, 辛夷, magnolia flower, 130, 136

Magnoliae Officinalis Cortex, *hòu pò*, 厚朴, officinal magnolia bark, 19-20, 24-26, 37, 42, 50, 57-58, 60-61, 69-70, 103-104, 155-156, 161, 166, 194

mài mén dōng tāng, 麦门冬汤, Ophiopogon Decoction, 183, 198-199

mài mén dōng, 麦门冬, ophiopogon, Ophiopogonis Radix, 49-50, 67, 124, 183, 198-199

mài yá, 麦芽, barley sprout, Hordei Fructus Germinatus, 37, 84

Major Center-Fortifying Decoction, *dà jiàn zhōng tāng*, 大建中汤, 156

malaria, 24, 178

malt sugar, *yí táng*, 饴糖, Maltosum, 131, 156-157

Maltosum, *yí táng*, 饴糖, malt sugar, 131, 156-157

màn jīng zǐ, 蔓荆子, vitex, Viticis Fructus, 27, 100, 130

máo gēn tàn, 茅根炭, charred imperata, Imperatae Rhizoma, 200

Marsileae Herba, *píng*, 苹, clover fern, 8, 19, 24, 26, 36-37, 49-50, 52, 83, 134, 145, 154, 157, 159, 175, 178, 188

Massa Medicata Fermentata, *shén qū*, 神曲, medicated leaven, 37, 161

mealy fangji, *fěn fáng jǐ*, 粉防己, Stephaniae Tetrandrae Radix, 175

Medical Formulas Gathered and Explained, *yī fāng jí jiě* (1682 (Qīng), Wāng Áng 汪昂), 68

Medical Insights, *yī xué xīn wù* (1732 (Qīng), Chéng Guó-Péng 程國彭), 27

Medical Remedies Researched, *yī fāng kǎo* (1584 (Míng), Wú Kūn 吳崑), 48, 93

medicated leaven, *shén qū*, 神曲, Massa Medicata Fermentata, 37, 161

Mel, *fēng mì*, 蜂蜜, honey, 67, 84

menstruation, 4, 10, 19, 116-118, 121, 198, 202

Menthae Herba, *bò hé*, 薄荷, mint, 62, 68

mǐ tāng, 米汤, rice decoction, Oryzae Decoctio, 175, 176

millet sprout, *gǔ yá*, 谷芽, Setariae Fructus Germinatus, 187-188, 190

millet, *sù mǐ*, 粟米, Setariae Semen, 188, 191

Minor Center-Fortifying Decoction, *xiǎo jiàn zhōng tāng*, 小建中汤, 156

mint, *bò hé*, 薄荷, Menthae Herba, 62, 68

mix-fried licorice, *zhì gān cǎo*, 炙甘草, Glycyrrhizae Radix cum Liquido Fricta, 26-27, 42, 89, 91, 100, 102, 103, 107-109, 124, 129-131, 143, 145, 155-157, 166-167

mix-fried turtle shell, *zhì biē jiǎ*, 炙鳖甲, Trionycis Carapax cum Liquido Frictus, 41 *mò hàn lián*, 墨旱莲, eclipta, Ecliptae Herba, 118

mò, 墨, ink, Atramentum, 57, 118

moderate pulse, 23, 34

moisten the intestines, 48, 50

moisten the intestines and free the stool, 50

Mori Cortex, *sāng bái pí*, 桑白皮, mulberry root bark, 91, 144

Mori Fructus, *sāng shèn*, 桑椹, mulberry, 91, 144

mounting qì, 20

Moutan and Gardenia Free Wanderer Powder, *dān zhī xiāo yáo sǎn*, 丹栀逍遥散, 68

Moutan Cortex, *mǔ dān pí*, 牡丹皮, moutan, 41, 42, 68, 69, 146

moutan, *mǔ dān pí*, 牡丹皮, Moutan Cortex, 41-42, 68-69, 146

mouth and tongue sores, 47, 49, 52, 54

mouth sores, 47, 54, 129, 138

move and transform the essence of grain and water, 96, 112

move dampness, 31

move qì, 101

move water, 163

movement and transformation failure, 28, 29

movement and transformation of the spleen and stomach, 40

moxibustion, 37, 73

mǔ cǎo, 母草, crustacean lindernia, Linderniae Crustaceae Herba, 118

mǔ dān pí, 牡丹皮, moutan, Moutan Cortex, 41-42, 68-69, 146

mù guā, 木瓜, chaenomeles, Chaenomelis Fructus, 26, 166, 196

mù tōng, 木通, trifoliate akebia, Akebiae Trifoliatae Caulis, 63, 69

mù xiāng, 木香, costusroot, Aucklandiae Radix, 19-20, 25-26, 36-37, 57-58, 83, 87-89, 103, 118, 124, 130, 144, 155-156, 161, 166, 175

mugwort, *ài yè*, 艾叶, Artemisiae Argyi Folium, 118

mulberry root bark, *sāng bái pí*, 桑白皮, Mori Cortex, 91, 144

mulberry, *sāng shèn*, 桑椹, Mori Fructus, 91, 144

Mume Fructus, *wū méi*, 乌梅, mume, 108, 113, 118

mume, *wū méi*, 乌梅, Mume Fructus, 108, 113, 118

Myristicae Semen, *ròu dòu kòu*, 肉豆蔻, nutmeg, 108, 182

nasal congestion, 5, 10, 127-128, 130, 136

nausea, 23, 30, 56-57, 66, 69, 117, 120, 142, 155, 162

nausea and retching, 69

nausea and vomiting, 56, 57, 66, 117, 120, 142, 155, 162

Nelumbinis Folium, *hé yè*, 荷叶, lotus leaf, 190, 200

Nelumbinis Fructus, *shí lián zǐ*, 石莲子, lotus fruit, 83-84, 188, 194

Nelumbinis Rhizoma, *ǒu*, 藕, lotus root, 200

Nelumbinis Rhizomatis Nodus, *ǒu jié*, 藕节, lotus root node, 200

Nelumbinis Semen, *lián ròu*, 莲肉, lotus seed, 83-84, 188, 190, 200-201

Nelumbinis Semen, *lián zǐ ròu*, 莲子肉, lotus seed, 83-84, 188, 190, 200, 201

Nelumbinis Semen, *lián zǐ*, 莲子, lotus seed, 83, 84, 188, 190, 194, 200-201

network vessel, 39, 41, 93, 126, 165

night sweating, 197, 198, 199, 201

nine orifices, 1, 111, 125-126, 135

niter, *xiāo shí*, 硝石, Nitrum, 42

Nitrum Rubrum, *chì xiāo*, 赤硝, red niter, 42

Nitrum, *xiāo shí*, 硝石, niter, 42

niú xī, 牛膝, achyranthes, Achyranthis Bidentatae Radix, 196

no desire for food and drink, 14, 120

no pleasure in eating, 33, 64, 74, 189

no thought of food, 160, 185

no thought of food and drink, 81, 92, 94, 142, 153

non-glutinous rice, *gēng mǐ*, 粳米, Oryzae Semen, 175-176, 189-190, 199-200

non-transformation of food, 79, 82

nosebleed, 4, 10, 117-118, 121, 198-199, 202

Notoginseng Radix, *sān qī*, 三七, notoginseng, 118

notoginseng, *sān qī*, 三七, Notoginseng Radix, 118

Notopterygii Rhizoma et Radix, *qiāng huó*, 羌活, notopterygium, 26-27

Notopterygium Dampness-Overcoming Decoction, *qiāng huó shèng shī tāng*, 羌活胜湿汤, 26

notopterygium, *qiāng huó*, 羌活, Notopterygii Rhizoma et Radix, 26-27

nourish the heart, 99

numbness, 46, 93, 122, 123, 138

nuò mǐ, 糯米, glutinous rice, Oryzae Glutinosae Semen, 176, 199

nutmeg, *ròu dòu kòu*, 肉豆蔻, Myristicae Semen, 108, 182

obesity, 2, 9, 31, 35, 80

Officinal Magnolia Bark Center-Warming Decoction, *hòu pò wēn zhōng tāng*, 厚朴温中汤, 24, 155

officinal magnolia bark, *hòu pò*, 厚朴, Magnoliae Officinalis Cortex, 19-20, 24-26, 37, 42, 50, 57, 58, 60-61, 69-70, 103-104, 155-156, 161, 166, 194

old rice, *chén cāng mǐ*, 陈仓米, Oryzae Semen Vetum, 200

On Blood Patterns, *xuè zhèng lùn* (1884 (Qīng), Táng Róng-Chuān 唐容川), 117, 151, 184, 186, 198-199

On Cold Damage and Miscellaneous Diseases, *shāng hán zá bìng lùn* (Eastern Hàn, Zhāng Jī 张机 [Zhòng-Jǐng 仲景]), 7, 29, 50, 58, 60, 79, 90, 149, 155-156, 165, 167, 176, 183, 193, 194

On the Spleen and Stomach, *pí wèi lùn*, 31, 36, 75, 79, 96-97, 99-101, 111, 123, 129, 133, 135, 139, 144, 150, 174

On Warm Epidemics, *wēn yì lùn* (1642 (Míng), Wú Yǒu-Xìng 吳有性 [Yòu-Kě 又可]), 112

Ophiopogon Decoction, *mài mén dōng tāng*, 麦门冬汤, 183, 199

ophiopogon, *mài mén dōng*, 麦门冬, Ophiopogonis Radix, 49-50, 67, 124, 183, 198-199

Ophiopogonis Radix, *mài mén dōng*, 麦门冬, ophiopogon, 49-50, 67, 124, 183, 198-199

oppression in the chest, 20, 22, 31, 35-36, 49, 88, 95, 99

oral putrescence, 129, 131

Origin and Indicators of Disease, *zhū bìng yuán hòu lùn* (610 (Suí), Cháo Yuán-Fāng 巢元方), 159

original qì, 7, 38, 74, 80, 99, 127, 129, 136, 140, 150, 169

original qì vacuity, 136

Oryzae Aqua, *gēng mǐ gān*, 粳米泔, rice water, 106, 115

Oryzae Decoctio, *mǐ tāng*, 米汤, rice decoction, 175, 176

Oryzae Glutinosae Semen, *nuò mǐ*, 糯米, glutinous rice, 176, 199

Oryzae Semen Vetum, *chén cāng mǐ*, 陈仓米, old rice, 200

Oryzae Semen, *gēng mǐ*, 粳米, non-glutinous rice, 175-176, 189-190, 199-200

ǒu jié, 藕节, lotus root node, Nelumbinis Rhizomatis Nodus, 200

ǒu, 藕, lotus root, Nelumbinis Rhizoma, 200

outpour diarrhea, 7, 155

overcome dampness, 64

overwork, 105, 127, 128

Paeoniae Radix Alba, *bái sháo yào*, 白芍药, white peony, 20, 26, 37, 67-68, 100, 130-131, 145, 156, 166, 189-190, 194, 196, 199

Paeoniae Radix Alba, *bái sháo*, 白芍, white peony, 19-20, 24-27, 32, 37, 41, 49-50, 57-58, 67, 68, 70, 84, 87, 89, 91, 100, 130-131, 145, 156, 166, 176, 182, 189-190, 194, 196, 199

Paeoniae Radix Rubra, *chì sháo yào*, 赤芍药, red peony, 41

Paeoniae Radix Rubra, *chì sháo*, 赤芍, red peony, 41

Paeoniae Radix, *sháo yào*, 芍药, peony, 19-20, 24-27, 32, 37, 41-42, 49-50, 57,-58, 67-68, 70, 84, 87, 89, 91, 100, 130-131, 145, 156, 166, 176, 182, 189-190, 194, 196, 199

Pain and Diarrhea Formula, *tòng xiè yào fāng*, 痛泻要方, 20

pain in the abdomen, 14

pain in the limbs, 86, 95

pain in the stomach duct and abdomen, 154, 156, 178

pain in the underside of the foot, 17

pain in the urethra, 66

painful tongue, 54

pale lips, 174, 181

pale tongue, 126, 139

pale white facial complexion, 3, 9, 139, 174, 181

palpitations below the heart, 88, 95, 163

panting, 2, 9, 31, 34-35, 139-140, 144, 163-164

panting and cough, 31, 164

panting and fullness, 163

pào fù zǐ, 炮附子, blast-fried aconite, Aconiti Radix Lateralis Tosta, 26

pào jiāng, 炮姜, blast-fried ginger, Zingiberis Rhizoma Praeparatum, 26, 174-175

papules, 184, 190-191

paralysis, 122, 138

parched lips, 47, 49, 52

Passer, *què*, 雀, sparrow, 90

patchouli, *guǎng huò xiāng*, 广藿香, Pogostemonis Herba, 49, 84, 87

Pathoconditions: Causes, Pulses, and Treatments, *zhèng yīn mài zhì* (1641 (Míng), Qín Jǐng-Míng 秦景明), 56, 60, 103, 134, 170

peach kernel, *táo rén*, 桃仁, Persicae Semen, 19, 25, 27, 37, 41-42, 58, 124, 167

pèi lán, 佩兰, eupatorium, Eupatorii Herba, 50-51

peony, *sháo yào*, 芍药, Paeoniae Radix, 20, 26, 37, 41-42, 50, 67-68, 100, 130-131, 145, 156, 166, 189-190, 194, 196, 199

Persicae Semen, *táo rén*, 桃仁, peach kernel, 19, 25, 27, 37, 41-42, 58, 124, 167

perspiration, 62, 66, 174

Peucedani Radix, *qián hú*, 前胡, peucedanum, 50

peucedanum, *qián hú*, 前胡, Peucedani Radix, 50

Phellodendri Cortex, *huáng bǎi*, 黄柏, phellodendron, 60-61, 130, 196

phellodendron, *huáng bǎi*, 黄柏, Phellodendri Cortex, 60-61, 130, 196

phlegm turbidity, 18, 31-34, 44

phlegm-damp, 6, 31

phlegm-drool, 93, 129, 169

phlegm-fire, 45

phlegm-rheum, 2, 9, 31-34, 44, 88, 93, 163, 169

phragmites, *lú gēn*, 芦根, Phragmitis Rhizoma, 57, 67, 70

Phragmitis Rhizoma, *lú gēn*, 芦根, phragmites, 57, 67, 70

pinellia, *bàn xià*, 半夏, Pinelliae Rhizoma, 32, 42, 50, 57-58, 60-61, 70, 87, 89-90, 102-103, 108-109, 112, 143, 145, 176, 199

Pinelliae Rhizoma, *bàn xià*, 半夏, pinellia, 32, 42, 50, 57-58, 60-61, 70, 87, 89-90, 102-103, 108-109, 112, 143, 145, 176, 199

píng wèi sǎn, 平胃散, Stomach-Calming Powder, 19, 24, 26, 36

píng, 苹, clover fern, Marsileae Herba, 8, 19, 24, 26, 36-37, 49-50, 52, 83, 134, 145, 154, 157, 159, 175, 178, 188

placenta, *zǐ hé chē*, 紫河车, Hominis Placenta, 199

Plantaginis Herba, *chē qián*, 车前, plantago, 26, 69, 167, 196

Plantaginis Semen, *chē qián zǐ*, 车前子, plantago seed, 26, 69, 167, 196 plantago seed, *chē qián zĭ*, 车前子, Plantaginis Semen, 26, 69, 167, 196

plantago, *chē qián*, 车前, Plantaginis Herba, 26, 69, 167, 196

Platycladi Cacumen, *cè băi yè*, 侧柏叶, arborvitae leaf, 118

platycodon, *jié gěng*, 桔梗, Platycodonis Radix, 83-84, 108-109, 188

Platycodonis Radix, *jié gěng*, 桔梗, platycodon, 83-84, 108-109, 188

Pogostemonis Folium, *huò xiāng yè*, 藿香叶, patchouli leaf, 49, 84, 87

Pogostemonis Herba, *guăng huò xiāng*, 广藿香, patchouli, 49, 84, 87

Pogostemonis Herba, *huò xiāng*, 藿香, patchouli, 49-51, 62, 84, 87, 175

polygala, *yuăn zhì*, 远志, Polygalae Radix, 118, 144

Polygalae Radix, *yuăn zhì*, 远志, polygala, 118, 144

Polygonati Odorati Rhizoma, *yù zhú*, 玉竹, Solomon's seal, 67, 189

Polygonati Rhizoma, *huáng jīng*, 黄精, polygonatum, 67, 194

polygonatum, *huáng jīng*, 黄精, Polygonati Rhizoma, 67, 194

Polygoni Multiflori Radix, *hé shŏu wū*, 何首乌, flowery knotweed, 124

polyporus, *zhū líng*, 猪苓, Polyporus, 25, 62, 91, 101-102, 167

Polyporus, *zhū líng*, 猪苓, polyporus, 25, 62, 91, 101-102, 167

poor appetite, 86, 95, 179

poor hearing, 99, 114

poor qì transformation, 163, 178

Poria Alba, *bái fú líng*, 白茯苓, white poria, 26

Poria cum Pini Radice, *fú shén*, 茯神, root poria, 49, 190

Poria Five Powder, *wŭ líng săn*, 五苓散, 90, 167

Poria Rubra, *chì fú líng*, 赤茯苓, red poria, 50

poria skin, *fú líng pí*, 茯苓皮, Poriae Cutis, 62, 91

Poria, Cinnamon Twig, White Atractylodes, and Licorice Decoction, *líng guì zhú gān tāng*, 苓桂术甘汤, 163, 165

poria, *fú líng*, 茯苓, Poria, 24-27, 32, 42, 49-50, 60-62, 68, 83-84, 87, 89-91, 101-103, 109, 112, 118, 130-131, 143-146, 156, 163, 165-167, 175, 187-188, 190, 196, 200

Poria, *fú líng*, 茯苓, poria, 24-27, 32, 42, 49-50, 60-62, 68, 83-84, 87, 89-91, 101-103, 109, 112, 118, 130-131, 143-146, 156, 163, 165-167, 175, 187-188, 190, 196, 200

Poriae Cutis, *fú líng pí*, 茯苓皮, poria skin, 62, 91

postpartum diarrhea, 169

precipitate qì, 198

predilection for strange foods, 36

premature ejaculation, 104

processed aconite, *zhì fu zĭ*, 制附子, Aconiti Radix Lateralis Praeparata, 25, 27, 146, 157, 165-167, 175-176

profuse dreaming, 143

profuse menstruation, 4, 10, 117-118, 121, 198, 202

profuse sweating, 63

prolapse of the rectum, 3, 9, 105, 115

prolapse of the uterus, 113, 115

Prolonging Life and Preserving the Origin, *shòu shì băo yuán* (17th century (Míng), Gōng Tíng-Xián 龚廷贤), 116

propping fullness in the chest and rib-side, 163, 171

pseudostellaria, *tài zĭ shēn*, 太子参, Pseudostellariae Radix, 188

Pseudostellariae Radix, *tài zĭ shēn*, 太子参, pseudostellaria, 188

psoralea, *bŭ gŭ zhī*, 补骨脂, Psoraleae Fructus, 182

Psoraleae Fructus, *bŭ gŭ zhī*, 补骨脂, psoralea, 182

pú huáng, 蒲黄, typha pollen, Typhae Pollen, 118

pubescent angelica, *dú huó*, 独活, Angelicae Pubescentis Radix, 27

pudendal itch, 107, 115

pueraria, *gé gēn*, 葛根, Puerariae Radix, 58, 87, 130, 175, 194

Pueraria, Scutellaria, and Coptis Decoction, *gé gēn qín lián tāng*, 葛根芩连汤, 58

Puerariae Radix, *gé gēn*, 葛根, pueraria, 58, 87, 130, 175, 194

puffy face, 164

puffy swelling, 23, 25, 63, 90, 151

pure heat, 48, 53

pyrrosia, *shí wéi*, 石韦, Pyrrosiae Folium, 41

Pyrrosiae Folium, *shí wéi*, 石韦, pyrrosia, 41

qì accumulation, 178

qì ascent, 144, 198, 201

qì aspect, 62

Qí Bó, 53, 122

qì counterflow, 7, 155, 199

qì depression, 15, 17, 20, 31, 60, 112, 115, 164

qì drum, 170

qì glomus, 115

qì impediment, 64

qì reversal, 80

qì shortage, 135

qì stagnation, 39-41, 43, 48, 60, 70, 82, 86, 92, 98, 101, 103, 112, 114, 142, 153-154, 162, 173, 181, 192

qì stagnation and blood stasis, 43, 70

qì timidity, 120

qì transformation, 56-57, 153, 163-164, 178

qì vacuity, 75, 79-81, 86, 90, 92, 99, 113, 116-118, 120, 140-142, 144, 145, 202

qì vacuity fall, 113

qì vacuity heat, 138, 140-141

qī wèi bái zhú săn, 七味白术散, Seven-Ingredient White Atractylodes Powder, 7, 86-87, 174-175

qiàn căo gēn, 茜草根, madder, Rubiae Radix, 118

qián hú, 前胡, peucedanum, Peucedani Radix, 50

qiàn shí, 芡实, euryale, Euryales Semen, 67, 84, 109, 167, 188, 194

Qián Yĭ, 14, 47, 74

qiān, 铅, galenite, Galenitum, 14, 46, 74, 79, 122-123, 134, 149, 155, 163, 173

qiāng huó shèng shī tāng, 羌活胜湿汤, Notopterygium Dampness-Overcoming Decoction, 26-27

qiāng huó, 羌活, notopterygium, Notopterygii Rhizoma et Radix, 26-27

qiāng láng, 蜣螂, dung beetle, Catharsius, 42

Qì-Boosting Sharp and Bright Decoction, *yì qì cōng míng tāng*, 益气聪明汤, 127, 130

qín jiāo, 秦艽, large gentian, Gentianae Macrophyllae Radix, 175

qīng pí, 青皮, unripe tangerine peel, Citri Reticulatae Pericarpium Viride, 113

qing1 pi2, 青皮, unripe tangerine peel, Citri Reticulatae Pericarpium Viride, 19-20, 25, 27, 32, 37, 58, 61, 167

qū mài, 瞿麦, dianthus, Dianthi Herba, 42

quality of voice and enunciation, 172

què, 雀, sparrow, Passer, 90

rapid pulse, 57, 199

raving, 34

raw chaenomeles, *shēng mù guā*, 生木瓜, Chaenomelis Fructus, 26, 166, 196

rectify the spleen, 199

red dysentery, 46

red niter, *chì xiāo*, 赤硝, Nitrum Rubrum, 42

red peony, *chì sháo yào*, 赤芍药, Paeoniae Radix Rubra, 41

red peony, *chì sháo*, 赤芍, Paeoniae Radix Rubra, 41

red poria, *chì fú líng*, 赤茯苓, Poria Rubra, 50

red tangerine peel, *jú hóng*, 橘红, Citri Reticulatae Exocarpium Rubrum, 84, 188, 190, 200

red tongue, 67

reddish urine, 56, 66

reduced eating, 2-3, 9, 23, 30-31, 35, 80-83, 90, 94-95, 101, 143-144, 153, 155, 162, 186-187, 189-192

rehmannia, *dì huáng*, 地黄, Rehmanniae Radix, 67, 69, 124, 145-146, 196

Rehmanniae Radix Exsiccata seu Recens, *shēng dì huáng*, 生地黄, dried/fresh rehmannia, 67, 69, 124, 196

Rehmanniae Radix Praeparata, *shú dì huáng*, 熟地黄, cooked rehmannia, 145-146

Rehmanniae Radix Recens, *xiān dì huáng*, 鲜地黄, fresh rehmannia, 69, 124

Rehmanniae Radix, *dì huáng*, 地黄, rehmannia, 67, 69, 124, 145-146, 196

Rehmanniae Radix, *gān dì huáng*, 干地黄, dried rehmannia, 67, 69, 124, 145-146, 196

rén shēn, 人参, ginseng, Ginseng Radix, 26, 42, 83-84, 87, 89, 91, 100, 102-103, 107-109, 118, 124, 129-130, 136, 140, 143-145, 155-157, 166-167, 175-176, 182, 187-188, 190, 194, 199

repletion heat, 46, 49

restraining (five phases), 60, 90, 160

retching, 21, 184

retching counterflow, 33, 64, 157, 161

retracted testicles, 173

reversal of the extremities, 178

Revised Popular On Cold Damage, *chóng dìng tōng sú shāng hán lùn*, 178

Rhei Radix et Rhizoma, *dà huáng*, 大黄, rhubarb, 41, 49-50, 60, 194

Rhinopitheci Adeps seu Caro, *róng*, 狨, snub-nosed langur, 75, 151, 184, 198-199

rhubarb, *dà huáng*, 大黄, Rhei Radix et Rhizoma, 41, 49-50, 60, 194

rib-side, 20, 22, 52, 59, 66, 68, 145

rib-side distention, 52

rib-side pain, 68

rice decoction, *mǐ tāng*, 米汤, Oryzae Decoctio, 175-176

rice water, *gēng mǐ gān*, 粳米泔, Oryzae Aqua, 106, 115

rice-paper plant pith, *tōng cǎo*, 通草, Tetrapanacis Medulla, 58, 62

right qì, 173-174, 178

róng, 狨, snub-nosed langur, Rhinopitheci Adeps seu Caro, 75, 151, 184, 198-199

root of earlier heaven, 127

root of the tongue, 8, 33, 47, 52

root poria, *fú shén*, 茯神, Poria cum Pini Radice, 49, 190

ròu dòu kòu, 肉豆蔻, nutmeg, Myristicae Semen, 108, 182

ròu guì, 肉桂, cinnamon bark, Cinnamomi Cortex, 146, 175

rough stagnant stool, 193

Rubiae Radix, *qiàn cǎo gēn*, 茜草根, madder, 118

rumbling in the abdomen, 154

rumbling intestines (borborygmus), 2, 7-8, 31, 74, 79, 82, 88, 95, 97, 149, 153-155, 159-160, 173

runny nose, 127, 130

Saigae Tataricae Cornu, *líng yáng jiǎo*, 羚羊角, antelope horn, 175

Sal, *yán*, 盐, salt, 41, 118, 143, 149, 164, 166

salt, *yán*, 盐, Sal, 41, 118, 143, 149, 164, 166

sān qī, 三七, notoginseng, Notoginseng Radix, 118

sandalwood, *tán xiāng*, 檀香, Santali Albi Lignum, 188

sāng bái pí, 桑白皮, mulberry root bark, Mori Cortex, 91, 144

sāng shèn, 桑椹, mulberry, Mori Fructus, 91, 144

sanguisorba, *dì yú*, 地榆, Sanguisorbae Radix, 118

Sanguisorbae Radix, *dì yú*, 地榆, sanguisorba, 118

Santali Albi Lignum, *tán xiāng*, 檀香, sandalwood, 188

saposhnikovia, *fáng fēng*, 防风, Saposhnikoviae Radix, 20, 27, 49, 175

Saposhnikoviae Radix, *fáng fēng*, 防风, saposhnikovia, 20, 27, 49, 175

scaling of the skin, 134

scallion, *cōng*, 葱, Allii Fistulosi Herba, 127, 130

scant sticky phlegm, 198, 201

scant urine, 164165, 172

Schema of Miscellaneous Patterns, *zá zhèng mó*, 92, 97, 99, 104-107, 120, 153, 160

schisandra, *wǔ wèi zǐ*, 五味子, Schisandrae Fructus, 107-108, 113, 145, 182

Schisandrae Fructus, *wǔ wèi zǐ*, 五味子, schisandra, 107-108, 113, 145, 182

schizonepeta, *jīng jiè*, 荆芥, Schizonepetae Herba, 26, 167

Schizonepetae Herba et Flos Carbonisatae, *jīng jiè tàn*, 荆芥炭, charred schizonepeta, 167

Schizonepetae Herba, *jīng jiè*, 荆芥, schizonepeta, 26, 167

scorch-fried crataegus, *jiāo shān zhā*, 焦山楂, Crataegi Fructus Ustus, 84, 188

Scutellaria and Talcum Decoction, *huáng qín huá shí tāng*, 黄芩滑石汤, 62

scutellaria, *huáng qín*, 黄芩, Scutellariae Radix, 41, 49-50, 58, 62-63, 69

Scutellariae Radix, *huáng qín*, 黄芩, scutellaria, 41, 49-50, 58, 62-63, 69

sea cucumber, *hǎi shēn*, 海参, Stichopus Japonicus, 201

sea of blood (the thoroughfare vessel liver or SP-10), 116

Secret Treasure of the Orchid Chamber, *lán shì mì cáng* (1276, Lǐ Gǎo 李杲 [Dōng-Yuán 東垣]), 165

secure, 5, 117, 154, 174

seminal efflux, 112

seminal emission, 105, 115

seminal emission and premature ejaculation, 104

separation of the clear and turbid, 154

Sepiae Endoconcha, *hǎi piāo xiāo*, 海螵蛸, cuttlefish bone, 118

Setariae Fructus Germinatus, *gǔ yá*, 谷芽, millet sprout, 187-188, 190

Setariae Semen, *sù mǐ*, 粟米, millet, 188, 191

seven affects, 6, 18, 33, 40

Seven-Ingredient White Atractylodes Powder, *qī wèi bái zhú sǎn*, 七味白术散, 7, 86, 174

severe pain, 156, 173, 175, 181

sexual intercourse, 96

sexual taxation, 106, 170

shā rén, 砂仁, amomum, Amomi Fructus, 36-37, 62, 83-84, 88-89, 103, 108-109, 130, 155, 161, 176, 188

shā shēn, 沙参, adenophora/glehnia, Adenophorae seu Glehniae Radix, 67, 189

shān yào, 山药, dioscorea, Dioscoreae Rhizoma, 26, 67, 83-84, 107-109, 113, 146, 166, 183, 187-188, 190-191, 199, 201

shān zhā, 山楂, crataegus, Crataegi Fructus, 37, 60-61, 84, 187-188

shān zhī zǐ, 山栀子, gardenia, Gardeniae Fructus, 49, 57, 60, 68-70, 113

shān zhū yú, 山茱萸, cornus, Corni Fructus, 146

sháo yào, 芍药, peony, Paeoniae Radix, 20, 26, 37, 41-42, 50, 67-68, 100, 130-131, 145, 156, 166, 189-190, 194, 196, 199

shaved cinnamon bark, *guì xīn*, 桂心, Cinnamomi Cortex Rasus, 175

shé chuáng zǐ, 蛇床子, cnidium seed, Cnidii Fructus, 113

shè gān, 射干, belamcanda, Belamcandae Rhizoma, 41, 62

shēn líng bái zhú sǎn, 参苓白术散, Ginseng, Poria, and White Atractylodes Powder, 83, 130, 188

shén qū, 神曲, medicated leaven, Massa Medicata Fermentata, 37, 161

shēng dì huáng, 生地黄, dried/fresh rehmannia, Rehmanniae Radix Exsiccata seu Recens, 67, 69, 124, 196

shēng jiāng, 生姜, fresh ginger, Zingiberis Rhizoma Recens, 32, 37, 51, 87, 131, 156

shēng má, 升麻, cimicifuga, Cimicifugae Rhizoma, 49, 84, 87, 100-104, 107-109, 124, 129-130, 174, 175

shēng mù guā, 生木瓜, raw chaenomeles, Chaenomelis Fructus, 26, 166, 196

shí chāng pú, 石菖蒲, acorus, Acori Tatarinowii Rhizoma, 62, 70

shí gāo, 石膏, gypsum, Gypsum Fibrosum, 49, 175

shí hú, 石斛, dendrobium, Dendrobii Herba, 67, 188-189, 196

shì jì shēng, 柿寄生, hairy mistletoe, Loranthi Yadoriki Ramus, 118, 143, 149, 164, 166

shí lián zǐ, 石莲子, lotus fruit, Nelumbinis Fructus, 83-84, 188, 194

shí wéi, 石韦, pyrrosia, Pyrrosiae Folium, 41

short inhibited voidings of urine, 196

short voidings of reddish urine, 56

short voidings of scant urine, 164, 172

shortage of qì, 5, 10, 99, 114, 117, 151

shortness of breath, 82, 84, 88, 99, 105, 120, 139, 144, 163, 171

shú dì huáng, 熟地黄, cooked rehmannia, Rehmanniae Radix Praeparata, 145-146

shǔ fù, 鼠妇, wood louse, Armadillidium, 41

shǔ yù wán, 薯蓣丸, Dioscorea Pill, 183

shuǐ niú jiǎo, 水牛角, water buffalo horn, Bubali Cornu, 49

sì jūn zǐ tāng, 四君子汤, Four Gentlemen Decoction, 101, 130, 142-143, 191, 199

sì nì tāng, 四逆汤, Counterflow Cold Decoction, 149, 179

sì shén wán, 四神丸, Four Spirits Pill, 182

Sichuan fritillaria, *chuān bèi mǔ*, 川贝母, Fritillariae Cirrhosae Bulbus, 62

six bowels, 1, 116, 126, 142

six channels, 125

six excesses, 6, 14, 45, 73, 170, 185

Six Gentlemen Decoction, *liù jūn zǐ tāng*, 六君子 汤, 41, 87, 90, 91, 101, 142, 144, 146

six qì (wind cold fire summerheat dryness and dampness), 33

Six Spirits Decoction, *liù shén tāng*, 六神汤, 187-188

Six-Ingredient Yáng-Returning Beverage, *liù wèi huí yáng yǐn*, 六味回阳饮, 120

skin swelling, 23

sliminess in the mouth, 50

slimy tongue fur, 19, 36

slimy white tongue fur, 23

slippery pulse, 36

sloppy stool, 2, 8-9, 23-24, 30, 36, 57-58, 69, 82-83, 95, 126, 142-144, 145, 154, 165, 170, 172, 187-188, 191-192

smaller-abdominal pain, 20

snub-nosed langur, *róng*, 狨, Rhinopitheci Adeps seu Caro, 75, 151, 184, 198-199

Sojae Semen Atrum, *hēi dà dòu*, 黑大豆, black soybean, 201

Sojae Semen Praeparatum, *dàn dòu chǐ*, 淡豆豉, fermented soybean, 57, 70

Solomon's seal, *yù zhú*, 玉竹, Polygonati Odorati Rhizoma, 67, 189

somnolence, 5, 10, 14, 59, 140, 174, 193, 197

sore pharynx, 199

sore throat, 201

sores, 47, 49, 52, 54, 107, 109, 115, 129

Sorghi Semen, *běi shú mǐ*, 北秫米, sorghum, 55

sorghum, *běi shú mǐ*, 北秫米, Sorghi Semen, 55

sparrow, *què*, 雀, Passer, 90

Spatholobi Caulis, *jī xuè téng*, 鸡血藤, spatholobus, 124

spatholobus, *jī xuè téng*, 鸡血藤, Spatholobi Caulis, 124

Special Achievement Powder, *yì gōng sǎn*, 异功散, 83, 101, 142

spiny jujube, *suān zǎo rén*, 酸枣仁, Ziziphi Spinosi Semen, 118, 144, 196

Spirit Gate, 7

spirit qì, 5

spleen accumulation, 40

spleen distention, 14

spleen heat, 46, 48

spleen qì failing to bear upward, 98

spleen qì fall, 3, 96-97, 105-107, 112-113

spleen qì vacuity, 44, 79-81, 90, 92-93, 112-113, 116-118, 120-122, 126, 128-129, 135, 142, 144, 149, 151, 202

spleen vacuity engendering phlegm, 86, 88

spleen yáng vacuity, 44, 118, 142, 149-151, 153-155, 159-161, 163-165, 173, 179-181

spleen yīn vacuity, 75-76, 142, 183-187, 191, 193-194, 198-199, 201-202

spleen-kidney yáng vacuity, 182

Spleen-Returning Decoction, *guī pí tāng*, 归脾汤, 118, 143, 185

spleen-stomach damp-heat, 67, 68

spleen-stomach qì vacuity, 75, 81

spleen-stomach vacuity, 90, 174

spleen-stomach vacuity cold, 153

spleen-stomach yáng vacuity, 75, 155

spleen-stomach yīn vacuity, 67, 190, 202

splenic pure heat, 48, 53

splenic transformation failure, 38

spontaneous bleeding of the flesh, 4, 117-118, 198-199, 202

spontaneous diarrhea, 151, 160

spontaneous sweating, 5, 179

spontaneous tearing, 163

spotting, 4, 10, 117-118, 121

squirrel's droppings, *wǔ líng zhī*, 五灵脂, Trogopteri Faeces, 41

stagnant diarrhea, 64

stasis turbidity, 65

static blood, 4, 18, 39, 40, 44

steam-wash, 113

stellaria, *yín chái hú*, 银柴胡, Stellariae Radix, 199

Stellariae Radix, *yín chái hú*, 银柴胡, stellaria, 199

Stephaniae Tetrandrae Radix, *fáng jǐ*, 防己, fangji, 175

Stephaniae Tetrandrae Radix, *fěn fáng jǐ*, 粉防己, mealy fangji, 175

Stichopus Japonicus, *hǎi shēn*, 海参, sea cucumber, 201

stiff tongue, 33, 173, 178

stir-fried barley sprout, *chǎo mài yá*, 炒麦芽, Hordei Fructus Germinatus Frictus, 84

stirring palpitation, 88

stomach cold, 164

stomach disease, 6, 36, 75, 97, 184

stomach fire, 184, 194

stomach qì, 3, 14, 20, 56-57, 66, 75, 80, 82, 92, 97, 99, 111-112, 120, 122, 136, 139-140, 142, 154-155, 161, 165, 174, 179, 191, 193

stomach qì vacuity, 75, 111, 120, 165

stomach reflux, 34, 74

stomach vacuity, 90, 127, 133, 150, 160, 174

stomach vacuity cold, 153

stomach yáng vacuity, 75, 136, 155

stomach yīn vacuity, 189, 202

Stomach-Calming Poria Five Decoction, *wèi líng tāng*, 胃苓汤, 24

Stomach-Calming Powder, *píng wèi sǎn*, 平胃散, 19, 24, 26, 36

straitened spleen, 193

stringlike pulse, 19, 20

strings and aggregations, 39

sù mǐ, 粟米, millet, Setariae Semen, 188, 191

suān zǎo rén, 酸枣仁, spiny jujube, Ziziphi Spinosi Semen, 118, 144, 196

summerheat-damp, 14, 133

Supplement to the Classified Case Histories of Famous Physicians, *xù míng yī lèi àn*, 62

Supplemented Six Gentlemen Decoction, 加味六君汤, *jiā wèi liù jūn zǐ tāng*, 87

susceptibility to the common cold, 174, 181

sweating, 5, 10, 29, 57, 61-63, 82, 99, 139, 141, 174, 179-181, 185, 197-199, 201

Sweet Dew Toxin-Dispersing Elixir, *gān lù xiāo dú dān*, 甘露消毒丹, 62

swelling of the feet, 40

swill diarrhea, 36, 74, 79, 82, 97, 106

swollen cheek (mumps), 8

swollen lips, 48

swollen throat, 49
swollen tongue, 47
Systematized Identification of Warm Diseases, *wēn bìng tiáo bian* (1798 (Qīng), Wú Táng 吳 瑭 [Jú-Tōng 鞠通]), 58, 62, 184, 187, 194
Systematized Patterns with Clear-Cut Treatments, *lèi zhèng zhì cái* (1839 (Qīng), Lín Pèi-Qín 林 佩琴), 29, 101, 161, 186, 189

tài zǐ shēn, 太子参, pseudostellaria, Pseudostellariae Radix, 188
Tài-Píng Imperial Grace Pharmacy, 19, 24, 83, 145, 157, 188
Tài-Píng Imperial Grace Pharmacy Formulas, *tài píng huì mín hé jì jú fāng*, 19, 24, 83, 145, 157, 188
talcum, *huá shí*, 滑石, Talcum, 58, 62-63
Talcum, *huá shí*, 滑石, talcum, 58, 62-63
tán xiāng, 檀香, sandalwood, Santali Albi Lignum, 188
Táng Róng-Chuān, 75, 151, 184, 198-199
tangerine peel, *chén pí*, 陈皮, Citri Reticulatae Pericarpium, 19-20, 24-26, 32, 37, 42, 50, 57-58, 60-61, 83-84, 87, 89-91, 100, 102-103, 107-109, 113, 124, 129, 143, 145, 156, 167, 188, 190, 200
tangerine, *jú*, 橘, Citri Fructus, 19-20, 24-26, 32, 37, 42, 50, 58, 61, 83-84, 87, 89-91, 100, 102-103, 107-109, 124, 129, 143, 145, 156-157, 167, 188, 190, 200
táo rén, 桃仁, peach kernel, Persicae Semen, 19, 25, 27, 37, 41-42, 58, 124, 167
taxation damage, 164, 169
taxation fatigue, 6, 38, 64, 80, 99, 105, 111, 120, 139-141, 160, 185
tea, *chá yè*, 茶叶, Theae Folium, 22, 54
tearing, 163
ten questions (in the enquiry examination), 177
Testudinis Carapax et Plastrum, *guī bǎn*, 龟版, tortoise shell, 199
tetany, 23
Tetrapanacis Medulla, *tōng cǎo*, 通草, rice-paper plant pith, 58, 62
Theae Folium, *chá yè*, 茶叶, tea, 22, 54
thin sloppy stool, 82, 95, 154
thin stool, 19, 22
thirst, 29, 46, 48, 53, 56-57, 62, 66, 139, 144, 149, 163, 172, 178, 181, 183
thirst with a liking for hot drinks, 172, 178, 181
thirst without large fluid intake, 62, 66
Thorough Knowledge of Medicine, *yī guàn* (1687 (Qīng), Zhào Xiàn-Kě 趙獻可), 55
Thousand Gold Pieces Formulary, *qiān jīn fāng*, 173
Thousand Gold Pieces Prescriptions, *qiān jīn yào fāng* (full title *Bèi Jí Qiān Jīn Yào Fāng* 備急千金要方), 14, 46, 74, 79, 122, 123, 134, 149, 155
throughflux diarrhea, 24, 46
tiān mén dōng, 天门冬, asparagus, Asparagi Radix, 124

tiáo zhōng yì qì tāng, 调中益气汤, Center-Regulating Qì-Boosting Decoction, 123, 124
tight pulse, 49
tíng lì zǐ, 葶苈子, lepidium/descurainiae, Lepidii/Descurainiae Semen, 42
tinnitus, 99, 114, 126-127, 130, 135, 138, 145
tōng cǎo, 通草, rice-paper plant pith, Tetrapanacis Medulla, 58, 62
tōng mài sì nì tāng, 通脉四逆汤, Vessel-Freeing Counterflow Cold Decoction, 179
tòng xiè yào fāng, 痛泻要方, Pain and Diarrhea Formula, 20
tongue body, 52, 54, 128, 139, 172
tongue fur, 20
tongue sore, 47, 49, 52, 54
torpid intake, 2-3, 9, 24, 36, 38-39, 59, 68-69, 81, 83, 90, 94-95, 143-145, 153, 155, 186-187, 189, 191
torpid stomach intake, 18, 81, 101, 115
tortoise shell, *guī bǎn*, 龟版, Testudinis Carapax et Plastrum, 199
Trachycarpi Petiolus Carbonisatus, *zōng tàn*, 棕 炭, charred trachycarpus, 118
Trachycarpi Petiolus, *zōng lǘ pí*, 棕榈皮, trachycarpus, 118
Trachycarpi Stipulae Fibra Carbonisata, *zōng lǘ tàn*, 棕榈炭, charred trachycarpus, 118
trachycarpus, *zōng lǘ pí*, 棕榈皮, Trachycarpi Petiolus, 118
transform dampness (eliminate), 24
transform into fire, 45, 185
transform into heat, 55, 185
transform qì (move qì and transform stagnation), 198
Transforming Yellow Powder, *yì huáng sǎn*, 易黄散, 8
Trapae Fructus et Radix, *líng*, 菱, water caltrop, 4, 17, 21, 24-28, 32, 41-42, 50, 52, 60-62, 68, 74, 79, 83-84, 87, 89-91, 96, 101-103, 109, 112, 118, 123, 127-128, 130-131, 143-146, 149, 156, 159, 163, 165-167, 175, 183, 187-188, 190, 196, 200
trifoliate akebia, *mù tōng*, 木通, Akebiae Trifoliatae Caulis, 63, 69
Trionycis Carapax cum Liquido Frictus, *zhì biē jiǎ*, 炙鳖甲, mix-fried turtle shell, 41
Trionycis Carapax, *biē jiǎ*, 鳖甲, turtle shell, 41
Tritici Semen, *xiǎo mài*, 小麦, wheat, 189
Trogopteri Faeces, *wǔ líng zhī*, 五灵脂, squirrel's droppings, 41
true yáng, 135, 164, 170
true yīn, 170
Tsaoko Fructus, *cǎo guǒ*, 草果, tsaoko, 26, 166
tsaoko, *cǎo guǒ*, 草果, Tsaoko Fructus, 26, 166
turbid qì, 48, 56, 82, 102, 112
turbid urine, 57, 106, 107
turbid yīn, 107, 136
Turtle Shell Decocted Pill, *biē jiǎ jiān wán*, 鳖甲煎丸, 41
turtle shell, *biē jiǎ*, 鳖甲, Trionycis Carapax, 41

Two Matured Ingredients Decoction, *èr chén tāng*, 二陈汤, 32, 34

typha pollen, *pú huáng*, 蒲黄, Typhae Pollen, 118

Typhae Pollen, *pú huáng*, 蒲黄, typha pollen, 118

ulcerating sore, 107

uncaria, *gōu téng*, 钩藤, Uncariae Ramulus cum Uncis, 190

Uncariae Ramulus cum Uncis, *gōu téng*, 钩藤, uncaria, 190

unclean food, 36

Unified Treatise on Diseases, Patterns, and Remedies According to the Three Causes, *sān yīn jí yī bìng zhèng fāng lùn* (1174 (Sòng), Chén Yán 陈言 [Wú-Zé 無擇]), 19, 106

uninhibited clear stool and urine, 103

unquiet sleep, 21

unripe bitter orange, *zhǐ shí*, 枳实, Aurantii Fructus Immaturus, 19-20, 24-27, 32, 34, 37, 41-42, 50, 57-58, 84, 87, 89, 91, 102, 104, 143, 145, 166, 184, 194

unripe tangerine peel, *qīng pí*, 青皮, Citri Reticulatae Pericarpium Viride, 19, 20, 25, 27, 32, 37, 58, 61, 113, 167

upbear the clear, 18, 34, 56-57, 96, 99, 104-106, 111-112, 122-123, 127, 134-136

upbear the clear and downbear the turbid, 101

upflow nausea, 23, 30, 56, 66

urinary block, 4, 13

urinary incontinence, 113

uterine network vessels, 105, 113

uterus, 105, 113, 115

vacuity and repletion, 7-8, 74

vacuity cold, 28, 105, 142, 149, 153-155, 173-174

vacuity cold diarrhea, 154

vacuity desertion, 129

vacuity detriment, 14, 73, 75, 120, 189, 191, 193

vacuity distention, 103

vacuity fall, 105, 113, 150

vacuity fire flaming upward, 198

vacuity glomus, 101

vacuity heat, 139-140, 185, 197-199, 201

vacuity rumbling in the abdomen, 154

vacuity swelling, 170

vacuity taxation, 185, 190

vagina, 106, 113, 164

vaginal discharge, 2, 9, 23, 25, 30, 86, 95, 164, 166, 170, 172

Vespae Nidus, *lù fēng fáng*, 露蜂房, hornet's nest, 42

Vessel-Freeing Counterflow Cold Decoction, *tōng mài sì nì tāng*, 通脉四逆汤, 179

vexation, 6-8, 21, 46, 48-49, 52, 139, 155, 185, 198, 201

vexation and fullness, 185, 198

vexation and oppression, 8, 49

vexation in the limbs, 21

vexing heat in the five hearts, 141, 199, 201

Vinum seu Spiritus, *jiǔ*, 酒, liquor, 22, 33, 37, 46, 54, 73

Virgate Wormwood Decoction, *yīn chén hāo tāng*, 茵陈蒿汤, 60

Virgate Wormwood, Atractylodes, and Aconite Decoction, *yīn chén zhú fù tāng*, 茵陈朮附汤, 27

virgate wormwood, *yīn chén hāo*, 茵陈蒿, Artemisiae Scopariae Herba, 27, 60, 63

visceral cold, 149, 160

visiting evil, 112

vitex, *màn jīng zǐ*, 蔓荆子, Viticis Fructus, 27, 100, 130

Viticis Fructus, *màn jīng zǐ*, 蔓荆子, vitex, 27, 100, 130

vomiting, 7-8, 23, 29, 33-34, 38, 40, 44, 46, 56-57, 66, 73-74, 105, 117, 120, 142, 149, 153, 155, 161-163

vomiting and diarrhea, 23, 29, 38, 40, 73-74, 120

wán dài tāng, 完带汤, Discharge-Ceasing Decoction, 25-26, 166

Wáng Hào-Gǔ, 150

wáng shì lián pò yǐn, 王氏连朴饮, Wang's Coptis and Officinal Magnolia Bark Beverage, 57

Wáng Shū-Hé, 7

Wang's Coptis and Officinal Magnolia Bark Beverage, *wáng shì lián pò yǐn*, 王氏连朴饮, 57

warm and supplement the spleen and stomach, 117

warm and transform, 163, 164, 172, 178, 182

warm disease school, 14, 184

warm diseases, 8, 58, 62, 184, 187, 194

warm epidemic, 112

water buffalo horn, *shuǐ niú jiǎo*, 水牛角, Bubali Cornu, 49

water caltrop, *líng*, 菱, Trapae Fructus et Radix, 4, 17, 21, 24-28, 32, 41-42, 50, 52, 60-62, 68, 74, 79, 83-84, 87, 89-91, 96, 101-103, 109, 112, 118, 123, 127-128, 130-131, 143-146, 149, 156, 159, 163, 165-167, 175, 183, 187-188, 190, 196, 200

water qì, 2, 6, 17, 63, 89-90, 122, 163

water shield, *chún*, 莼, Braseniae Caulis et Folium, 29, 59, 184, 196

water swelling, 2, 9, 40, 44, 63-64, 86, 90, 94-95, 163-164, 166, 170, 182

water-damp, 22, 23, 25, 30-31, 54, 61, 81, 85-86, 88, 90, 92,-95, 151, 163-164, 169, 170-172, 182

Water-Damp Failing to Transform, 30, 81, 85, 95, 151, 163, 169, 171

water-humor, 81, 163, 164, 182

weak constitution, 190

weak pulse, 8, 139

wèi líng tāng, 胃苓汤, Stomach-Calming Poria Five Decoction, 24-25

wheat, *xiǎo mài*, 小麦, Tritici Semen, 189

White Atractylodes Powder, *bái zhú sǎn*, 白朮散, 83, 130, 188

white atractylodes, *bái zhú*, 白朮, Atractylodis Macrocephalae Rhizoma, 7, 20, 25-27, 32, 34, 42, 68, 83-84, 86-87, 89, 91, 100, 102-103, 107-109, 112, 118, 120, 124, 129-130, 143-145, 155, 157, 163, 165-167, 174-176, 182, 184, 187-188, 194

white facial complexion, 3, 9, 139, 174, 176, 179, 180, 181

white peony, *bái sháo*, 白芍, Paeoniae Radix Alba, 19-20, 24-27, 32, 37, 41, 49-50, 57-58, 67-68, 70, 84, 87, 89, 91, 100, 130-131, 145, 156, 166, 176, 182, 189-190, 194, 196, 199

white poria, *bái fú líng*, 白茯苓, Poria Alba, 26

white tongue fur, 20, 23

white turbidity, 23, 30, 97, 109, 112

white vaginal discharge, 164, 166, 170, 172

whittling of the flesh, 133

wilting of the legs, 52

wind evil, 64

wind strike (stroke), 111, 134

wind-cold, 133, 139, 141

wind-damp (rheumatism), 14

withered hair, 193, 197

withered-yellow facial complexion, 170

wood louse, *shǔ fù*, 鼠妇, Armadillidium, 41

Wú Kūn, 48

wǔ líng sǎn, 五苓散, Poria Five Powder, 90-91, 167

wǔ líng zhī, 五灵脂, squirrel's droppings, Trogopteri Faeces, 41

wū méi, 乌梅, mume, Mume Fructus, 108, 113, 118

wǔ pí yǐn, 五皮饮, Five-Peel Beverage, 91

wǔ wèi zǐ, 五味子, schisandra, Schisandrae Fructus, 107-108, 113, 145, 182

wū yào, 乌药, lindera, Linderae Radix, 19, 41, 103-104

wú zhū yú, 吴茱萸, evodia, Evodiae Fructus, 157, 182

Xanthii Fructus, *cāng ěr zǐ*, 苍耳子, xanthium, 130

Xanthii Herba, *cāng ěr*, 苍耳, xanthium stem and leaf, 130

xanthium stem and leaf, *cāng ěr*, 苍耳, Xanthii Herba, 130

xanthium, *cāng ěr zǐ*, 苍耳子, Xanthii Fructus, 130

xì xīn, 细辛, asarum, Asari Herba, 175

xiān dì huáng, 鲜地黄, fresh rehmannia, Rehmanniae Radix Recens, 69, 124

xiān hè cǎo, 仙鹤草, agrimony, Agrimoniae Herba, 118

xiāng fù zǐ, 香附子, cyperus, Cyperi Rhizoma, 19, 37, 41, 157

xiāng shā liù jūn zǐ tāng, 香砂六君子汤, Costusroot and Amomum Six Gentlemen Decoction, 88-89, 103, 130, 161

xiāng shā píng wèi sǎn, 香砂平胃散, Costusroot and Amomum Stomach-Calming Powder, 36-37

xiāng yuán, 香橼, citron, Citri Fructus, 20

xiǎo jiàn zhōng tāng, 小建中汤, Minor Center-Fortifying Decoction, 156

xiǎo mài, 小麦, wheat, Tritici Semen, 189

xiāo shí, 硝石, niter, Nitrum, 42

xiāo, 鸮, Glaucidii Caro, 42, 62, 68, 118

xiè huáng sǎn, 泻黄散, Yellow-Draining Powder, 7, 8, 47, 49

xiè, 蟹, crab, Eriocheiris Caro et Viscera, 7-8, 20, 25, 27, 47, 49-50, 68-69, 84, 91, 101-102, 131, 146, 167

xīn yí, 辛夷, magnolia flower, Magnoliae Flos, 130, 136

xìng rén huá shí tāng, 杏仁滑石汤, Apricot Kernel and Talcum Decoction, 58

xìng rén, 杏仁, apricot kernel, Armeniacae Semen, 50, 58, 175, 194

xìng zǐ, 杏子, apricot, Armeniacae Fructus, 50, 58, 175, 194

xù duàn, 续断, dipsacus, Dipsaci Radix, 118

xuè yú tàn, 血余炭, charred hair, Crinis Carbonisatus, 200

xuè yú, 血余, hair, Crinis, 111, 123, 138, 144, 193, 197, 200

yán hú suǒ, 延胡索, corydalis, Corydalis Rhizoma, 41

yán, 盐, salt, Sal, 41, 118, 143, 149, 164, 166

yáng collapse, 99

yáng jaundice, 46

yáng qì vacuity, 106-107, 116

yáng vacuity, 75, 117-118, 141-142, 149-151, 155, 164, 173, 178-179, 182

Yellow Emperor, 79

yellow face, 14, 34

yellow facial complexion, 170

Yellow-Boosting Powder, *yì huáng sǎn*, 益黄散, 8

Yellow-Draining Powder, *xiè huáng sǎn*, 泻黄散, 7, 8, 47, 49

yellowing, 29, 40, 59, 60, 64, 66

yì gōng sǎn, 异功散, Special Achievement Powder, 83, 101, 142, 143

yì huáng sǎn, 易黄散, Transforming Yellow Powder, 8

yì mǔ cǎo, 益母草, leonurus, Leonuri Herba, 118

yì qì cōng míng tāng, 益气聪明汤, Qi-Boosting Sharp and Bright Decoction, 127, 130

yí táng, 饴糖, malt sugar, Maltosum, 131, 156, 157

yì yǐ rén, 薏苡仁, coix, Coicis Semen, 83-84, 86-87, 188

yì zhì rén, 益智仁, alpinia, Alpiniae Oxyphyllae Fructus, 107-108, 161

yīn and yáng, 14, 150, 165, 174, 187, 194

yín chái hú, 银柴胡, stellaria, Stellariae Radix, 199

yīn chén hāo tāng, 茵陈蒿汤, Virgate Wormwood Decoction, 60

yīn chén hāo, 茵陈蒿, virgate wormwood, Artemisiae Scopariae Herba, 27, 60, 63

yīn chén zhú fù tāng, 茵陈朮附汤, Virgate Wormwood, Atractylodes, and Aconite Decoction, 27

yīn depletion, 173

yīn desertion, 106

yīn exuberance, 173

yīn fire, 193

yīn humor, 67, 142, 193, 198

yīn jaundice, 23, 24, 27

yīn vacuity, 76, 185, 201-202

yīn within yīn, 160

yù jīn, 郁金, curcuma, Curcumae Radix, 19, 20, 25, 27, 32, 58, 167

yù zhú, 玉竹, Solomon's seal, Polygonati Odorati Rhizoma, 67, 189

yuǎn zhì, 远志, polygala, Polygalae Radix, 118, 144

Zanthoxyli Pericarpium, *huā jiāo*, 花椒, zanthoxylum, 157, 176

zanthoxylum, *huā jiāo*, 花椒, Zanthoxyli Pericarpium, 157, 176

zé xiè, 泽泻, alisma, Alismatis Rhizoma, 25, 27, 69, 84, 91, 101-102, 131, 146, 167

Zhāng Jīng-Yuè, 64, 75, 97, 150

Zhāng Yuán-Sù, 75

Zhāng Zhòng-Jǐng, 74, 149, 183

zhè chóng, 蟅虫, ground beetle, Eupolyphaga seu Steleophaga, 42

zhì biē jiǎ, 炙鳖甲, mix-fried turtle shell, Trionycis Carapax cum Liquido Frictus, 41

zhì fù zǐ, 制附子, processed aconite, Aconiti Radix Lateralis Praeparata, 25, 27, 146, 157, 165-167, 175-176

zhì gān cǎo, 炙甘草, mix-fried licorice, Glycyrrhizae Radix cum Liquido Fricta, 26, 27, 42, 89, 91, 100, 102-103, 107-109, 124, 129,-131, 143, 145, 155-157, 166-167

zhǐ qiào (ké), 枳壳, bitter orange, Aurantii Fructus, 34, 37, 41, 50, 57-58, 60-61, 84, 103, 108-109, 188, 194

zhǐ shí, 枳实, unripe bitter orange, Aurantii Fructus Immaturus, 19-20, 24-27, 32, 34, 37, 41-42, 50, 57-58, 84, 87, 89, 91, 102, 104, 143, 145, 166, 184, 194

zhǐ zhú wán, 枳术丸, Unripe Bitter Orange and White Atractylodes Pill, 184, 194

Zhū Dān-Xī, 183

zhū líng, 猪苓, polyporus, Polyporus, 25, 62, 91, 101-102, 167

zhú rú, 竹茹, bamboo shavings, Bumbusae Caulis in Taenia, 50

zǐ hé chē, 紫河车, placenta, Hominis Placenta, 199

zǐ wǎn, 紫菀, aster, Asteris Radix, 145

zǐ wēi gēn, 紫葳根, campsis, Campsitis Radix, 42

Zingiberis Rhizoma Praeparatum, *pào jiāng*, 炮姜, blast-fried ginger, 26, 174-175

Zingiberis Rhizoma Recens, *shēng jiāng*, 生姜, fresh ginger, 32, 37, 51, 87, 131, 156

Zingiberis Rhizoma, *gān jiāng*, 干姜, dried ginger, 25-27, 32, 37, 41, 51, 87, 91, 131, 155-157, 166-167, 174-176, 182

Zingiberis Rhizoma, *jiāng*, 姜, ginger, 25-27, 32, 37, 41, 51, 87, 91, 131, 151, 155-157, 166-167, 174-176, 182

Zingiberis Rhizomatis Cortex, *jiāng pí*, 姜皮, ginger skin, 91

Ziziphi Spinosi Semen, *suān zǎo rén*, 酸枣仁, spiny jujube, 118, 144, 196

zōng lǘ pí, 棕榈皮, trachycarpus, Trachycarpi Petiolus, 118

zōng lǘ tàn, 棕榈炭, charred trachycarpus, Trachycarpi Stipulae Fibra Carbonisata, 118

Own the set!

Pathomechanisms of the Five Viscera

by Yán Shí Lín 严石林

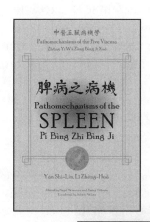

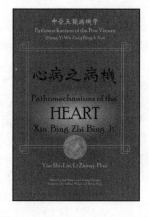

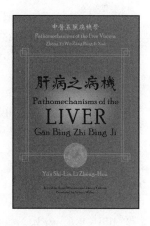

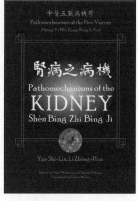

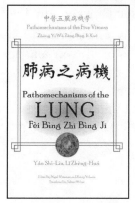

Published by Paradigm Publications, Taos, NM, USA
www.paradigm-pubs.com
Distributed by Redwing Book Company, Taos, NM, USA
www.redwingbooks.com

About the Author

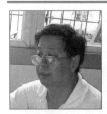 **Yàn Shí Lín** is a professor and Ph.D. advisor at Chengdu University of Traditional Chinese Medicine. He has enjoyed a distinguished professional career spanning more than 40 years with a specialization in pathomechanisms research and pattern differentiation. Among his Chinese published contributions he has written as Editor-in-Chief of the Diagnosis Chapter of the medical volume of the *Chinese Medical Encyclopedia,* the Pulse Diagnosis portion of the *Chinese Medical Classics* Series, and the *Study Guide Series for Self-Study Tests in Chinese Medicine.* He also contributed to the compilation of both the 6th and the 7th edition of the *Chinese National Standardized Textbooks* and the accompanying study guides, as well as many other national textbook projects. Additionally, he has published more than 80 academic papers in the field of Chinese medicine.

Academically, he has been the first to raise important theories such as cold-fire, sunken qì of liver and spleen, and qì stagnation caused by middle jiāo vacuity. He has undertaken a thorough and detailed study of the pathomechanisms of the five zang as well as micro-modeling of zàng fǔ pattern differentiation in Chinese medicine that has contributed greatly to researching patterns in Chinese medicine.